Children's Respiratory Nursing

Children's Respiratory Nursing

Edited by

Janice Mighten RGN, RSCN, MSc, BMed Sci(Hons)

Children's Respiratory Nurse Specialist
Nottingham Children's Hospital

WILEY-BLACKWELL

A John Wiley & Sons, Ltd., Publication

Library of Congress Cataloging-in-Publication Data

Children's respiratory nursing / edited by Janice Mighten.
     p. ; cm.
   Includes bibliographical references and index.
   ISBN 978-1-4051-9775-5 (pbk. : alk. paper) – ISBN 978-1-118-27826-0 (ebook) –
   ISBN 978-1-118-27827-7 (epub) – ISBN 978-1-118-27825-3 (emobi)
I. Mighten, Janice.
[DNLM: 1. Respiratory Tract Diseases–nursing.   2. Child.   3. Pediatric Nursing. WY 163]
   616.2′004231–dc23
                                    2012022788

A catalogue record for this book is available from the British Library.

Wiley also publishes its books in a variety of electronic formats. Some content that appears in print may not be available in electronic books.

Cover image: © Leonid Ikan, Fotolia.com
Cover design by Meaden Creative

Set in 9/11.5pt Times by SPi Publisher Services, Pondicherry, India
Printed in Singapore by Ho Printing Singapore Pte Ltd

1   2013

Contents

Contributors

Jayesh Bhatt MD, DCH (Lond), FRCPCH
Consultant Respiratory Paediatrician,
Nottingham Children's Hospital, Nottingham

Conrad Bosman MBBS, MRCPCH
Paediatric Registrar, Nottingham Children's
Hospital, Nottingham

Phil Brewin BSc, MSc
Consultant Clinical Psychologist, Nottingham
Children's Hospital, Nottingham

Katherine Carter RSCN
Previously Advanced Nurse Practitioner,
Transplant Team, Great Ormond Street
Hospital for Children NHS Trust, London

Debra Forster RGN, RSCN, BSc(Hons)
Specialist Practitioner in Children's
Community Nursing, Children's Respiratory/
Allergy and Community Nurse, Nottingham
Children's Hospital, Nottingham

Chhavi Goel MBBS, MD, MRCPCH
Consultant Paediatrician, Burton Hospitals
NHS Foundation Trust, Burton on Trent

**Donna Hilton Dip HE Youth and
Community**
Youth Service Manager, Nottingham
Children's Hospital, Nottingham

**Janice Mighten RGN, RSCN, MSc, BMed
Sci(Hons)**
Specialist Practitioner in Children's
Community Nursing, Children's Respiratory/
Community Nurse Specialist, Nottingham
Children's Hospital, Nottingham

Ammani Prasad FCSP
CF Co-ordinator/Senior Research
Physiotherapist, Great Ormond Street Hospital
for Children NHS Trust, London

**Andrew Prayle BMedSci, BMBS,
MRCPCH**
Research Fellow, Division of Child Health,
School of Clinical Sciences, University of
Nottingham, Nottingham Children's Hospital,
Nottingham

**Alan R. Smyth MA, MBBS, MRCP,
MD, FRCPH**
Professor of Child Health, Division of Child
Health, School of Clinical Sciences,
University of Nottingham; Honorary
Consultant in Paediatric Respiratory
Medicine, Nottingham Children's Hospital,
Nottingham

**Helen Spencer MB, ChB, DCH,
MRCPCH, MD**
Consultant in Transplant and Respiratory
Medicine, Great Ormond Street Hospital for
Children NHS Trust, London

Sarah Spencer RN(Child), BSc(Hons)
Specialist Practitioner in Children's
Community Nursing, Nottingham Children's
Hospital, Nottingham

**David Thomas MB, CHB, DCH, MRCP
(UK), FRICPCH**
Paediatric Consultant, Nottingham Children's
Hospital, Nottingham

Harish Vyas FRCP, FRCPCH
Professor in PICU and Paediatric Respiratory
Medicine, Nottingham Children's Hospital,
Nottingham

Beverley Waithe BSc(Hons), RN(Child)
Children's Community Matron, Nottingham
Children's Hospital, Nottingham

Caroline Youle RGN, RSCN
Children's Respiratory Nurse Specialist,
Nottingham Children's Hospital, Nottingham

Foreword

I am delighted to write the foreword to this excellent book. It is a real honour for me as many of the authors work within the senior nursing and medical team at the Nottingham Children's Hospital. I know that nurses regularly working within this area of practice with children and young people will welcome this textbook which discusses all aspects of respiratory care. It will also be an *aide mémoire* for nurse specialists, doctors and allied health professionals, and will be a standard reference for nursing students. Particular attention has been paid to standards within national guidelines that can support practice.

The book has also been designed to adopt a systematic manner in which it is presented. My opinion is that the reader will greatly benefit from this, starting with Chapter 1 as a revision tool covering the anatomy and physiology of the respiratory system. Each chapter then increases the reader's knowledge, highlighting age-appropriate care. Transition to adult services is later covered in Chapter 14. Other professional nursing issues are also described in great detail which will improve the overall care for this patient group.

Children and young people are very different from adults. This is most evident to nurses when treating children diagnosed with illnesses similar to those of adults. For this reason, nurses need special skills when planning their care.

Congratulations first to the editor, Janice Mighten. Congratulations also to all the chapter authors, contributors and publisher.

The authors have given a wealth of knowledge that can only come from their extensive experience. Although this book is not meant to be exhaustive, it includes a wealth of information for all who are caring for children and young people with respiratory conditions.

This textbook will be a welcome addition to my collection.

Angela Horsley
Clinical Lead, Nottingham Children's Hospital

Preface

The ever-changing world of modern medicine has enabled healthcare professionals to provide good-quality care. The idea for this book was born out of experiences with a merger of children's respiratory services and the need to provide a unified service based on quality and high standards. It is beyond the scope of this book to discuss every aspect of paediatric respiratory medicine, although a variety of conditions will be covered alongside the role of the children's respiratory nurse specialist, working as an important member of the multidisciplinary team.

This book is aimed at qualified nurses caring for children with respiratory conditions. It may also be useful as a point of reference to nurse specialists and students from a variety of backgrounds such as nurses, doctors and allied health professionals. This is an essential text that will support your practice and is based on standards, including national guidelines. Also included are illustrations, images and case studies to aid learning.

How to use this book

The approach that has been adopted is straightforward to guide the reader through the book in a systematic manner.

The book is divided into three sections. Each chapter begins with learning objectives and some chapters will have case studies that share relevant experiences. Finally, most of the chapters conclude with questions and answers, to enable the reader to consolidate learning. A glossary is also included at the end of the book explaining some of the more complex medical terminology.

Section I begins with an introduction that provides an overview of the respiratory nursing role and how this has evolved over time. An insight is then given into the anatomy and physiology of the respiratory system for children in Chapter 1. The process of homeostasis and the effect on the respiratory system are outlined in Chapter 2. The significance of nursing assessment and history taking is discussed in Chapter 3. This concludes with consideration of collaborative working with professionals in primary and secondary care. Reference to this concept is also continued throughout the book.

Section II begins with an outline of investigations in Chapter 4; this provides an overview of the various investigations that aid diagnosis and treatment such as chest x-rays and bronchoscopy. The images allow the reader to gain an understanding of the exploratory nature of such investigations and the relevance to treatment options. The process of assessment continues in Chapter 5, providing an insight into the assessment of airflow, including the impact spirometry testing has on daily management of patients with respiratory conditions and the necessity of nursing support to facilitate the process. Chapter 6 takes the concept of airflow further in relation to oxygen therapy, assessment, monitoring and evaluation based on national guidelines. Chapter 7 pursues the theme of long-term ventilation for children. Although this focuses on physiological and practical aspects, consideration is also given to the ethical dilemmas associated with long-term ventilation for some children. The importance of adequate nursing support for the family is also a feature of this chapter.

Section III begins with Chapter 8 which introduces the topic of respiratory infection, providing an overview of the common infections in children such as bronchiolitis and pneumonia, again referring to national and local guidelines. Chapter 9 provides a brief overview of pharmacology and the drugs used in respiratory medicine. Chapter 10 provides current information surrounding the diagnosis, care and management of children with asthma, including reference to the most current version of the British Thoracic Society management guidelines. Some of the most common congenital abnormalities that affect children are the main focus of Chapter 11. The theme of long-term conditions continues in Chapter 12, with particular reference to genetically inherited diseases such as cystic fibrosis and primary ciliary dyskinesia. The concept of multidisciplinary working is illustrated explicitly and is also applied to many other disease processes throughout the book. Maximum treatment can eventually be ineffective for some children with chronic lung disease so lung transplantation needs to be considered as an option. This is covered in a comprehensive and systematic manner in Chapter 13, including all elements of nursing care.

Section IV moves away from the management of conditions and focuses on the pertinent issues that impact on practice for children's nurses. Chapter 14 provides an overview of transition from children's to adult services, with reference to youth work services that support transition. For all healthcare professionals, the legal context of practice and quality assurance is very much a necessity, and this is discussed in Chapter 15. Finally chapter 16 completes this theme with a very important overview of communication and the skills required for all professionals involved in caring for children and families, in particular with chronic and long-term conditions.

I hope that this book is a valuable read for all to enjoy.

Janice Mighten

Acknowledgements

There are so many people who have worked tremendously hard towards making this book happen. Firstly I would like to thank all the contributors who have given their time to make a fine contribution towards the development of this book, and the medical photography department at Nottingham University Hospital for their help with some of the images. The positive feedback and evaluation from the reviewers are also appreciated; many of their suggestions have been incorporated into the final text. To all friends, colleagues and family, thank you for your support throughout this long process, and thanks to the publishers who have facilitated the process throughout.

Introduction: the evolution of children's respiratory nursing

Janice Mighten

Children's Respiratory/Community Nurse Specialist, Nottingham Children's Hospital

The health service has progressed over the years largely due to advancements in technology, which define how we treat many diseases. The changes that have occurred in nursing have been responses not only to technology but also to political influences and standards outlined within quality assurance frameworks. Other developments within the National Health Service (NHS) have also emerged, such as the concept of regional centres, generating high costs and resources. Consequently, nurses with specialist knowledge and skills were required, to meet the demand.

Many models of practice originated from North America and had some impact on elements of nursing care within the United Kingdom. This included specialist areas of nursing practice, which were recognised as early as 1979, within the Merrison Report, which also made reference to the concept of clinical nurse specialists (Middleton 2005).

Project 2000, introduced in the 1990s, changed nursing education and the concept of specialist areas (Holland et al. 2008). This provided specific areas of nurse training, such as the children's branch, and also set the standard for changes within nurse education. This change has continued further with the important move towards nursing becoming an all-degree profession, with emphasis on quality and standards, as suggested by the Prime Minister's Commission (Department of Health 2010). Basford and Slevin (2003) allude to such changes in nurse education and suggest that they have lead to the emergence of practitioners with qualities that include competency, safety and effective communication , which the modern health service demands.

Within the realms of paediatric respiratory medicine, we have witnessed the development of many nursing positions. Specialist areas such as paediatric respiratory nursing have emerged through the interest of individuals practising within the field of general respiratory medicine. This began with long-term conditions, such as asthma, and lead on to many more health conditions.

Wooler (2001) outlines the importance of the children's respiratory nurse specialist in the management of children with asthma in both primary and secondary care. Wooler also highlights the opportunity that such a role provides for children's respiratory nurse specialists to broaden their skills within respiratory medicine.

A general medical placement provides the learner with the opportunity to gain experience when caring for children with a variety of respiratory conditions. A qualified nurse with a special interest in paediatric respiratory medicine can be presented with opportunities within this field. Such positions are very varied, from clinical nurse specialists and advanced nurse practitioners to nurse consultants.

Children's Respiratory Nursing, First Edition. Edited by Janice Mighten.
© 2013 Blackwell Publishing Ltd. Published 2013 by Blackwell Publishing Ltd.

Currently, there are very few nurses at consultant level within paediatric respiratory medicine. This suggests that the time is right to promote and encourage professional development for those who have the desire, passion and drive to reach such heights, even in these times of austerity. The ultimate aim will be to provide positive role models for the nurse specialists of the future.

References

Basford L, Slevin O. (2003) *Theory and Practice of Nursing. An integrated approach to caring practice*, 2nd edn. London: Campion Press.

Department of Health. (2010) *Front Line Care. Report by the Prime Minister's Commission on the Future of Nursing and Midwifery in England*. London: Department of Health.

Holland K, Jenkins J, Solomon J, Whittam S. (2008) *Applying the Roper, Logan and Tierney Model in Practice*, 2nd edn. Edinburgh: Elsevier.

Middleton C. (2005) Short journey down a long road: the emergence of professional bodies. In: Sidey A, Widdas D (eds) *Textbook of Community Children's Nursing*. London: Elsevier.

Wooler E. (2001) The role of the nurse in paediatric asthma management. *Paediatric Respiratory Reviews* **2(1)**, 76–81.

Section I

The fundamental principles of respiratory nursing

Chapter 1

Anatomy and physiology of the respiratory system

Conrad Bosman

Paediatric Registrar, Nottingham Children's Hospital

Learning objectives

After studying this chapter, the reader will have an understanding of:

- the anatomy of the upper and lower respiratory tract
- stages of lung development
- the development of the respiratory system
- physiology of the respiratory system.

Introduction

A solid understanding of the anatomy and physiology of the respiratory system is an essential part of children's respiratory nursing. Furthermore, some knowledge of the embryological origins of those respiratory structures allows understanding of the development of congenital pathology.

The function of the respiratory system is simple: to provide oxygenation to the blood and removal of carbon dioxide. In disease, the mechanisms allowing such gaseous exchange are impaired. Therefore knowledge of the physiology of the upper and lower respiratory structures allows an understanding of why impairment of ventilation and perfusion occurs in various disease states.

Anatomy of the upper respiratory tract

The respiratory tract begins at the tips of the nostrils (alae nasi), which are kept open by soft cartilage. Around the nostrils are the alar nasalis muscles which cause the nostrils to flare open during states of respiratory distress, and can reduce nasal airway resistance by up to 25% (Carlo et al. 1983). The nasal cartilage encloses the anterior nasal cavity called the nasal vestibule. The cells of the nasal vestibule are the same as skin and contain small hairs, vibrissae, which can help stop debris such as dust from entering. There is a large vascular capillary network in the anterior vestibule, commonly called Little's area, which is a common site of nosebleeds in children.

Children's Respiratory Nursing, First Edition. Edited by Janice Mighten.
© 2013 Blackwell Publishing Ltd. Published 2013 by Blackwell Publishing Ltd.

A midline nasal septum divides the nasal cavity into two. On the lateral walls lie three curved turbinate bones called conchae, which direct airflow. Air passing through the nasal cavity is warmed and humidified and prevents the airways from drying out. Ventilator humidifiers do the same thing when the nose is bypassed by an orotracheal tube. This is the beginning of the nasopharynx, the site where nasopharyngeal aspirates are taken. The cells in this area are ciliated respiratory epithelial cells, rather than squamous cells, and move any particulate matter towards the oropharynx where it can be swallowed.

It is notable that the lacrimal ducts drain into the nasal conchae and the eustachian tube, that equalizes pressure in the middle ear. The adenoids are located near this region of the nasopharynx, and during viral upper respiratory tract infections adenoidal hypertrophy can block the eustachian tube in some infants and children which can lead to otitis media with effusion (Wright et al. 1998).

The naso- and oropharynx lead to the pharnyx where the epiglottis protects the laryngeal opening from the tracheal aspiration of food and liquids. During swallowing, the epiglottis moves down

(a)

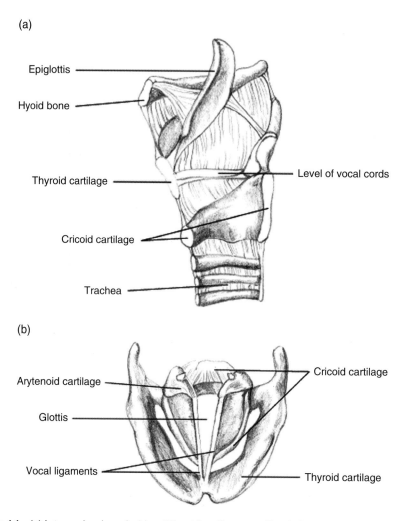

Epiglottis

Hyoid bone

Thyroid cartilage

Level of vocal cords

Cricoid cartilage

Trachea

(b)

Arytenoid cartilage

Cricoid cartilage

Glottis

Vocal ligaments

Thyroid cartilage

Figure 1.1 (a) Larynx showing cricoid and thyroid cartilages and level of vocal cords. (b) Vocal cords. Courtesy of Dr Phoebe Sneddon.

to close off the larynx. In epiglottitis, the epiglottis becomes very red and inflamed, swallowing becomes too painful, and the child drools.

The larynx is a complex structure that contains 'C'-shaped rings of cartilage and the vocal cords and muscles (Figure 1.1). The vocal cords and the space between them are commonly referred to as the glottis. Any abnormalities in this area will cause a variety of sounds, the most common being stridor. Below the vocal cords are the windpipe or trachea, which is part of the lower respiratory tract.

Anatomy of the lower respiratory tract

The trachea bifurcates at the carina to become the right and left main bronchi. The angles are slightly different, with the left main bronchi coming off at a more acute angle. Thus any inhaled foreign bodies tend to go down the right main bronchus. These bronchi then divide repeatedly into secondary and tertiary bronchi until finally dividing into the terminal bronchioles, respiratory bronchioles and finally alveoli.

The lung itself is covered by a pleural membrane which consists of the visceral and parietal pleura, with a small fluid-filled space in between. The visceral pleura covers the lung itself, while the parietal pleura is attached to the inner walls of the thorax. Infection and/or inflammation within the lung tissue can lead to accumulation of fluid or pus in this pleural space, respectively called a pleural effusion and empyema.

The work of breathing is done by the diaphragm and the intercostal muscles, located between the ribs. In poorly controlled respiratory conditions such as asthma, the diaphragm works much harder than usual and can deform the chest wall, as the muscle fibres attach to the lower part of the rib cage. This chronic deformity of the chest wall is called Harrison's sulci.

Surface anatomical landmarks

The ability to describe surface locations on the chest is important, and is usually described in terms of ribs or intercostal spaces and vertical lines drawn from anatomical landmarks. The second rib is located first by feeling for the sternal angle, then moving laterally. Other ribs can then be identified by counting downwards. The important vertical lines are the midclavicular and midaxillary. The midclavicular line passes straight down from the middle of the clavicle and the midaxillary line passes straight down from the axilla, when looking at the patient side on. In pneumothorax, needle thoracocentesis is performed by inserting a butterfly needle or venflon into the second intercostal space in the midclavicular line. Emergency chest drains are inserted into the fifth intercostal space in the midaxillary line.

Development of the respiratory system

Congenital defects of the upper airway originate from abnormalities of the embryological pharyngeal arches. Six arches are formed in the ventral surface of the hindbrain during the fourth to fifth weeks of embryological development, and give the embryo a characteristic appearance. These arches are derived from mesenchymal cells. The first pharyngeal arch mainly forms the lower jaw and anterior tongue, and defects can present as the Pierre Robin sequence with micrognathia, cleft palate and glossoptosis. The second pharyngeal arch gives rise to the root of the tongue, as well as other structures in the neck. Such a difference in embryological origin explains why the different

Table 1.1   Stages of human lung development

Stage	Age (weeks)	Structures
Embryonic	3–6	Trachea, lung buds, right and left main bronchi, lobar and segmental bronchi
Pseudoglandular	6–16	Bronchial tree to terminal bronchioles, pneumocyte precursors
Canicular	16–26	Terminal bronchioles, acini, type I and II pneumocytes
Saccular	26–36	Respiratory bronchioles, smooth-walled sacculi
Alveolar	36–maturity	Alveoli

parts of the tongue are innervated by different cranial nerves. The epiglottis forms from the fourth arch. The larynx opens in the 10th week of gestation. Incomplete opening at this point can lead to a laryngeal web, which can present in infancy as stridor.

The trachea and lower respiratory tract develop in the fourth week from the outpouchings of the embryological foregut, and thus are derivatives of endoderm. Incomplete separation from the gut leads to the condition of tracheo-oesophageal fistula. The lung buds divide in the fifth week, with three main divisions in the right bud and two in the left. These will eventually correspond to the three lobes of the right lung and the two of the left. By the end of the fifth week the embryonic stage of lung development is finished.

The diaphragm forms in the 6th week and failure of fusion can result in herniation of abdominal contents into the thorax – congenital diaphragmatic hernia. The left side is most commonly affected.

Following on from the embryonic stage are stages of lung development (Table 1.1) (Scarpelli 1990). Before 24 weeks' gestation, the lungs simply cannot function, even with exogenous surfactant. This stage of gestation is commonly seen as the limit of viability.

Changes in anatomy with age

In infancy, the narrowest point of the upper airway is the cricoid ring, rather than the vocal cords as in older children. Endotracheal intubation requires placing a suitably sized tube so as not to damage the vocal cords, whilst ensuring that any air leak is minimal. In younger children and infants the cricoid ring provides a seal, whereas in older children an endotracheal tube with an inflatable cuff is used. When the endotracheal tube passes through the vocal cords and is in the correct position, the cuff is inflated which creates a seal against the trachea and prevents air leak.

An important consideration in airway resistance is the change that occurs when the diameter is reduced due to mucus or inflammation. Poiseuille's law states that airway resistance is inversely proportional to the fourth power of the airway radius (Figure 1.2). Thus a 1 mm change in airway diameter in an older child will have little effect on resistance compared to that of a newborn or infant (Balfour-Lynn and Davies 2006).

Physiology of the respiratory system

The function of the lung is to oxygenate the blood and remove carbon dioxide. Air at sea level contains 21% oxygen, with inert nitrogen making up the remainder. In order for the oxygen to be delivered to the blood, flow of air into the lung must occur. To accomplish this, a pressure gradient

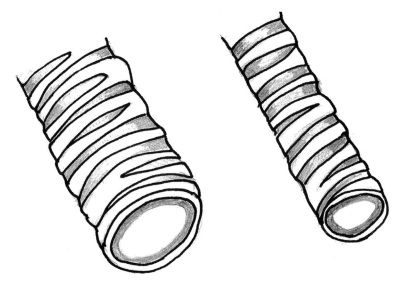

Figure 1.2   A similar amount of airway narrowing causes a much larger increase in airway resistance in smaller airways. Courtesy of Dr Phoebe Sneddon.

must be created between the terminal respiratory unit and the outside air. By contraction mainly of the diaphragm, against a thoracic cavity held rigid by the rib cage, a negative intrathoracic pressure is generated and flow of air occurs.

The anatomical 'dead space' consists of the terminal bronchioles, bronchi, trachea and upper airway. Although air passes through this dead space, no gas exchange occurs. Similarly, the tubes from a ventilator to the patient, including the endotracheal tube, extend this dead space. In neonatal ventilation, endotracheal tubes are kept as short as safely possible to reduce dead space.

During inspiration, the negative pressure exerts a force against the extrathoracic trachea and larynx, which instead of the rib cage relies on the cartilaginous rings to prevent collapse. During times of upper airway obstruction such as croup, increased effort to create flow will create further narrowing in the upper airway which is why inspiratory stridor occurs before expiratory stridor. In laryngomalacia the cartilage is not fully formed and stridor occurs as the larynx partially collapses with inspiration.

Involuntary breathing is controlled by centres in the brainstem which receive signals from chemoreceptors located in the medulla, carotid and aortic bodies. These chemoreceptors mainly respond to changes in acid–base balance which correspond to changes in blood carbon dioxide levels. Higher centres in the cortex can over-ride brainstem signals, allowing voluntary control of ventilation.

During exhalation, the diaphragm relaxes and the elastic recoil of the lungs creates a relative positive pressure within the airways to create flow of air out of the lungs. *Resistance* is the obstruction to airflow and is increased in conditions such as acute bronchiolitis and asthma. *Compliance* is the extent of lung inflation at a given inflation pressure. It is dependent on the production of surfactant by type II pneumocytes, which reduces the surface tension on the alveoli and prevents atelectasis. Low compliance is commonly referred to as a stiff lung.

The alveoli provide an enormous surface area for the diffusion of oxygen into the pulmonary blood and the removal of carbon dioxide. This assumes that the areas of the lung that are ventilated are also being perfused with pulmonary blood. In conditions such as asthma, in which mucous plugging occurs, areas of lung are not ventilated or perfused by blood. This is called *ventilation/perfusion* or *V/Q mismatching*.

Oxygen then transfers across the alveolar capillary membrane, binds to haemoglobin and is carried to the tissues, where it is made available for aerobic metabolism.

Conclusion

This chapter has provided an overview of the development of the respiratory system. This should enable readers to fully appreciate how ill health and congenital abnormalities can affect the function of the respiratory system.

Questions

1. What is the function of the alar nasalis muscle?
2. What is the function of the conchae?
3. The main reason why an inhaled foreign body would go down the right main bronchus much more easily than the left is?
4. What defects are present in Pierre Robin sequence?
5. An infant with a laryngeal web would present with what?
6. Why does inspiratory stridor occur before expiratory stridor?

References

Balfour-Lynn IM, Davies JC. (2006) Viral laryngotracheobronchitis. In: Chernick V (ed) *Kendig's Disorders of the Respiratory Tract in Children*. Philadelphia: Elsevier.

Carlo WA, Martin RJ, Bruce EN, Strohl KP, Fanaroff AA. (1983) Alae nasi activation (nasal flaring) decreases nasal resistance in preterm infants. *Pediatrics* **72**, 338–43.

Scarpelli EM. (1990) Lung cells from embryo to maturity. In: Scarpelli EM (ed) *Pulmonary Physiology. Fetus, Newborn, Child and Adolescent*, 2nd edn. Philadelphia: Lea and Febiger.

Wright ED, Pearl AJ, Manoukian JJ. (1998) Laterally hypertrophic adenoids as a contributing factor in otitis media. *International Journal of Pediatric Otorhinolaryngology* **45**, 207–14.

Chapter 2

Homeostasis and the respiratory system

Andrew Prayle

Research Fellow, Division of Child Health, University of Nottingham, and Nottingham Children's Hospital

---

Learning objectives

After studying this chapter, the reader will have an understanding of:

- the principles of homeostasis
- the respiratory rate, carbon dioxide and pH
- negative feedback mechanism
- how ill health disrupts homeostasis.

Introduction

We live in an ever-changing environment but despite this, the body needs to maintain its internal environment within strict limits. The process by which the body maintains internal consistency (or internal equilibrium) is termed *homeostasis* (Chiras 2002). Respiration is one of the many body systems which are regulated by homeostatic processes. This chapter describes this process and gives an example of how it can be affected by ill health.

Respiratory rate, carbon dioxide and pH

Blood pH needs to be held within a neutral range of approximately 7.35–7.45. A lower pH is too acid and a higher pH too alkaline. The body's metabolism naturally produces acids, most of which are ultimately excreted by the kidneys. Carbon dioxide is produced by all cells as they make energy, and is also acidic. However, carbon dioxide is an acidic gas and so it is removed from the bloodstream by the lungs through breathing. The rate of carbon dioxide removal from the body is proportional to the volume of each breath (bigger breaths remove more carbon dioxide) and the respiratory rate (faster breathing removes more carbon dioxide).

Children's Respiratory Nursing, First Edition. Edited by Janice Mighten.
© 2013 Blackwell Publishing Ltd. Published 2013 by Blackwell Publishing Ltd.

Carbon dioxide dissolved in the blood regulates the respiratory rate

The brain regulates the amount of carbon dioxide in the blood by altering the respiratory rate and depth (also termed the *tidal volume*). Chemical sensors termed chemoreceptors in the medulla of the brain can determine if carbon dioxide levels have increased by detecting the decreased blood pH caused by the increased carbon dioxide (Chiras 2002). A drop in blood pH is detected by the medulla which then stimulates nerves to the diaphragm and intercostal muscles, increasing the respiratory rate and tidal volume (West 2004). This leads to an increase in the rate of removal of carbon dioxide from the body, and the blood levels of carbon dioxide fall back to normal. This in turn returns the blood pH to its normal level, removing the stimulus which previously increased the respiratory rate and tidal volume, and the tidal volume and respiratory rate settle at this new level (Figure 2.1).

Control of respiratory rate is an example of a negative feedback mechanism

In a negative feedback mechanism, a stimulus causes a response which removes the original stimulus, thus 'turning off' the response. You will notice that raised carbon dioxide triggers an

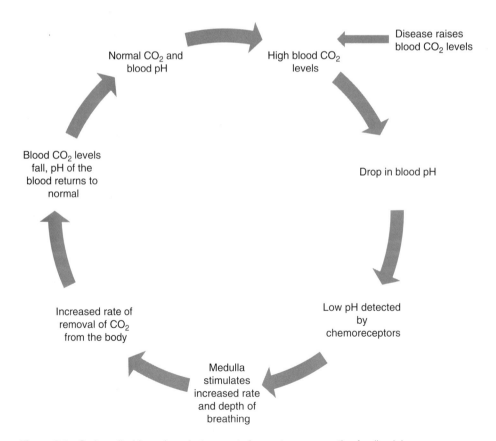

Figure 2.1   Carbon dioxide and respiratory control operate as a negative feedback loop.

increase in respiratory rate, which decreases the amount of carbon dioxide, and the respiratory rate falls again. So, control of breathing by carbon dioxide is an example of a negative feedback mechanism. There are several causes of increased carbon dioxide production, such as exercise or severe sepsis. Negative feedback is a common mechanism used by the body to regulate itself and maintain homeostasis (Clancy and McVicar 2009). Other examples are the control of blood sugar through regulating insulin release from the pancreas and maintenance of blood pressure by regulating the heart rate.

In disease homeostasis is disrupted

Disease processes affect the body's ability to regulate itself (Waugh and Grant 2010). This is particularly important in respiratory disease, as without adequate respiratory function patients quickly become acidotic (due to a rise in carbon dioxide) and hypoxic (due to a lack of oxygen).

An example of this is an acute severe asthma attack. An asthma attack is characterised by reversible narrowing of the airways (termed *bronchospasm*), which leads to the wheezing sound which asthmatics make. At the start of a severe asthma attack, a child will breathe more quickly to maintain arterial oxygen saturations. The increased rate of breathing often initially reduces the blood carbon dioxide levels. The patient usually looks unwell, sits upwards, has intercostal and subcostal recession and supports their breathing by using their accessory muscles, like an athlete would after a race. If the arterial oxygen saturation falls, supplemental oxygen is administered. However, if this situation persists without intervention (or even with intervention in severe cases), the child's respiratory muscles (the intercostal muscles and diaphragm) fatigue. They are unable to maintain the high respiratory rate necessary for gas exchange due to the increased work of breathing caused by the narrowed airways. The breathing depth and rate fall and carbon dioxide levels gradually rise. The brain detects this rise in carbon dioxide but is unable to increase the rate or depth of breathing and homeostasis is disrupted. The rise in carbon dioxide causes a respiratory acidosis and, with increasing severity, worsening hypoxia occurs due to lack of oxygen transfer. Without urgent intervention, this child would die (Figure 2.2).

The regulation of blood pH is called acid–base balance and is assessed with blood gas analysis

The control mechanisms of the respiratory system have a key role in maintaining acid–base balance of the blood. Acidosis (low pH) and alkalosis (high pH) are both damaging to the body. Table 2.1 summarises the blood gas findings which occur with a respiratory and metabolic acidosis. A blood gas test takes only a few minutes to perform and analyse, and is an invaluable part of the investigation of many respiratory disorders.

Table 2.1 demonstrates typical results found with various acid–base disorders. Approximate normal ranges are shown in brackets. The first step in the diagnosis is to look at the pH; if this is low an acidosis is present, if high an alkalosis. Next look at the carbon dioxide; if this is raised in an acidosis then this is a respiratory acidosis. If it is low or normal, then the acidosis is metabolic (due to increased acid production by the body, for example during sepsis). The respiratory system will usually try to compensate for a metabolic acidosis by increasing the respiratory rate and excreting more carbon dioxide. So sometimes in a metabolic acidosis (e.g. during a diabetic ketoacidosis) a low pH, low carbon dioxide, low bicarbonate and low base excess are all found; this is a metabolic acidosis with respiratory compensation.

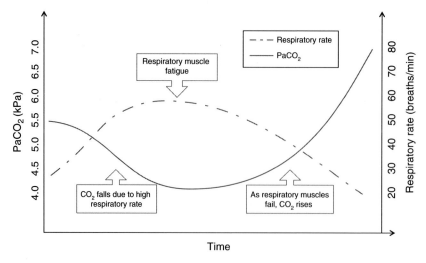

Figure 2.2   Blood carbon dioxide and respiratory rate during a severe asthma attack unresponsive to therapy. Initially carbon dioxide falls due to the high respiratory rate. Later, as the child tires, the blood carbon dioxide rises. The normal homeostatic mechanism which keeps the blood carbon dioxide within tight limits has failed due to the disease process.

Table 2.1   Blood gas analysis

	Respiratory acidosis	Metabolic acidosis	Respiratory alkalosis	Metabolic alkalosis
pH (7.35–7.45)	↓	↓	↑	↑
PaCO$_2$ (4.5–6.3 kPa)	↑	→ (or ↓)	↓	→
Bicarbonate (23–27 mmol/L)	→ (or ↑)	↓	→	↑
Base excess (−1 to +1)	→	↓	→	↑

Conclusion

The respiratory system is primarily responsible for the regulation of oxygen and carbon dioxide in the blood. Ill health results in disturbed homeostasis and the normal regulatory systems fail. Healthcare interventions can in a sense be seen as efforts to artificially maintain the body's homeostasis, when it cannot cope with an illness. Examples of this are discussed later in this book – drug therapy for asthma is discussed in Chapter 10, and oxygen delivery to maintain oxygen saturations is also discussed in the context of children with chronic lung disease of prematurity in Chapter 8.

Homeostatic mechanisms within the respiratory system maintain blood carbon dioxide and oxygen levels within tight limits. However, respiratory disease such as asthma can overwhelm the body's normal homeostatic mechanisms, and lead to low blood oxygen and high carbon dioxide levels. It is useful for nurses to have a basic understanding of homeostasis when caring for children with respiratory conditions. This can assist nurses with the continual assessment of sick children, especially nurses working in paediatric intensive care where blood gas analysis is an important aspect of management.

Questions

Answer true or false.

1. Increased carbon dioxide will cause the blood to become alkaline.
2. The blood pH is monitored by chemoreceptors in the medulla.
3. The respiratory rate will increase if carbon dioxide falls.
4. A high carbon dioxide level is a sign of serious illness in asthma.
5. Control of breathing rate by carbon dioxide levels is an example of a positive feedback mechanism.

References

Chiras DD. (2002) *Human Biology: health, homeostasis and the environment*, 4th edn. Sudbury, MA: Jones and Bartlett.

Clancy J, McVicar A. (2009) *Physiology and Anatomy for Nurses and Healthcare Practitioners: a homeostatic approach*, 3rd edn. London: Hodder Arnold.

Waugh A, Grant A. (2010) *Ross and Wilson Anatomy and Physiology in Health and Illness*, 11th edn. London: Elsevier.

West JB. (2004) *Respiratory Physiology: the essentials*, 7th edn. Philadelphia: Lippincott Williams and Wilkins.

Chapter 3

Nursing assessment, history taking and collaborative working

Janice Mighten

Children's Respiratory/Community Nurse Specialist, Nottingham Children's Hospital

---

Learning objectives

After studying this chapter, the reader will have an understanding of:

- the importance of a structured approach during a nursing assessment for the child with respiratory disease
- the significance of a paediatric early warning scoring system for respiratory assessments
- the significance of history taking and building relationships with parents
- the impact of presenting symptoms associated with respiratory disease on the activities of daily living
- the impact of collaboration on health.

Introduction

Comprehensive history taking, good consultation skills and a thorough assessment are the starting point of all patient care. This model of practice provides a framework for guidance, based on the activities of daily living for nurses, referred to by Roper, Logan and Tierney (2000) as the nursing process. This process emphasises nursing care based on the concept of assessment, planning, implementation and evaluation (Holland et al. 2008).

There is also a need within modern healthcare to use the concepts of critical analysis, including best practice (Basford and Slevin 2003) and available evidence such as the British guidelines on the management of asthma (BTS 2011). This will be covered in more detail in Chapter 10. This chapter will provide an overview of assessment, history taking and consultation skills for nurses. Consideration will also be given to the importance and benefits of assessment, when planning care for children with respiratory disease.

Assessment

When planning care following the Roper 1996 nursing model, a thorough assessment needs to be carried out in a systematic manner (Basford and Slevin 2003). This enables the identification of a

---

Table 3.1 Normal pulse and respiration

Age	Respiratory rate; breaths per minute	Pulse; beats per minute
Infants	30–60	100–220
3 months–2 years	25–35	80–150
3–7	20–30	70–100
8–18	20–25	55–90

Adapted from Huband and Trigg (2000).

problem with the ultimate aim of assisting a diagnosis. This approach can also be applied to many specialist areas such as children's respiratory nursing.

Using a framework such as the nursing process not only assists with assessment of the patient but also enables nurses to consider particular elements of the assessment, such as breathing. Naturally, respiration is relevant to respiratory disorders and is also essential for life. Any alteration in breathing affects other activities of daily living such as eating and drinking (Holland et al. 2008). Therefore a holistic approach to assessment is recommended, including prioritising nursing activity when planning care.

Recording the respiratory rate is the most significant observation in the respiratory system (Smyth 2001). A child in respiratory distress can present with grunting, head bobbing and recession (the use of accessory muscles). This clinical presentation is also highlighted within NICE guidelines (2007), which provides a comprehensive framework when assessing patients for respiratory distress.

It is important that nurses have a clear understanding of the normal values when monitoring vital signs such as pulse and respiratory rate (Table 3.1). This allows interpretation of observations which a child may present with when unwell. Also, the respiratory rate should not be taken when a child is crying as this ultimately affects the respiratory rate.

Assessment and recording of observations, with the use of a paediatric early warning scoring system (PEWS), are now an established part of clinical practice, following the introduction of NICE guidelines to assist the early detection of sick patients who have the potential to become critically ill (NICE 2007). The NHS Institute for Innovation and Improvement (2011) has also produced a 'paediatric trigger tool' in conjunction with healthcare professionals caring for children. The ethos of this was to assist practitioners to maintain patient safety with care delivery by using a scoring system.

Oliver et al. (2010) report that when caring for children, observations are not always recorded on a regular basis. This also included variation in which specific observations were actually recorded; for example, the pulse rate may be recorded but not the respiratory rate. Oliver et al. suggest that early warning scoring systems can help to address this problem, in areas that have yet to introduce this in practice.

The introduction of this concept is based on the traffic light system of red, amber and green when assessing clinical risk (NICE 2007). Thompson et al. (2009) found that a system of monitoring vital signs can be of value for both serious and less serious infection in children.

Therefore, the importance of recording height and weight should not be underestimated in children. Not only are they important for drug therapy and developmental milestones but they are important parameters for assessing states of dehydration and fluid requirement, needed to correct dehydration. This can be significant with infants who have bronchiolitis and present with symptoms such as tachypnoea, poor feeding and low oxygen levels.

At postregistration level, nurses have the extended knowledge that enables them to interpret what the observations are indicating. Oliver et al. (2010) observed in practice that respiration was the one

---

Box 3.1   Signs of cyanosis

Central cyanosis

Discoloration of lips, tongue and mucous membranes
Dyspnoea
Tachypnoea
Discoloration of fingers/toes

Peripheral cyanosis

Discoloration of affected area
Cold extremities
Discoloured nail bed
Mottled extremities

---

observation that was often omitted, despite the use of a scoring system. This indicates that nurses caring for children with respiratory conditions can benefit from support and education from experienced individuals, such as the respiratory nurse specialist. Oliver et al. reinforce this point by suggesting that the success of a paediatric early warning scoring system is reliant on nurses not only recording the observations but understanding and acting on such recordings for the sick child.

Essentially, nursing observations not only assist with diagnosis but can help prevent long-term complications. For example, post pneumonia, a child who continues to cough should undergo further investigations because this can be an indication of persisting atelectasis. If this is not treated then bronchiectasis can develop (Smyth 2001).

During observations, it is also useful to assess skin colour for signs of cyanosis. Cyanosis is caused by a high level of deoxygenated haemoglobin in the tissue (Ward et al. 2006). The skin has an abnormal discoloration and can have a greyish blue tinge. There are many causes of cyanosis, including impaired blood flow or circulatory shock. The presenting signs and symptoms are dependent on the underlying cause, which will determine whether it is central or peripheral cyanosis (Box 3.1). Central cyanosis occurs with heart and lung disease or haemoglobin that is abnormal. Peripheral cyanosis occurs as a result of blood flow that is impaired, causing reduced circulation and the removal of oxygen in the peripheral tissues (Ward et al. 2006).

Although cyanosis is more obvious in the lips or tongue, it can be difficult to assess, particularly in children. It is important that nurses understand how this can be much more difficult to assess in children with darker skin colour.

Although it is important to make an assessment of the respiratory system, it is also paramount to consider the psychological impact of ill health on the child's and family's quality of life and wellbeing.

History taking

Taking a history is not just a process of information gathering. History taking also requires interaction with all concerned and an acknowledgement of the problem (Smyth 2001). It is also important to use a systematic and structured approach, including various factors (listed in Box 3.2) that may affect patient care. This allows the opportunity for parents to provide information that may be vital. Equally as important is a discussion with the family about home life and other physiological issues such as lack of sleep. Therefore, when taking a history from parents, effective communication is key.

Box 3.2   Factors to consider when taking a history

History of symptoms
Past medical history
Cognitive development
Activities of daily living, i.e. nutrition
Lifestyle: smokers in the household
Environmental factors: housing, damp conditions, no central heating
Social issues

Table 3.2   Physical examination.

Site	Symptoms	Possible diagnosis
Chest	Crackles and reduced air entry on auscultation Breathless/cough	Pneumonia/consolidation Exacerbation of asthma
Skin	Dry, loss of elasticity	Dehydration, reduced urine output
Mucous membranes	Cyanosis Hypoxia/hypoxaemia	Pneumonia
Nail bed	Clubbing	Infection, progressive lung disease, cardiac problem

Communication in the form of a clear concise line of questioning is often demonstrated during an assessment. When establishing the primary problem, first impressions may be different from the information given by other healthcare professionals. Therefore Smyth (2001) maintains that it is important to establish what the family see as the problem, using a systematic approach, prior to any examination.

Medical assessments and examinations can reveal abnormalities such as noises in the chest, often referred to as crackles (Table 3.2). However, sometimes professionals can assume that families understand the terminology we use, for example what reduced air entry means (Fairhurst-Winstanley 2007). This is not always the case, so clear explanations of all terminology are required for good communication. During a nursing assessment, effective communication with the family can also assist families with their understanding of such terminology and any other information given to them. This enables the practitioner to get a clearer picture during the assessment.

At times children do not always present with the symptoms that parents report in a consultation. Therefore it can be useful for the respiratory nurse specialist to do a home visit, for further discussions within the home environment which can sometimes provide a fuller picture.

Consultation skills

Making a diagnosis based on information gathering and assessment forms the basis of clinical practice (Smyth 2001). Price (2010) defines consultation as a process that brings children and families together with professionals. Therefore communication skills are also an important element of all consultations.

The starting point of all consultations should be professionals introducing themselves to children and families. Equally important is the need to establish the identity of the adult attending the consultation with the child, because it is vital to have their co-operation. This is not always the child's parent and building a rapport is necessary for future continuity of care (Smyth 2001).

Nursing assessment and history taking should coincide with the medical team's assessment. When consulting with children and families in nurse-led clinics, respiratory nurse specialists will access information from medical notes. This will enable the nurse to gain an insight into previous medical assessments and further ensure consistency and continuity of care. In a randomised trial in relation to day case admissions, Rushforth et al. (2000) assessed the safety of nurse-led clerking in comparison to that of senior house officers. The study found that nurses demonstrated more accuracy during this process and had superior history-taking skills.

Children often present with a persistent cough which is a common problem. Asking appropriate questions such as when the symptoms began and the frequency of a cough enables a process of elimination before any proposed treatment. Equally it is also important to establish if this happens following food or drink, because inhalation of a foreign body quite often leaves a child with a persistent cough.

However, when reviewing a child with an established diagnosis, a different set of questions is required (Smyth 2001). For example, a cough is a common feature for some children with long-term conditions. Therefore, during an assessment it would be useful to ascertain if the frequency and nature of the cough have changed, which is helpful when planning treatment.

Physiological assessment is an important part of a conventional medical consultation, as well as accurately documenting medicines that the child may be taking. It is just as important for nurses taking a history to ask questions about medication and allergies. This can affect the overall treatment plan and can be crucial, especially in preschool children. Special consideration must also be given to social history, in particular with concerns about safeguarding.

Preschool children

Preschool children, whose cognitive ability is still developing, are often the most difficult group from whom to obtain an assessment. Consequently, building rapport and a trusting relationship by engaging with parents helps with both child and parental anxiety. Therefore it is necessary to make allowances for the child's cognitive development and acknowledge previous experiences with healthcare professionals, whether good or bad, because at times this can add to the anxiety.

Adolescents

Some young people may be reluctant to engage with healthcare professionals and do not always perceive the relevance of some issues or can be embarrassed. During consultations, the presence of parents can either be friendly or confrontational. This can affect the assessment process, including the young person's psychological perception of illness. Consequently, creating the right environment for an assessment is just as important as the assessment itself.

Young people should be part of the interactive process. This can be achieved by nurses using their experience to engage the young person in a topic of interest, for example sport, to help with building a rapport. Generally, young people are capable of giving their own account of how they feel. During a consultation, the nurse specialist would always clarify the information given with parents. However, consideration must always be given to the fact that some young people with chronic illness under-report symptoms, because of a fear of the need for a hospital admission (Smyth 2001).

Collaborative working

Successful healthcare for children and young people requires professionals to work together, in order to tailor care that meets their needs. This section will explore the notion of collaborative working when caring for children and young people with respiratory conditions.

According to Mead and Ashcroft (2005), collaboration means the ability to work together towards goals that are ultimately shared. Therefore health and social care relationships between practitioners are fundamental to collaborative working. Such relationships are driven by global modernisation policies which are redefining relations within healthcare. Overall this contributes to new ways of working.

Collaboration is not a new phenomenon but it is now used in practice more efficiently and is evolving all the time (Barratt et al. 2005). Such collaboration is delivered through the mechanism of interprofessional education and progress (Mead and Ashcroft 2005).

Health service provision has changed rapidly by trying to keep up with the pace of change in society. Therefore care delivery for patients within the heath service also needs to reflect these changes. Barratt et al. (2005) maintain that health changes in the 21st century now increase the need for integrated services through the notion of collaborative working. For healthcare practitioners this is becoming more evident in our everyday practice.

Children with an acute respiratory illness such as viral-induced wheeze or bronchiolitis will encounter various professionals during their hospital stay. With long-term conditions a multidisciplinary approach is required to deliver care that supports the child and family by professionals from both primary and secondary care. Consequently collaboration plays a major role in clinical outcomes when planning and implementing health.

When children are cared for in hospital, nurses are at the forefront of communicating with key individuals, in order to deliver the care that is required. It is important for learners to understand the concept of multidisciplinary working for such care delivery. This can be facilitated by placements with a respiratory nurse specialist to gain an insight into the dynamics of multidisciplinary team working and the importance of collaboration, in order for children and families to receive appropriate care.

Promoting independence and empowering parents, for example from a neonatal unit in the hospital to home, require collaboration. When caring for a child with health needs at home, it is vital that professionals from primary and secondary care communicate effectively. This will ensure that the family can be confident that their child's healthcare will be managed appropriately. Lineham (2010) suggests that professionals who include young people with chronic illness when planning a package of care highlight how collaboration can work well.

Elements of the government's modernisation agenda have also focused on collaborative working, with initiatives such as NHS Direct and Sure Start, now superseded by children's centres (Barratt et al. 2005). Respiratory nurses also need to be instrumental in providing training and education to colleagues in areas such as NHS Direct. This will ensure that practitioners are provided with adequate knowledge to support the care of children who access such services.

We have also witnessed increased migration to the UK, with migrants from European and other countries who are often homeless and prone to contracting tuberculosis (TB). Adults with TB will often transmit the disease to children. In areas of the UK where the number of children with TB is greater, they will have access to a children's respiratory nurse specialist but those areas with small numbers will not. Generally many children with TB are cared for by adult nurse specialists, who have much more expertise in TB management because it is more prevalent in adults.

Collinson and Ward (2010) describe an effective collaboration with TB services, which provides a multidisciplinary outreach service for adults. This collaboration adopted a practical approach which included working with other agencies who help the homeless. The aim of this collaboration was not only to provide a service for the homeless with TB, but also to ensure that they complete all their treatment.

Hodges et al. (2007) also looked at service provision for children in school with severe allergy, using the process of audit and a service review. This highlighted the need for a collaborative approach from a multidisciplinary perspective, including the involvement of school personnel. The results of this audit identified that there was a lack of management and education for children in school with severe allergy. The ultimate aim is to improve the healthcare for these children in school.

Although the concept of collaborative working is one that benefits healthcare, it can also have risks by association. This is demonstrated, for example, with poor communication when collaborative working is not effective (Mead and Ashcroft 2005). Professionals working with children have witnessed such poor practice with a detrimental outcome, for example as highlighted by the inquiry into the death of Victoria Climbié (2003). As previously discussed, each individual has professional responsibility and accountability for their own practice and without this, collaborative working can also be ineffective.

Collaboration is key to the progress of the modernised health services (Mead and Ashcroft 2005), which ultimately contributes to a holistic approach to healthcare. This section has provided a brief overview of how health can be promoted by fostering a culture that encourages independence, with effective communication.

Conclusion

This chapter has provided some information on factors such as assessment and evaluation that contribute to the basic principles of paediatric respiratory nursing. The ultimate aim is to establish good relationships with families, in order to promote self-management skills for parents and young people with respiratory disorders. At the forefront of this is collaborative working with health professionals and parents, to optimise respiratory function (Fairhurst-Winstanley 2007).

Questions

Answer true or false.

1. When taking a history, it is important to allow the parents to tell their story in order to get a clear picture of the perceived problem.
2. The respiratory rate is not the most significant observation to record.
3. Signs of respiratory distress include tachypnoea, grunting, tracheal tug and cyanosis.
4. A paediatric early warning score (PEWS) provides a framework to monitor, record and act on vital signs in a timely fashion.
5. Cyanosis is a sign of hypoxia and can be difficult to assess in children with dark skin.

References

Barratt G, Sellman D, Thomas J. (2005) *Interprofessional Working in Health and Social Care: professional perspectives*. Basingstoke: Palgrave Macmillan.

Basford L, Slevin O. (2003) *Theory and Practice of Nursing: an integrated approach to caring practice*, 2nd edn. London: Campion Press.

British Thoracic Society (BTS). (2011) *British Guideline on the Management of Asthma: a national clinical guideline*. London: British Thoracic Society.

Collinson S, Ward R. (2010) A nurse led response to unmet needs of homeless migrants in inner London. *British Journal of Nursing* **19**(1), 36–41.

Fairhurst-Winstanley W. (2007) Caring for a patient with a respiratory disorder. In: Walsh M, Crumbie A (eds) *Watson's Clinical Nursing and Related Sciences*, 7th edn. London: Elsevier.

Hodges B, Clack G, Hodges I. (2007) Severe allergy: an audit and service review. *Paediatric Nursing* **19(9)**, 26–31.

Holland K, Jenkins J, Solomon J, Whittam S. (2008) *Applying the Roper, Logan and Tierney Model in Practice*, 2nd edn. Edinburgh: Elsevier.

Huband S, Trigg E. (2000) *Practices in Children's Nursing: guidelines for hospital and community; Section 3 assessment*. London: Churchill Livingstone.

Lineham K. (2010) Caring for young people with chronic illness: a case study. *Paediatric Nursing* **22(1)** , 20–3.

Mead G, Ashcroft J. (2005) *The Case for Interprofessional Collaboration*. Oxford: Blackwell.

National Institute for Health and Clinical Excellence (NICE). (2007) *Feverish Illness in Children: assessment and initial management in children younger than 5 years*. London: National Institute for Health and Clinical Excellence.

NHS Institute for Innovation and Improvement. (2011) Safer care: improving patient safety. The paediatric trigger tool. Available at: www.institute.nhs.uk/safer_care/paediatric.

Oliver A, Powell C, Edwards D, Mason B. (2010) Observations and monitoring: routine practices on the ward. *Paediatric Nursing* **22(4)**, 28–32.

Price B. (2010) Techniques to use when consulting families about child health services. *Paediatric Nursing* **22(5)**, 26–34.

Roper N, Logan W, Tierney AJ. (2000) *The Roper-Logan-Tierney Model of Nursing*. Edinburgh: Churchill Livingstone.

Rushforth H, Bliss A, Burge D, Glasper EA. (2000) A pilot randomised controlled trial of medical versus nurse clerking for minor surgery. *Archives of Diseases in Childhood* **83(3)**, 223–6.

Smyth A. (2001) Taking a history. In: Silverman M, O'Callaghan C (eds) *Practical Paediatric Respiratory Medicine*. London: Arnold.

Thompson M, Coad N, Harden A, Mayon-White R, Pereral R, Mant D. (2009) How well do vital signs identify children with serious infections in paediatric emergency care? *Archives of Disease in Childhood* **94**, 888–93.

Ward JP, Ward J, Leach R, Weiner C. (2006) *The Respiratory System at a Glance*, 2nd edn. Oxford: Blackwell.

Section II

Respiratory investigations and assessments

Chapter 4

Investigations

Alan R. Smyth,[1] Conrad Bosman[2] and Janice Mighten[3]

[1]*Professor of Child Health, School of Clinical Sciences, University of Nottingham; Honorary*
  Consultant in Paediatric Respiratory Medicine, Nottingham Children's Hospital
[2]*Paediatric Registrar, Nottingham Children's Hospital*
[3]*Children's Respiratory/Community Nurse Specialist, Nottingham Children's Hospital*

Learning objectives

After studying this chapter the reader will have an understanding of:

- the rationale for chest x-ray and computed tomography scan
- the need for cautionary measures with x-rays
- investigations such as bronchoscopy
- the assessment of alveolar specimens
- preoperative nursing management
- the importance of monitoring vital signs postoperatively.

Chest x-ray

X-rays are a form of electromagnetic radiation with a very high frequency and short wavelength. This allows them to penetrate certain solid objects. The degree of penetration depends on the electron density of the object through which the x-rays pass. Bones are composed mainly of calcium, which absorbs a high percentage of the x-ray photons. Soft tissues allow much more of the x-rays through. This allows an image to be created when radiographic film is placed behind a subject.

Cautionary measures for x-rays

It must be remembered that although very useful in diagnosing pathology, x-rays are ionising radiation and increase the chances of lymphoma in later life. As such, careful consideration of whether the investigation is really necessary must be made before ordering tests.

Just like shadows from a light source, the size of the radiographic image is dependent on the distance from the source of the x-rays to the subject, and then to the film. Even when these distances are optimised, the fact that the body is not flat means that the structures furthest from the film will be magnified to a degree.

In order to reduce this magnification effect on structures such as the heart, the usual practice in older children and adolescents is for them to stand upright with the front of their chest pressed

---

Children's Respiratory Nursing, First Edition. Edited by Janice Mighten.
© 2013 Blackwell Publishing Ltd. Published 2013 by Blackwell Publishing Ltd.

against the x-ray film, with the x-rays passing through them from back to front. This standard type of chest x-ray is called a *posteroanterior* (PA) film.

In an *anteroposterior* (AP) film, the x-ray film is placed behind the patient's back and x-rays are beamed from front to back. This is the type of chest x-ray performed in babies and young infants, and also in bed-bound children. As the heart is anterior, there will be a magnification effect which must be considered when assessing for cardiomegaly. Other views include the lateral view, which is not routine in the UK, and taking the image in different states of inspiration or expiration (which can help diagnose inhaled foreign bodies).

Storage of x-rays

Images are stored in a picture archiving and communication system (PACS), which has replaced hard copy films. When accessing such a system, the process of querying the patient name and film has largely removed errors in assuming that the film you are looking at is indeed of the correct patient. However, it is still good practice when interpreting any x-ray to confirm that it is correct one.

Systematic interpretation

Any obvious abnormality on the chest x-ray should be noted immediately. Once this is done, a structured method of interpretation should be followed, so as not to miss any subtle abnormalities. One common system (of many) involves checking the *ABC* before looking at the airways and lung fields.

A: adequacy, alignment and apparatus

Adequate exposure of the image relates to whether too much or too little radiation was used to create the x-ray (Figure 4.1). The intervertebral disc spaces are just visible when the correct exposure is used. They are not visible at all in an underexposed film. In an overexposed film, the disc spaces will be visible but the whole film will be very dark. The alignment is next assessed by looking for symmetry in the clavicles and anterior ribs. Any tubes, lines or drains should be commented on.

B: bones

A quick survey of the bones is mandatory if healing fractures are not to be missed. Such fractures can be a sign of child abuse, or osteopenic bones.

C: cardiac

The cardiac silhouette, cardiophrenic and costophrenic angles must be inspected. The cardiac silhouette (shadow) should be clear both right and left, and orientated towards the left (Figure 4.2). An indistinct shadow can be a sign of consolidation. An estimation of cardiac size can be made by measuring the cardiothoracic ratio, which is the ratio of the widest diameter of the heart shadow over the diameter of the chest at the same level. It should be less than 0.6 in children and less than 0.5 in an adult.

Loss of the normal costophrenic angle indicates a pleural effusion. Such effusions may be very large, and an ultrasound of the thorax is often required to distinguish an effusion from an empyema. The radiologist will place a mark or cross on the chest wall indicating a suitable position for a chest drain if a large effusion or empyema is found.

Finally inspection of the trachea, right and left main bronchi, perihilar regions and lung fields completes the survey.

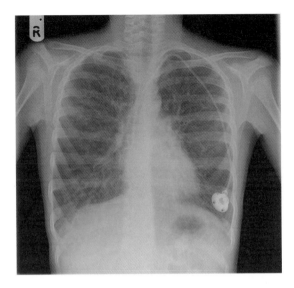

Figure 4.1 A 12-year-old boy with cystic fibrosis and bronchiectasis. Note the well-aligned, adequately exposed film. There is a portacath *in situ*, with the tip in the lower superior vena cava. A gastrostomy button can just be seen below the stomach bubble. There is hyperinflation and generalised marked bronchial wall thickening.

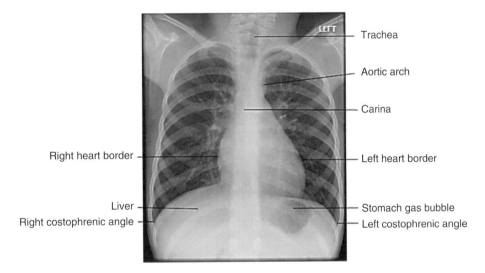

Figure 4.2 A normal chest x-ray of a 7-year-old girl.

Consolidation

The chest x-ray findings in bacterial pneumonia vary from subtle patchiness or obliteration of a heart border to a white-out of an entire lung field. The x-ray changes are called *consolidation* and correspond to the accumulation of pus and inflammatory cells in and around the parenchyma of the lung (Figure 4.3). Thus in early pneumonia, before the immune system has had a chance to react, there can be little or no consolidation, even when clinical signs are present.

(a)   (b)

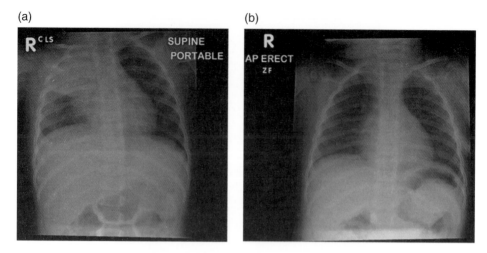

Figure 4.3   (a) Consolidation on the chest x-ray of a child with a right upper and middle lobe pneumococcal pneumonia. (b) Resolution 6 weeks later.

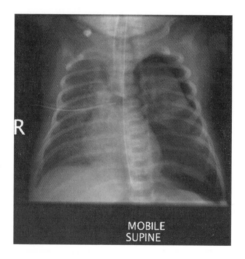

Figure 4.4   An intubated premature infant with a right-sided chest drain. Note the left-sided tension pneumothorax. A nasogastric tube is in the stomach.

It can sometimes be very difficult to distinguish consolidation from the right upper lobe aspiration that commonly occurs in infants with acute bronchiolitis.

Hyperinflation

Chest x-rays taken of infants and children with air-trapping states such as bronchiolitis and asthma frequently show hyperinflation. This can be seen as an increase in the lung fields, with flattening of the diaphragm. Within the radiolucent lung field, at least 10 posterior ribs can be counted. The mediastinum is narrowed and a normal heart may appear small.

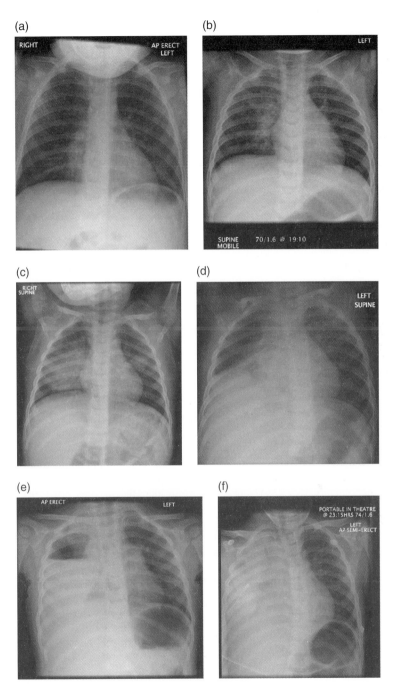

Figure 4.5 (a) Indistinct right heart border indicating consolidation in the medial segment of the right middle lobe. (b) Right middle lobe consolidation. (c) Rounded consolidation in the right lower lobe and left upper lobe. (d) Right middle and lower lobe consolidation. (e) Large right-sided hydropneumothorax. (f) Right necrotising pneumonia.

Box 4.1   Other investigations

Corticosteroid reversibility testing for 2 weeks: justify continuous use of inhaled steroids
Blood profile: immunoglobulin levels (IgE)
Laryngoscopy: test to diagnose vocal cord dysfunction
pH study: gastro-oesophageal reflux
  Skin tests
  Exercise testing
Blood gas analysis: CO_2 monitoring

Air leaks

The lung is encased within the visceral pleura. The chest wall is lined by the parietal pleura. The space between contains a small amount of fluid which helps avoid friction during respiration. Air within the pleural space is called a pneumothorax and if enough is present, it can be seen on a chest x-ray. The air can enter either via the lung or from a penetrating chest injury. When enough air is in the pleural space, the mediastinum will deviate towards the opposite side, causing a tension pneumothorax (Figures 4.4, 4.5). Air under the diaphragm in an erect chest x-ray is seen with a perforated bowel.

Limitations of the plain chest x-ray

Each x-ray is two-dimensional. To help confirm if a shadow noticed on a plain PA chest x-ray is intrapulmonary or extrapulmonary, a lateral film can help. However, high-resolution computed tomography (HR-CT) scan can provide three-dimensional information, and at much higher resolution. This aids in confirming the location of pathology and provides much improved visualisation. Inflamed bronchi, for example, easily seen on HR-CT, are not easily seen on plain chest x-ray. The disadvantage is in the increased radiation dose, and in smaller children and infants, sedation is usually required.

It is beyond the scope of this chapter to discuss all the investigations that may be performed for children with respiratory disease but some other investigations that may requested are identified in Box 4.1.

Bronchoscopy and bronchial lavage

Flexible bronchoscopy is a procedure whereby a flexible telescope is passed through the vocal cords into the lungs, usually under general anaesthetic. This procedure has been used for decades in adult patients, where it may be helpful in the diagnosis of lung cancer through biopsies performed with the aid of the bronchoscope. In recent years, the procedure has been used increasingly in children, to allow visual inspection of the airway, collection of samples by lavage (washing) the airway and occasionally biopsy (Midulla et al. 2003).

The arrangement of equipment and patient for flexible bronchoscopy is shown in Figure 4.6. The bronchoscope may be passed into the trachea, using a largyngeal mask airway (LMA) which sits above the vocal cords (Smyth et al. 1996) or a endotracheal tube which passes between the cords (see Figure 4.7). The bronchoscope must be disinfected in glutaraldehyde before and after each procedure. This must only be performed by suitably trained personnel and the cleaning must be done well in advance to allow the procedure to commence on time.

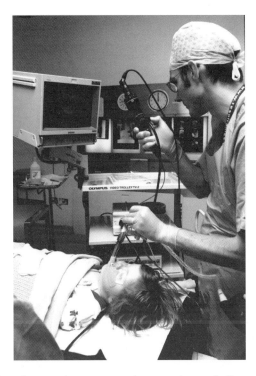

Figure 4.6   Flexible bronchoscopy in progress under general anaesthetic.

(a)   (b)

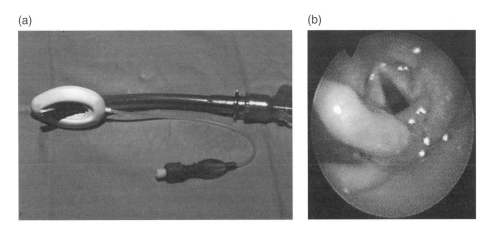

Figure 4.7   (a) The laryngeal mask airway, with the bronchoscope *in situ*. (b) The appearance of the vocal cords (vocal folds) through the flexible bronchoscope.

Technique

The bronchoscope has a suction channel through which 0.9% saline may be flushed into the airways (Figure 4.8). The saline is then sucked back, along with respiratory cells and in some cases pathogens (such as *Pneumocystis jiroveci* (see below) or bacteria). This procedure is called bronchial

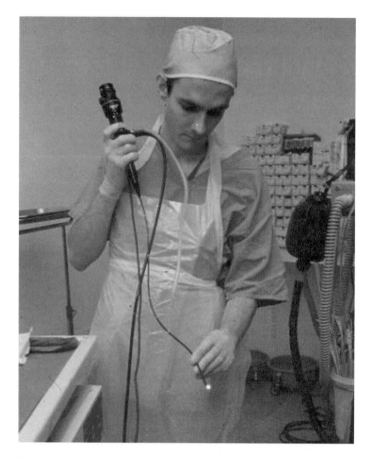

Figure 4.8   The equipment used for flexible bronchoscopy.

lavage or, when the bronchoscope is in the periphery of the lung, bronchoalveolar lavage (BAL). A maximum of 2 mL/kg of 0.9% saline is used per procedure. In most cases, the first specimen taken is bronchial and the second and third are alveolar. An alveolar sample can be analysed for *P. jiroveci* and viruses. The alveolar specimen may also be assessed to determine whether the cells which clear up debris (macrophages) contain fat globules (lipid-laden macrophages), suggesting that milk may have refluxed from the stomach and been inhaled. This is an important cause of lung disease in some babies.

Some situations in which flexible bronchoscopy might be helpful

Stridor (rasping breathing) in a young infant

Some babies are born with pressure on the windpipe (e.g. from an abnormal blood vessel) or abnormalities of the vocal cords (e.g. laryngomalacia or 'floppy larynx'). This leads to a rasping noise or stridor, usually when breathing in, which may be accompanied by laboured breathing. The bronchoscopy may help make the diagnosis. Treatment may be needed (such as surgery for an abnormal blood vessel) or the parents may be reassured that the problem will settle on its own (as with laryngomalacia).

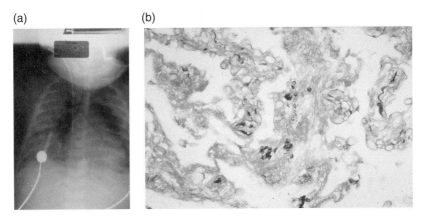

(a)   (b)

Figure 4.9 (a) Chest x-ray and (b) bronchoalveolar lavage specimen from an infant with HIV infection. The lavage specimen is stained with silver stain to show *Pneumocystis jiroveci*.

Persistent cough or wheeze

Children who cough over a long period may have a foreign body in the airway (see below). Alternatively the airway may be floppy (tracheomalacia or bronchomalacia), leading to cough and a harsh wheeze when breathing out. A floppy trachea is common in children who have had surgery for an abnormal connection between the trachea and the oesophagus (tracheo-oesophageal fistula or TOF). The TOF may be very noticeable ('TOF cough').

Haemoptysis (coughing up blood)

This may be seen where there is a foreign body in the airway, in children with TB or bronchiectasis and with some airway abnormalities where there is an abnormal connection between the arteries and veins (arteriovenous malformation).

Persistent collapse of one or more lung lobes

This may be seen in inhaled foreign body (see below). Occasionally bronchoscopy may be therapeutic, e.g. removal of a mucus plug.

Pneumonia in a child with immune deficiency or immune suppression

In children with immune deficiency (e.g. HIV infection) or immune suppression (e.g. children treated for cancer), unusual infections may occur such as *Pneumocystis* pneumonia (PCP; see Glossary), caused by the fungal organism *Pneumocystis jiroveci*. Bronchoscopy and lavage is the most effective method of diagnosis (Figure 4.9). Specific treatment (high-dose co-trimoxazole) is indicated and additional steroid treatment may be given.

Suspected inhaled foreign body (combine with rigid bronchoscopy)

Occasionally a small foreign body can lodge in a lobar bronchus (Figure 4.10). Such items include peanuts, raisins and pencil rubbers. In the lower airway foreign bodies give rise to chronic cough and wheeze is heard on one side only. A chest x-ray may show collapse of the obstructed lobe and

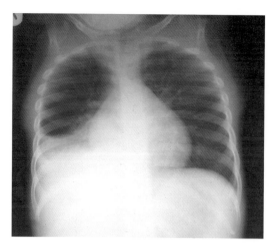

Figure 4.10   A foreign body in the bronchus intermedius on the right (not visible on x-ray). The image also illustrates collapse of the obstructed lobe and hyperinflation of adjacent lobes.

(a)   (b)

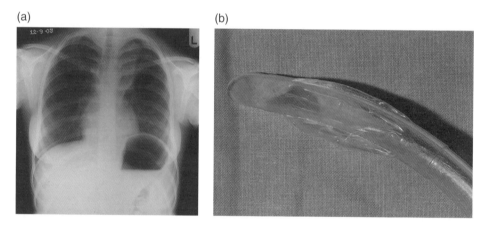

Figure 4.11   Mucus plugging has led to the collapse of the left upper lobe in a teenager with cystic fibrosis. (a) Partial collapse of the left upper lobe due to a mucus plug. (b) The mucus plug has been removed using the bronchoscope, but has occluded the endotracheal tube. The tube was changed during the procedure and the lobe subsequently re-expanded.

hyperinflation of adjacent lobes (see Figure 4.10). A foreign body in the lower airway must be removed by rigid bronchoscopy, undertaken by an ear, nose and throat (ENT) surgeon. The flexible scope may help locate the foreign body (under the same anaesthetic). Care must be taken with foreign bodies which have been in the lower airway for a week or more as friable granulation tissue may have formed, leading to bleeding. This is a particular problem with peanuts. The oil which coats the peanuts is irritant, causing arachis bronchitis.

Cystic fibrosis: to obtain specimens or attempt mucus plug removal

Patients with cystic fibrosis (CF) may develop plugs of thick mucus which can block the airway, leading to the collapse of the lung beyond the obstruction (Figure 4.11). In some cases the mucus plug can be removed using the bronchoscope. Where this is impossible, a drug which breaks down mucus plugs, such as dornase α, can be instilled through the bronchoscope.

Tracheostomy assessment and difficult intubation

The bronchoscope can be passed through a tracheostomy tube to examine the trachea and other airways below the tracheostomy tube. In some cases, where intubation is difficult, the endotracheal tube can be passed over the bronchoscope, the bronchoscope passed through the vocal cords and then the endotracheal tube slid into place to secure the airway.

Diagnosis of an H-type fistula

This is an abnormal communication between the trachea and oesophagus which may be diagnosed late because there is no interruption to the oesophagus (no oesophageal atresia). If an endoscope is placed in the oesophagus and a bronchoscope in the trachea, then bubbles of air can be passed from the oesophagus into the trachea, diagnosing the fistula.

Diagnosis of interstitial lung disease (biopsy required)

Rarely, children may develop inflammation of the lung tissue which is not due to infection (interstitial pneumonitis). This shows itself as laboured breathing, an oxygen requirement and growth faltering. A combination of high-resolution CT scan of the chest and bronchoscopy with biopsy helps make the diagnosis.

Flexible bronchoscopy should not be performed if the child has a problem with blood clotting or has very low oxygen levels.

While this can be a very useful investigation, it is also paramount that children are supported in an environment with appropriate nursing expertise.

Nursing management

Naturally, tests and investigations will increase anticipatory anxiety in child and parent. Therefore it is important to acknowledge that both will display anxiety when accessing hospital services.

It is vital to explain the process thoroughly to the child and family prior to any procedure to ensure that they are adequately prepared. In preparation for a bronchscopy, it is important that the child and parents understand the significance of preoperative care, including the need for a general anaesthetic, which will later be reinforced by a doctor. Nurses can also ensure that doctors have obtained consent for any photography during the procedure.

Preoperative preparation also includes communicating to the child and family basic information, such as no food to be given for 4 h and clear fluids only for 2 h before the procedure (BTS 2001).

During the procedure, monitoring and maintaining the patient's oxygen saturation levels above 90% are recommended as good practice by the British Thoracic Society (BTS 2001), because cardiac arrhythmias can be a problem during and after the procedure. Children with chronic lung disease are more susceptible to such complications so in the initial postoperative period, supplementary oxygen is recommended to minimise the risk (Connett 2005).

Postoperative nursing management following bronchoalveolar lavage and bronchcoscopy

There are many complications that can occur following a bronchoscopy; some of these are listed in Box 4.2. Therefore, following a bronchoscopy, or any surgical procedure, children will require monitoring of vital signs. This will ensure that complications can be recognised as soon as possible.

Box 4.2   Possible complications following a bronchoscopy

Fever
Bronchospasm or laryngospasm
Reaction to sedation
Respiratory depression
Pneumonia
Hypoxia
Nausea and vomiting
Sore throat

Children with severe lung disease occasionally require postoperative management in a paediatric high-dependency unit. A 24-h period of observation enables close monitoring and the opportunity for nurses to report complications to the doctors in a timely fashion. The high-dependency environment is also the most appropriate area in which to nurse the child if there are concerns about cardiac arrhythmias, and monitoring with an electrocardiogram (ECG) is required.

If a biopsy has been performed, there is an increased risk of bleeding from the site and leakage of air known as a pneumothorax (BTS 2001). Therefore monitoring of vital signs such as respiratory rate, breath sounds and colour is also paramount. Other possible complications include infection. Some patients will have intravenous antibiotics before the procedure, thus reducing the risk of infection. However, fever is the most common adverse effect following bronchoscopy and BAL. Therefore temperature should be monitored and treated appropriately.

Other complications that can occur at the time of the procedure and after are listed in Box 4.2. However, the BTS guidelines (2001) state that at the time of the procedure, complications such as swelling can occur to the larynx or trachea. This is noted to occur at the initial stages of the procedure. Consequently it is important to monitor the patient until the gag reflex returns, sedation wears off and the patient's breathing returns to normal respiration (BTS 2001). It is also good practice, as part of airway management, not to offer food until the patient is swallowing adequately to ensure safety (Ramsay 1989). Once it has been established that the gag reflex has returned, the introduction of fluids and food should be a gradual process. This is because it is also common for nausea and vomiting to occur.

Parents and children need to be informed that it is normal to have a sore throat after the procedure, even though a local anaesthetic is applied to the throat.

For many children with respiratory disease, cough is also a common feature. Post procedure, this can be exacerbated for up to 48 h, sometimes with a wheeze. It is important that observations are recorded and reported to medical staff, in particular if the cough persists and causes respiratory distress.

Postbronchoscopy complications which are rare but more severe and possibly life threatening are listed in Box 4.2. However, hypoxia and hypoxaemia are more common when BAL is performed.

Most children will be admitted as a day case and discharged home following the procedure. Sometimes it is necessary for children to stay overnight if they present with the following problems.

- Unable to take food or fluids.
- Breathing difficulties.
- Continues to have a temperature.
- Still drowsy following anaesthetic.
- Needs further treatment such as intravenous (IV) fluids.

On discharge, parents should be reminded that their child may cough more than usual for some weeks.

Case study

Kate was an 8-year-old girl with CF who experienced a sudden change in her condition. Her symptoms included cough, sore throat, production of green sputum and pyrexia that did not respond to paracetamol.

On examination Kate was found to have mild intercostal recession, enlarged tonsils and reduced air entry within the left lung. A chest x-ray revealed that she had left lower lobe collapse (atelectasis) with consolidation and presence of a mucus plug in the airways.

Kate's treatment included IV antibiotic therapy and nebulised dornase α, to reduce the viscosity of her sputum. This would enable Kate to expectorate sputum more easily with physiotherapy.

Despite aggressive treatment, Kate did not appear to be improving. Therefore to improve the ateletasis a bronchoscopy was performed. This revealed that the bronchus in the left lower lobe was occluded by a mucus plug.

This occlusion was resolved by BAL and dornase α was instilled at the end of the procedure.

Following the bronchoscopy and completion of a 2-week course of IV antibiotics, Kate made a good recovery and was discharged home on dornase α without any further recurrence of the problem. This case study illustrates how investigations such as bronchoscopy and BAL can improve clinical outcome.

Conclusion

Modern medicine has provided healthcare professionals with greater options for tests and investigations that inform diagnosis and treatment. Advancements in technology also ensure that children receive care which is provided by knowledgeable nurses with specialist skills based on best practice.

Questions

Answer true or false.

1. Flexible bronchoscopy in children:
   a. is used routinely in the diagnosis of asthma
   b. is usually performed under general anaesthetic
   c. may be used to help locate an inhaled foreign body
   d. may be useful in the diagnosis of congenital stridor
   e. is useful in the diagnosis of cystic fibrosis.

2. Flexible bronchoscopy in children is useful in treatment:
   a. where there is congenital stridor
   b. where there is mucus plugging and lobar collapse in cystic fibrosis
   c. where dornase α may be instilled down the bronchoscope
   d. where co-trimoxazole may be instilled down the bronchoscope
   e. through removal of an inhaled foreign body with the flexible bronchoscope.

3. Flexible bronchoscopy in children should *not* be performed:
   a. where opportunistic infection is suspected
   b. without thorough disinfection of the bronchoscope
   c. where clotting is prolonged
   d. where there is haemoptysis
   e. where there is a high and increasing oxygen requirement.

4. A structured method of interpretation when reviewing chest x-rays enables:
  a. any abnormalities to be detected
  b. an assessment of alignment by looking at symmetry in the clavicles
  c. an assessment of the bones; it is important not to miss fractures or bone disease
  d. measurement of the stomach
  e. the nerves supplying the heart to be assessed.

5. Cautionary measures taken when carrying out x-rays include:
  a. only requesting x-rays when necessary, thus minimising exposure and reducing the risk of lymphoma in later life
  b. performing a posteroanterior film which reduces magnification and possible adverse effects on structures such as the heart
  c. no consideration of magnification when assessing for cardiomegaly
  d. no particular consideration of the position of the x-ray film for babies
  e. adopting a lateral view when performing x-rays.

6. Complications following flexible bronchoscopy include:
  a. swelling of the trachea
  b. sore throat
  c. bronchodilation
  d. low temperature
  e. the inability to swallow food or drink.

7. The reasons for admitting a patient overnight following bronchoscopy would be:
  a. breathing difficulties
  b. intravenous fluids not required
  c. continues with a fever
  d. is able to take food and fluids
  e. continues to be drowsy after anaesthetic.

References

British Thoracic Society (BTS). (2001) *Guidelines on Diagnostic Flexible Bronchoscopy*. London: British Thoracic Society.

Connett G. (2005) Monitoring and investigations: bronchoscopy. In: Peebles A, Maddison J, Gavin J, Connett G (eds) *Cystic Fibrosis Care: a practical guide*. London: Elsevier, pp.143–5.

Midulla F, de Blic J, Barbato A, *et al.* (2003) Flexible endoscopy of paediatric airways. *European Respiratory Journal* **22**, 698–708.

Ramsey J. (1989) *Nursing the Child with Respiratory Problems*. London: Chapman and Hall.

Smyth AR, Bowhay AR, Heaf LJ, Smyth R. (1996) The laryngeal mask airway in fibreoptic bronchoscopy. *Archives of Diseases in Childhood* **75**, 344–5.

Chapter 5

Assessment of defects in airflow and lung volume using spirometry

Harish Vyas[1] and Caroline Youle[2]

[1] *Consultant in Paediatric Respiratory Medicine*
[2] *Children's Respiratory Nurse Specialist, Nottingham Children's Hospital*

Learning objectives

After reading this chapter the reader will have an understanding of:

- the importance of history and assessment prior to spirometry testing
- spirometry tests and interpretation
- bronchodilator tests using spirometry
- nursing assessment
- criteria and contraindications for spirometry testing.

Respiratory assessment

The respiratory assessment of a child is complex. It involves careful history taking, clinical evaluation and evaluation of pulmonary function when possible and indicated. In order to obtain a diagnosis, the presence of symptoms, pattern of illness and precipitating factors are very important.

History

The majority of children would develop symptoms of asthma in the first 5 years of life but diagnosis in infants is often difficult and many remain undiagnosed for long periods of time. A positive family history of asthma or atopy may help in early identification. It is always important to identify the frequency and onset of symptoms; further details will be discussed in Chapter 10. Asthma is seasonal, with symptoms being brought on by viral illnesses in winter and exposure to pollen and moulds in summer and autumn. In the older child, running or playing sports will bring on bouts of coughing and shortness of breath and a trial of β-agonists may be of benefit.

The majority of children will have intermittent symptoms, often with long periods of being completely well. However, in some chronically symptomatic patients, acute exacerbation may be punctuated by worsening of symptoms often requiring hospital admission.

Asthma is a clinical diagnosis but spirometry and other pulmonary function tests are very useful in establishing airflow obstruction and demonstrating evidence of reversibility.

Children's Respiratory Nursing, First Edition. Edited by Janice Mighten.
© 2013 Blackwell Publishing Ltd. Published 2013 by Blackwell Publishing Ltd.

Peak expiratory flow

The availability of portable spirometry has eclipsed the use of peak expiratory flow (PEF) measurement routinely for evaluation of airway obstruction. PEF is suboptimal as an investigation for evaluating airways obstruction and has poor reproducibility. There are no recognised reference values for many populations and PEF may underestimate airway obstruction, especially in muscular individuals. It should not be used on its own to diagnose asthma.

Spirometry

Pulmonary function tests are used to ascertain the severity of lung disease and trend changes in response to therapy. Asthma is defined by reversibility of airways obstruction and spirometry is particularly useful in demonstrating this effectively by the use of bronchodilators. It is a test which is increasingly recommended in children over 5 years of age. It should also be borne in mind that there may a discrepancy between the clinical severity of asthma and spirometry findings. It is also common practice to use spirometry for other respiratory conditions such as non-cystic fibrosis (CF) bronchiectasis, cystic fibrosis and primary cilary dyskinesia.

Spirometry measurements

Forced vital capacity (FVC) is the total amount of air exhaled after maximal inspiration. Forced expiratory volume in 1 second (FEV1) is the volume of air exhaled in the first second and is the most commonly used respiratory function test (Cooper and Mitchell 2003; Cotes 1979). It has excellent repeatability and extensive information is available in normal as well as diseased states. Decline in FEV1 reflects reduction in total lung capacity, loss of lung recoil and muscle weakness. However, its most common use is in evaluating intrathoracic airways obstruction. It is also used to evaluate and monitor severity of airways obstruction over time (ATS 1995). Spirometry can be routinely considered in all children aged over 5 years although with suitable training, preschool children may be able to perform spirometry.

Airflow obstruction is defined as FEV1 of less than 80% of predicted value and FEV1/FVC ratio of less than 0.8 (80%) (Nunn 1987). There are reference values available based on race, age, height and sex. The majority of new spirometers are computer based and will produce the ratios automatically. FEV1/FVC is a sensitive measure of impairment but FEV1 is a better indicator of future worsening.

In obstructive disorders, e.g. asthma, FEV1, forced expiratory flow (FEF)25–75 (representing small airways) and peak expiratory flow rate (PEFR) are decreased. The FEF25–75 is a parameter which is not effort dependent and may be useful in mild symptom-free patients with normal FEV1. FVC is reduced in restrictive disorders, e.g. severe scoliosis. In severe restriction, FEV1/FVC ratio will be elevated over 85%. In extrathoracic obstruction a distinctive pattern in flow–volume curves will be seen with a 'square box' symmetrical pattern of maximum inspiratory and expiratory flow.

Calibration

Modern medicine demands health and safety guidelines based on best practice and quality assurance measures. Practices such as spirometry also require safety mechanisms, so in order to record volumes of air inhaled and exhaled precisely, the spirometer needs to be calibrated and checked prior to each clinic, at 4-hourly intervals and if there is a change in the room temperature of 5°C, if practically possible (Education for Health 2005). In order to maintain such safe practices, the manufacturer's instructions for calibration should be adhered to. Some spirometers allow adjustment of the calibration immediately, e.g. Fleisch pneumotachograph, whilst others require correction by an engineer.

Calibration is done by using a 1 L or 3 L syringe to pump air into the spirometer. The syringe also needs to provide an accurate measurement, the 1 L syringe being accurate to 5 mL and the 3 L syringe to 15 mL. Periodically, the syringe needs checking for leaks by pushing the pistol of the syringe whilst the outlet is occluded (Booker 2008). The calibration check is performed with the filters on, in case any resistance alters the figures, thus ensuring that the correct syringe volume is entered into the data. The calibration readings produced should be within 3% of the syringe volume. Spirometers which calculate the calibration accept a response in the range of 0.97–1.03 (3%) before prompting to update the calibration (Booker 2008).

Spirometers moved from building to building will need time to adjust to the new room temperature before the calibration check is done, because spirometers are sensitive to temperature. Ideally spirometry should be performed at 20–25°C but definitely in the range of 17–40°C (Education for Health 2005).

The syringe should also be kept with the spirometer to provide the same temperature and humidity. It should be kept away from direct heat and sunlight. Some spirometers require the temperature and barometer recordings to be entered, whilst others will have sensors which automatically gather the information (Booker 2008; Miller et al. 2005a).

A printout or written calibration results should be kept for future reference in case of discrepancies, which could potentially lead to inaccurate results. Also documentation of any repairs, servicing and updates of the spirometer should be kept, which is an important element of health and safety (Miller et al. 2005a,b).

What to record

Before asking the child to perform the test, it is always best to demonstrate the manoeuvre to ensure that they understand the procedure. Important measurements are required such as the child's age, height and weight. The child should be preferably seated to limit movements. However, if the child prefers to stand then this is acceptable.

The process involved in spirometry testing will be discussed later in this chapter. Ideally a minimum of three manoeuvres is required. The success of the test relies on the skill of the person performing the test, as suggested by Cooper (2006). With flow–volume curves and/or volume–time curves being displayed on the screen, the best blows can be identified and poor blows excluded. Most spirometers have an incentive on the computer screen to optimise exhalation. This may take a few seconds. A clip may be put on to the nose to make sure that no air escapes from the nose. This process can be repeated to obtain the best result. Reproducibility (consistency) is important. Therefore during spirometry testing, it is important to continue to coach and cajole the patient with phrases such as 'come on, keep blowing', 'don't stop, keep blowing'.

There are five major criteria for accepting the test.

- There should be a good start to the test. It should be rapid and forceful.
- If the patient starts coughing during the procedure, the blow should be discarded.
- There should be no variable flow. Often children either start with a forceful breath but stop or take another breath during the manoeuvre.
- There should be no early termination.
- There should be reproducibility.

Associated problems

Lack of reproducibility

A child's poor technique on inspiration/expiration may result from a lack of understanding of the procedure or boredom from performing repeated tests. Verbal encouragement and praising the child for their correct technique may help them succeed with further blows.

Patients with vocal cord dysfunction may display variations in their results. Vocal cord dysfunction (VCD) occurs when the vocal cords do not open and close properly during speech and breathing (Mobeireek et al. 1995). The normal function of the vocal cords is to allow the flow of air into the trachea and the lungs.

Goldman and Muers (1991) outline the associated problems with airflow, which occur with both inspiration and expiration. Essentially, the vocal cords constrict on inspiration, often referred to as 'adduction'. The opening of the vocal cords then becomes smaller, restricting airflow into the trachea and lungs, causing difficulties with breathing.

When instructing a patient to do a flow–volume loop, it is important that the respiratory nurse has the experience to recognise abnormal sounds during the procedure and abnormal values when producing a report. It has been well documented that VCD can mimic and present with symptoms similar to bronchial asthma (Mobeireek et al. 1995). Therefore it is also necessary to save all the tests, especially the inspiration attempts, and to be aware of the medical history. Both the results and the history can assist in making a potential diagnosis and prevent long-term treatment for asthma (Mohiddin and Morris 2006).

Air leaks

Either an instrumental leak or air leaking from the mouth can be seen on the volume/time trace as a downward tilt. The correct positioning of the mouthpiece to prevent air leaks should be addressed during the procedure.

Slow start to the forced expiratory manoeuvre

Some children will take a good breath in and then not blow straight away, causing a slow start to the test (Figure 5.1). A delay of 4–6 s or a slow inbreath may reduce the FEV1 and PEF results (Miller et al. 2005a). Therefore it is necessary to give encouragement to blow hard and fast immediately after a deep breath in.

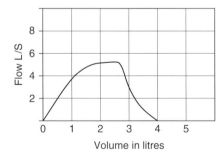

Figure 5.1   Rounded shape indicating poor start.

Cough

A wavy line appears on the trace when the patient coughs (Figure 5.2). If this occurs within the first second it should be discounted. Keep all the traces and obtain a good medical history. The patient will need adequate rest in between each blow. Abandon the tests if necessary.

Extra blows

Extra blows may occur with an enthusiastic child trying to obtain the best results, or a lack of understanding of the technique. Removing the mouthpiece before another breath is taken may help (Figure 5.3).

Early termination of the blow

The child may stop blowing too early (Figure 5.4). This sometimes occurs when the child is concentrating on the inspiratory part of the technique in flow–volume loops. Give encouragement until they cannot blow any more, and then ask them to breathe in. Young children may perform better if only the expiration trace is done. Early termination traces can still be used for the report.

Spirometry worsens with each effort

Spirometry is effort dependent and non-reproducible tests indicate variable effort (Figure 5.5). A forced blow may cause bronchospasm, with falling of the FEV1 and FVC. Overlapping traces help to detect this. In some children spirometry-induced bronchospasm will make each subsequent

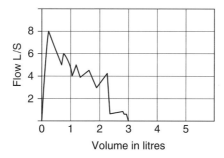

Figure 5.2 Coughing during spirometry.

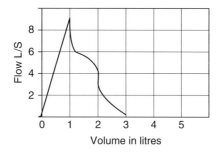

Figure 5.3 Variable flow rates.

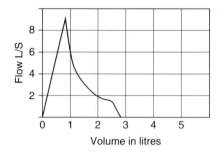

Figure 5.4   Early termination of exhalation.

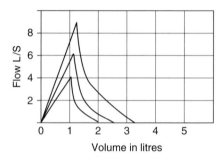

Figure 5.5   Spirometry worsens with each effort.

breath worse. In that situation, the first (best) test should be accepted. If this occurs, the testing is stopped and bronchodilators given if required or if needed for reversibility testing. The traces are labelled in time order.

Incomplete inspiratory curve

Young children may have difficulty performing this procedure, when they are expected to perform the expiratory curve as well. Pointing out where the inspiratory curve needs to join up with the expiratory one might help.

Bronchodilator challenge

Spirometry should be performed before and after administration of a bronchodilator to assess for airway reversibility. This is known as bronchodilator response. In clinical practice, lung function tests are carried out without withholding regular controller medications. For the purpose of clinical evaluation it is important that the patient has withheld a short-acting bronchodilator for at least 6 h and long-acting β-agonist for at least 12 h prior to the study. Salbutamol 400 µg is administered via a spacer and the patient is re-tested 15 min later. Significant reversibility is indicated by an increase in FEV1 of ≥ 12% suggesting asthma.

Bronchial challenge tests

These tests provoke a bronchial hyper-reactive response. They can be chemical, e.g. methacholine, exercise or cold air. These tests should be performed in a specialist laboratory in the presence of clinicians experienced in managing severe airway obstruction. A nebuliser with salbutamol should be prepared and oxygen should also be available. Naturally these tests should be avoided during an acute asthma attack.

Methacholine

This works on the parasympathetic nervous system, causing stimulation of smooth muscle, which can be found in the bronchioles. It is mainly used as a research tool (Liem et al. 2008). The test involves a stepwise increase in inhaled methacholine concentrations. FEV1 measurements are taken following each inhaled test. The concentration of methacholine required to produce a 20% reduction in FEV1 is referred to as PC20. There is an inverse relationship between the dosage and hyper-reactivity. PC20 at a low dose indicates significant hyper-responsive airways.

Exercise and cold air challenge

This is more widely used as it is better tolerated. The child is exercised on a treadmill until 85% of maximal heart rate for age is reached (usually for 6–8 min). Following the exercise, spirometry is performed repeatedly at frequent intervals for a maximum of 20 min. A 10% drop in FEV1 within that period is considered a positive challenge. Cold air challenge is performed similarly with the patient hyperventilating cold air. Once again, a drop in FEV1 of greater than 10% is considered positive.

Airway resistance

In asthma, airway resistance increases during an acute attack and falls following administration of β-agonist inhaler treatment. Measurement of airway resistance in the past has been difficult, requiring body plethysmography. However, recently introduction of interrupter resistance technique has made the measurement very easy. The technique is easy to use in preschool children. Its use in bronchodilator challenge is still not well established.

Lung volume measurement in children

The measurement of lung volumes usually refers to measurement of total lung capacity (TLC), residual volume (RV) and functional residual capacity (FRC) (Figure 5.6). These measurements are useful in identifying restrictive lung disorders and conditions associated with air trapping.

The two common methods used for these measurements are whole-body plethysmography and gas dilution using either helium or nitrogen washout. Whole-body plethysmography involves sitting the child inside a 'body box' which is tightly sealed. The child then breathes normally through a mouthpiece. Children with neuromuscular disease may have difficulty using this. In children with scoliosis, reference values should be determined using the arm span which is normally equal to height. In such cases or situations where the child is unable to stand, the arm span can be used (height = arm span divided by 1.06) (Miller et al. 2005b). The child is asked to breathe normally at tidal volume (TV). By using Boyle's law, FRC is calculated. It is a useful investigation for obstructive conditions. Some children find the experience frightening and the investigation may have to be abandoned. Gas dilution technique is ideal for measuring FRC.

Infant lung function

The investigation of lung function in infants is normally carried out in specialised laboratories. The reason for assessing pulmonary functions in infants is either research or clinical. Infant pulmonary

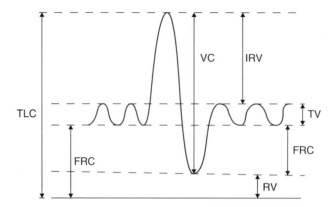

Figure 5.6   Lung volumes measured with a spirometer, only changes in lung volume can be measured with a spirometer. FRC, functional residual capacity; FRV, functional reserve volume; IRV, inspiratory reserve volume; RV, reserve volume; TLC, total lung capacity; TV, tidal volume; VC, vital capacity.

function tests are used for evaluating the impact of early events such as smoking, prematurity or ventilation on lung growth. In addition, these tests are used for evaluating medical interventions such as surfactant or steroid administration. Clinical applications include early recognition of diseases such as cystic fibrosis, effect of treatment, e.g. steroids, and impact of surgery.

Summary

Spirometry is a useful diagnostic tool. It is particularly useful for monitoring progression of lung disease and for ongoing assessment following lung transplantation. Respiratory nurses make a valuable contribution to preparing children and young people and facilitating parental understanding of this process.

Nursing management

As previously mentioned, spirometry testing is suitable for children 5 years and over. In preschool children spirometry performance may be inaccurate. This may also interfere with their inhaler technique and reference values will not be accurate in order to provide a comparison. Therefore it is important to adapt a consistent approach with spirometry testing to ensure accuracy, as suggested by the American Thoracic Society (ATS 2005).

The environment can also have some influence on how well children co-operate with spirometry testing. It is well documented that children should ideally be seen in a child-friendly environment, where toys are provided. This should also include individuals who are experienced in caring for children and young people, which should also be the case in a clinic or laboratory where spirometry testing is performed.

Priority of patients

Spirometry may be requested as an urgent referral or used in CF and asthma clinics as a routine occurrence. When planning the order of patients to be seen, there is the need to consider the infection risk to or from the patient. Therefore children who are immunocompromised should be delegated a position early on the list when the equipment has been freshly sterilised (Booker 2008;

Table 5.1   Time gap between medication administration and testing

Medication	Time gap
Inhaled β2-agonists Short-acting (SABA, i.e. salbutamol)	4–8 h
Long-acting (LABA, i.e. Serevent)	24 h
Anticholinergics	6 h
Theophylline twice-daily preparations	24 h

Education for Health 2005). Children with a respiratory infection ideally should not perform spirometry but if this is necessary, they should be placed last on the list and equipment cleaned afterwards. It is good practice to use a mouthpiece that contains a bacterial filter, with all spirometry equipment. Ideally a spirometry machine should be purchased that contains separate flow heads. This can also be used to reduce the risk of cross-infection from different bacteria.

Routine referrals for diagnostic purposes

These patients would ideally benefit from preinvestigation information, stating what the procedure involves and preparation instructions. Typically a child is asked:

- not to eat a large meal for 2 h before the test, as a full stomach can hinder the lung capacity
- to avoid wearing tight clothing which may restrict breathing
- not to climb the stairs but use the lift within half an hour of the appointment time
- to visit the toilet
- not to take salbutamol, ipratropium bromide or terbutaline inhalers prior to the test unless they cannot be avoided
- to take other inhalers/oral medications unless instructed not to by the requesting doctor
- to bring all inhalers presently used to the appointment.

(Adapted from ARTP 2000; Booker 2008; Miller et al. 2005b.)
Teenagers should refrain from smoking for 1 h before the test.

The reasons for withholding medications depend on the questions that need to be answered. Table 5.1 lists the time gaps required between medications and spirometry testing.

Spirometry checklist for use prior to testing

As spirometry requires considerable effort to obtain meaningful results; consideration is given to previous/present medical history. Contraindications include the following.

- Operations of the eyes, chest and abdomen in the last 3 months.
- High blood pressure, history of aneurysms and pneumothorax, coughing up blood and chest infections.
- Infection risk – coughs and colds and other infectious illnesses.
- Record if the child has taken bronchodilators and any other information which would interfere with the accuracy of the results.

Ensure that the child is comfortable prior to the test. Other factors to consider, such as needing to go to the toilet, feeling nauseated, vomiting, having diarrhoea, being in pain, having just eaten, all would hinder the child from blowing hard and putting effort into the blow (ARTP 2000; Booker 2008; Education for Health 2005).

Other important parameters include the need to accurately weigh and measure the child in metric units, making sure that outdoor clothing and shoes are removed. It is also vital to ensure that measurements and patient details are entered into the correct box on the spirometer. Some spirometers will not work unless the weight is entered. The weight becomes important if the Body Mass Index is over 34.

Some doctors request that spirometry results are based on the child's height or the child's arm span if the patient has scoliosis, for example. Muirhead and Conner (1985) emphasized the importance of lung function testing in children with scoliosis preoperatively. They suggested that lung function demonstrates a restrictive pattern but lung capacity is not always abnormal in this client group.

Performing the spirometry tests

Spirometry in children can be a challenge, and obtaining reliable spirometry results depends on the child having a good technique. This is not age related because a 5-year-old child's technique may be better than that of a teenager.

For safety reasons, the patient may be advised to be seated in a chair with arm rests (BTS 1994). This is in case the child feels faint or light-headed. Some spirometer instructions, however, request the patient to be standing. Therefore it is important to risk assess each patient and follow individual hospital/clinic protocol. Sitting may prevent an obese child with significant weight around their middle from breathing in deeply and thus may lower the results. For repeated studies, the previous position should be selected to provide consistency and to allow comparison of the results.

Spirometry testing in children often includes forced vital capacity, relaxed vital capacity and flow–volume loops as discussed earlier.

Each test requires a different technique. Trying to perform the different types of test all at once could confuse the young child. Being aware of the child's age, ability and medical history would help determine which test would be the most appropriate. The medical history would reveal any underlying conditions or contraindications for performing the test.

Different spirometry machines display visual aids to promote prolonged blowing. Incentives may include a clown with a bell, blowing bubble gum, etc. However Gracchi et al. (2003) suggest that computer incentives do not necessarily improve results. They found that in some cases spirometry results were worse when an incentive was utilised but maintain that practitioners should use clinical judgement when using the computer incentives available.

It is important to tell the parent and child why the test is being done. The respiratory nurse should always ensure that the reasons are the same as those given by the doctor. Provide a simple explanation of the technique. For example, 'take a deep breath in, place the mouthpiece into the mouth and seal your lips around the mouthpiece'. Using a suitable sized mouthpiece positioned in between the teeth with the lips sealed around it and avoiding the tongue obstructing the mouthpiece will give more accurate results than a child blowing into it like a trumpet.

A useful analogy is to instruct the child to imagine that they are blowing out the candles on a birthday cake in one long breath, until the candles are all out. This often helps younger children to grasp the concept of sustaining the blow for as long as possible. Participating parents, siblings and an enthusiastic technician could improve the child's results. However, a teenager who may be embarrassed would benefit from being alone with the technician.

Relaxed vital capacity

Relaxed vital capacity (RVC) is usually performed in adults. It helps to detect air trapping. This is less common in children and the relaxed vital capacity is not always needed. This procedure needs to be done before a forced vital capacity. The child is asked to take a deep breath in until no more air can be inhaled. The mouthpiece is placed in between the teeth with the lips tight around it. The child is instructed to breathe out nice and steady until they cannot blow out any more.

Breathing out too slowly can give a low recording of the vital capacity (Miller et al. 2005a). The wearing of a nose clip can prevent nasal breathing; quite often children do not like wearing these. A maximum of four RVC tests is suggested with a minimum of two reproducible tests. A relaxed inspiratory capacity result can also be affected by an inbreath that is too slow, not breathing in straight away or not taking a full breath in.

Forced vital capacity

The child is asked to take a fast big breath in, growing tall to fill the lungs with air, and then straight away blow hard and fast until they cannot blow any longer. The child is encouraged to keep blowing for 3 s if under 10 years old and for 6 s or longer if over 10 years (Miller et al. 2005).

Flow–volume loop

The same procedure is followed as the FVC. Once the air is exhaled completely, the child is asked to breathe in rapidly until the lungs are full again. Some spirometers start the test with tidal breathing, so follow the manufacturer's instructions. Although nose clips should be worn, not all children will tolerate them. They could pinch their nose instead.

Observe the child for:

- immediately exhaling from a full inspiration
- any coughing
- the amount of effort put into the blow
- whether the inbreath was adequate prior to the blow
- how long the child blew for
- position; was there any bending over at the waist?
- adequate rest taken between each blow
- accuracy of performance
- a good mouth seal; children with weakness or palsy at the mouth may require jaw support to prevent air escaping
- a dental brace that may hinder the performance, and write on the report if they have one.

It is important to check the traces between each blow to detect errors and to ensure all the figures are obtained and help the child to correct the technique.

Perfecting a child's technique may take more than three goes. A maximum of eight is recommended per session. Consideration should be given to the following.

- Whether the child requires reversibility testing.
- Is the child getting tired?
- Is the child bored and losing concentration so that they do not want to blow any more?
- Is the FEV1 dropping and the child becoming bronchoconstricted? If this happens the tests should stop and a bronchodilator be given if required.
- Is adequate rest provided in between each blow?

Give the child verbal praise, and point out which part of the technique they did really well, so that they do not feel criticized when attempts to adjust the technique are made. Written messages on the computer screen may also pop up when the child has done well. At the end of the test the child may be rewarded with stickers and a certificate.

Acceptable results

Maximum effort in expiration and inspiration should produce a trace which is smooth, steep and close to the vertical axis and a descent which tapers off until it reaches the horizontal axis and the inspiratory curve rejoins the starting point in a normal spirometry. Ideally three acceptable blows should be performed, two of which are reproducible within 100 mL of each FEV1 and FVC. The highest FVC and FEV1 of those are reported on, even if they are from different blows (Education for Health 2005).

The child needs to breathe out for at least 1 s until a plateau presents on the volume–time trace. Not every child can blow reproducible results without any errors. This should be taken into consideration when reporting, as it may be the child's best effort.

Technical errors include the following.

- Poor calibration: the syringe volume does not tally with the corresponding data entry on the computer.
- Height and weight entered into the wrong boxes.
- Wrong sex entered on the computer.
- Ethnicity/mixed race not taken into consideration.
- Spirometer set to give the best result, so other data are lost.
- Some spirometers will only give the best result.
- Some spirometers will not accept age and height in the younger age groups.
- Inability to examine trace because some spirometers do not produce traces.
- Inaccurate measurements of the arm span.

Reversibility testing

Once acceptable reproducible baseline spirometry tests are produced, the traces are examined. Signs of an obstructive pattern may warrant reversibility testing. Arrangements to proceed with reversibility testing vary from clinic to clinic but may include:

- doctors reporting on the results first
- prewritten bronchodilator prescriptions, allowing competent technicians to read the results and proceed
- technicians having Patient Group Directions for bronchodilator prescriptions.

Being aware of the child's medical history could help predict the outcome of the bronchodilator response. A child with mild or asymptomatic asthma may have little or no response to the bronchodilator whereas moderate asthma would show a good response. In severe asthma, where inflammation is present, the response may be limited (ARTP 2000).

Ascertain whether the patient is allergic to the bronchodilators or has cardiac problems that the medication may affect. The child is given a prescribed dose of salbutamol through a spacer device, as discussed earlier. The delivery technique is explained, checked and adjusted as required to provide maximum drug deposition. Using different delivery devices for bronchodilators could make the deposition of the drug vary and make comparison of previous results difficult. A 15–20-min wait will ensure a maximum response to the salbutamol, before repeating the spirometry tests, although a delay of up to 2 h is possible. If testing with terbutaline, give 500–1000 µg through the turbohaler. With ipratropium bromide, give the prescribed dose and wait 45 min. The maximum response would be seen at around 2–3 h. It is not advisable to test with ipratropium bromide and salbutamol in the same session as the results could be confusing (ARTP 2000; Education for Health 2005).

The accuracy of the spirometry technique is observed and adjusted accordingly, to produce two acceptable results. A combined total of eight pre- and postbronchodilator forced blows is allowed, as a forced manoeuvre can cause fatigue.

What to report

The report should consist of:

- name, identification number
- spirometry traces
- predicted values based on the child's height, weight, sex, race, age
- baseline values
- child's spirometry technique
- time when the last bronchodilators and other medication which will affect the results, e.g. prednisolone, was given
- present relevant medications
- name of bronchodilator for reversibility testing, dose, delivery method and technique
- postbronchodilator results
- other factors which could affect the results: upper respiratory tract infection, dental brace, mouth weakness
- record of whether the results lack reproducibility
- whether sitting or standing.

(Adapted from ARTP 2000; Education for Health 2005.)
Some spirometers are able to provide traces of blows on one chart. This allows assessment for reproducibility, any bronchoconstriction, deviation from the predicted trace and comparing pre- and postbronchodilator results. However, the number of traces printed on one chart may be limited. Trending of previous results is available on some machines.

Further testing

To gain a good comparison of results with further testing, the conditions ideally need to be consistent, i.e. the same technician, machine, location, preparation method, and same time of the day within 2 h.

Cleaning of the spirometer

Prior to purchasing a spirometer, consideration should be given to the suitability of the cleaning, disinfecting and sterilisation procedure in your own setting. For example, a Fleisch requires time to dry properly between clinics. It is advisable to follow the manufacturer's instructions and local protocol for cleaning, disinfecting and sterilising the spirometer. Afterwards check flow sensors for any holes or obstructions and allow thorough air drying. The volume measuring spirometers need to be checked for leaks to reduces the infection control risks.

Disposable antiviral and antibacterial expiratory and/or inspiratory filters are available for single patient use. Nose clips for individual patients are also supplied. A good hygiene routine of hand washing and cleaning of the external housing unit of the spirometer between each patient should be adopted to reduce the infection risk.

Maintaining a log of patients who have performed tests, with times and dates, provides a mechanism for tracing patients if a patient with an infectious illness has been tested prior to a diagnosis being made, thus maintaining an audit trail. It is advisable to avoid testing patients with known infections such as tuberculosis. Naturally, equipment needs sterilising if used on infectious patients; infection control staff should be contacted for advice and local procedures followed (Education for Health 2005).

Conclusion

Spirometry has a significant role to play in paediatric respiratory medicine. Equally nurses have a valuable contribution to make when supporting and teaching other colleagues about the practicalities of the process and the importance of the procedure, as well as fully informing children, young people and their parents. Consideration must always be given not only to reporting accuracy of the tests but also maintaining safe practice.

Questions

1. What is airflow obstruction?
2. What values will be affected during spirometry for obstructive conditions such as asthma?
3. List three criteria required for the acceptance of a spirometry test.
4. How can nurses encourage children when carrying out spirometry?
5. What infection control measures need to be considered before performing spirometry?

References

American Thoracic Society (ATS). (1995) Standardization of spirometry. *Am J Respir Crit Care Med* **152**, 1107–36.

Association for Respiratory Technology and Physiology (ARTP). (2000) *ARTP Spirometry Handbook*. Birmingham: Association for Respiratory Technology and Physiology.

Booker R. (2008) *Vital Lung Function*. London: Class Publishing, pp. 41–56.

British Thoracic Society (BTS). (1994) *Spirometry in practice: a practical guide to using spirometry in primary care*. London: British Thoracic Society (1994) *Spirometry in practice*; A practical guide to using spirometry in primary care 1st edition, BTS London.

Cooper BG. (2006) Performing good quality spirometry. Available at www.evidence.nhs.uk.

Cooper K, Mitchell P. (2003) Procedure for the assessment of lung function with spirometry. *Nursing Times* **99(23)**, 57–60.

Cotes JE. (1979) *Lung Function Assessment and Application in Medicine*, 4th edn. Oxford: Blackwell.

Education for Health. (2005) *Spirometry for Practice*. Warwickshire: Salvo.

Goldman J, Muers M. (1991) Editorial: vocal cord dysfunction. *Thorax* **46(6)**, 401.

Gracchi B, Boel M, van der Laag J, van der Ent C. (2003) Spirometry in young children: should computer animation programs be used during testing? *European Respiratory Journal* **21(5)**, 872–5.

Liem JJ, Kozyrskyj AL, Donald W, Cockcroft D, Allan B, Becker MD. (2008) Diagnosing asthma in children: what is the role of methacholine bronchoprovocation testing? *Pediatric Pulmonology* **43(5)**, 481–9.

Miller MR, Hankinson J, Brusasco V, *et al.* (2005a) Standardisation of spirometry. *European Respiratory Journal* **26**, 319–38.

Miller MR, Crapo R, Hankinson J, *et al.* (2005b) General considerations for lung function testing. *European Respiratory Journal* **26**, 153–61.

Mobeireek A, Alhamad A, Al-Subaei A, Alzer A. (1995) Psychogenic vocal cord dysfunction simulating bronchial asthma. *European Respiratory Journal* **8**, 1978–81.

Mohiddin S, Morris MJ. (2006) Vocal cord dysfunction and asthma; US espiratory care. Available at: www.touchrespiratory.com.

Muirhead A, Conner A. (1985) The assessment of lung function in children with scoliosis. *British Editorial Society of Bone and Joint Surgery* **67(5)**, 699–702.

Nunn JF. (1987) *Applied Respiratory Physiology*, 3rd edn. London: Butterworth.

Chapter 6

Oxygen therapy

Jayesh Bhatt[1] and Sarah Spencer[2]

[1] Consultant Respiratory Paediatrician
[2] Specialist Practitioner in Children's Community Nursing, Nottingham Children's Hospital

---

Learning objectives

By studying this chapter, the reader will:

- understand the importance of adequate oxygenation and its effects on the respiratory system in children
- learn about the methods used for and the significance of monitoring oxygen levels
- learn about the causes of low oxygen levels
- become familiar with home oxygen therapy and monitoring
- understand the importance of community nursing support.

Pathophysiology of oxygenation

The word oxygen (derived from Greek *oxys* acid, *genes* producer) is required for oxidative metabolism to produce energy for the tissues and the product of this is carbon dioxide (CO_2), an acidic gas (Davies and Carl 2003). The purpose of the lung is gas exchange and its primary function is to allow oxygen from inspired air to move into and carbon dioxide to move out of the blood, as discussed in Chapter 1. Problems can lead to low oxygen levels which will be discussed next.

Hypoxaemia/hypoxia

The terms 'hypoxia' and 'hypoxaemia' are sometimes used interchangeably but they represent different concepts. Hypoxia is an inadequate amount of oxygen available at the tissue level (this cannot be measured) whereas hypoxaemia is an inadequate amount of oxygen in the blood (this can be measured). Hypoxia occurs for a variety of reasons.

Children's Respiratory Nursing, First Edition. Edited by Janice Mighten.
© 2013 Blackwell Publishing Ltd. Published 2013 by Blackwell Publishing Ltd.

Pulmonary causes

- Alveolar hypoventilation, when there is inadequate respiratory effort secondary to respiratory depression or neuromuscular disease, for example.
- Diffusion defects at the alveolar-capillary level, for example in interstitial lung disease where the diseased interstitium is preventing adequate gas exchange.
- Ventilation-perfusion (V/Q) mismatch is the most common cause. This occurs (1) when areas of the lung that are receiving the blood supply, known as perfusion, are not moving the air in and out, known as ventilation, and (2) there are areas of the lung that are better ventilated than perfused, due to airway obstruction.

Non-pulmonary causes

- Reduced blood flow: myocardial infarction, shock and anaemia.
- Non-functioning haemoglobin (the element of the blood that transports oxygen): haemoglobin can become bound to other substances, such as carbon dioxide and cyanide. In order to cope with this, the body has compensatory mechanisms to prevent and correct hypoxia. The respiratory system will increase the minute ventilation by increasing the respiratory rate and/or the tidal volume, and will change the blood flow to optimize the V/Q ratio. The heart rate and contractility will increase, and selective vasoconstriction and vasodilation will take place to pump oxygenated blood to the priority organs.

With the exception of the kidneys' response, all the compensatory mechanisms to correct hypoxemia increase the tissue demand for oxygen, thus increasing workload, which can result in respiratory failure.

Respiratory failure

Respiratory failure exists when the respiratory system cannot transfer oxygen into or CO_2 out of the blood. This can happen acutely, for example with severe respiratory syncytial virus or bronchiolitis, or more insidiously in a child with neuromuscular disease. In the latter category, an intercurrent illness may tip these children over into acute or chronic respiratory failure.

It is helpful to consider respiratory failure as arising from various situations (Box 6.1).

Oxygen therapy is required for hypoxemic respiratory failure. For the purposes of this chapter, only long-term oxygen supplementation in a non-acute setting will be considered.

Long-term oxygen therapy

Long-term oxygen therapy (LTOT) is the provision of oxygen therapy for continuous use at home for patients with chronic hypoxaemia (due to any cause), in order to maintain oxygen saturation (SpO_2) at or above 92%. Measurement depends on the type of oximeter or arterial oxygen tension (PaO_2) above 8 kPa. LTOT may be required 24 h a day or during periods of sleep only. Any child likely to require continuous or intermittent oxygen therapy for more than 2–3 weeks should be considered for discharge home on LTOT. The principal aims of LTOT are to prevent harm from chronic hypoxaemia and to improve any relevant symptoms (Box 6.2) (Balfour-Lynn et al. 2009).

When considering LTOT, it is useful to include the following five fundamental questions, the first two of which will be discussed next. The last three questions will be covered in the section below on home oxygen guidelines.

Box 6.1   Causes of respiratory failure

- **Failure of control of respiration:** central nervous system diseases, e.g. conditions such as congenital central hypoventilation syndrome, drugs, encephalitis
- **Failure of the pump:** due to diseases of the spinal cord, e.g. spinal muscular atrophy, nerves, e.g Guillain–Barré syndrome, chest wall deformities, e.g. severe kyphoscoliosis
- **Lung diseases:** infections, e.g. severe bronchiolitis, pneumonia, upper or lower airway obstruction, e.g. acute laryngotracheobronchitis (croup) or acute severe asthma
- **Congenital lung disease:** e.g. pulmonary hypoplasia, diaphragmatic hernia

---

Box 6.2   Indications for long-term oxygen therapy (including ambulatory)

- Chronic neonatal lung disease
- Other oxygen-dependent neonatal lung conditions
- Pulmonary hypertension
- Infants and children who have recurrent cyanotic-apnoeic episodes, severe enough to require cardiopulmonary resuscitation
- Interstitial lung disease, obliterative bronchiolitis
- Hypoxic children with cystic fibrosis
- Obstructive sleep apnoea
- Hypoventilation (assuming the child is optimally ventilated)
- Sickle cell disease
- Palliative care

- Why give oxygen?
- Who needs home oxygen?
- How much oxygen should be given?
- What equipment is required?
- When is it no longer necessary?

Why give oxygen?

Poets (1998) reviewed the literature to ascertain if infants required supplentary oxygen, suggesting that chronic hypoxaemia can lead to pulmonary hypertension. This is initially a reactive phenomenon and can be reversible. If chronic hypoxia persists, structural changes happen in the pulmonary vasculature leading to permanent changes and established pulmonary hypertension.

Babies with chronic neonatal lung disease (CNLD) tend to have more reactive pulmonary vasculature, and small changes in oxygenation seem to produce significant changes in pulmonary artery pressure. Also repeated episodes of hypoxia seem to have a greater effect than isolated episodes. Pulmonary hypertension can develop in any case of chronic hypoxaemia, including severe advanced cystic fibrosis, sickle lung disease or obstructive sleep apnoea. It is important to recognise and correct chronic hypoxaemia in these disorders to prevent the occurrence of pulmonary hypertension.

As previously mentioned, CNLD infants have an increased risk of this complication. Teague et al. (1998) discussed increased airway resistance in CNLD babies. When SpO_2 of 89% on room air was corrected to 94–96% with supplemental oxygen, airway resistance decreased, dynamic compliance improved and work of breathing decreased. It is well documented that decreased oxygen levels have adverse effects on cognition and behaviour in babies with CNLD. For older children, growth and development will also be affected in the long term.

It may be difficult to separate out the effects of the stormy neonatal course and associated complications related to prematurity and the effects of chronic hypoxaemia on neurocognition and behaviour. Sleep-disordered breathing can lead to poor neurocognitive outcomes. It can be associated with gas exchange abnormality but there is also sleep fragmentation and both can lead to learning difficulties.

An increased risk of apparent life-threatening events in babies with CNLD occurs when target oxygen saturations are maintained at below 90%; failure to grow is another consequence of this. However, growth velocity improves and catch-up growth occurs when babies are supplemented with oxygen while the growth rate declines if oxygen is discontinued. Also, maintaining target oxygen saturation less than 90% leads to poor sleep quality in babies with CNLD, and this improves when supplemental oxygen is given.

Who needs home oxygen?

Current British Thoracic Society (BTS) guidelines make recommendations in relation to best practice for children who require supplemental oxygen (Balfour-Lynn et al. 2009). It should be remembered that the clinical conditions for which infants and children require home oxygen are very different from adults though there is an overlap between older children and young adults. The important factors that need to be considered are that the prognosis in infancy is usually good and many children only need oxygen for a limited period, although this may be for some years. As previously discussed, growth and neurodevelopment are important. Assessment of this is different at different gestational ages and consideration needs to be given particularly to the difficulty of arterial blood sampling as part of the assessment process prior to discharge home.

Monitoring oxygen therapies

The amount of oxygen in the blood can be measured in three different ways: the partial pressure of oxygen (PaO_2), oxygen content (CaO_2), and direct measurement of oxygen in the blood (SaO_2). SpO_2 involves an indirect measurement of the oxygen saturation level using a probe and pulse oximeter. SpO_2 obtained from the pulse oximeter is approximately equal to SaO_2 (arterial haemoglobin saturation from a blood gas).

- **PaO_2** is the pressure (P) exerted by oxygen dissolved in the arterial blood (a). 30% total oxygen.
- **CaO_2** is the number of millilitres of oxygen carried by 100 mL of whole blood.
- **SaO_2** is the percentage (%) of oxygen that the haemoglobin is carrying.

The greater portion of oxygen (about 97%) is chemically bound to haemoglobin as oxyhaemoglobin. The PaO_2 reflects gas exchange in the lung and is the driving force behind haemoglobin saturation.

In children, PaO_2 is obtained by performing an arterial blood gas measurement though this is usually only done when the child is on the intensive care unit and has an indwelling arterial line. A normal range for PaO_2 on room air is 70–100 mmHg. This measurement can be affected by age. As people age, their 'normal' PaO_2 decreases. Also, the higher the altitude, the lower the pressure to push oxygen into the blood.

Haemoglobin carries oxygen around the body. The haemoglobin molecule consists of two pairs of polypeptide chains (α and β) and each of the polypeptide chains has a haem group attached. Each haem group has one iron atom attached. Oxygen is attached to and detached from the haem groups during its transport around the body. As these haem groups 'fill up' with oxygen, the amount of light they absorb changes. This is why arterial blood tends to be bright red and venous blood tends to be darker. This is the basic principle used in pulse oximetry.

Pulse oximetry

Pulse oximetry measures the oxygen saturation of the arterial blood flow through the extremity on which the probe has been placed (Figure 6.1). A pulse oximeter will display oxygen saturation (SpO_2) and heart rate, with a plethysmographic waveform (Chandler 2000) showing the pulsatile nature of the arterial blood flow through the extremity. A pulse oximeter also displays a motion indicator showing the signal quality and whether the displayed saturation and heart rates can be considered accurate.

The basic principle of pulse oximetry is that a light is passed through the arteriolar bed (feet in small babies or an ear lobe) and measured on the other side. Therefore it is important that the light source and detector are opposite each other.

Correct positioning of the probe is very important in obtaining an accurate measure of the oxygen saturation. An appropriate probe for the size of the patient should be placed in an appropriate position (Table 6.1). It can run on battery or mains power and will have audible alarms which can be set with both an upper and a lower limit.

Red and infrared light are transmitted alternately from the light source. The absorption of light by haemoglobin varies with the level of oxygenation. Pulse oximetry requires a pulsatile flow between the light source and photodetector. There is a relationship between SpO_2 and PaO_2 (Table 6.2) and it is important to understand this, especially when trying to understand the lower normal limits during emergency situations.

The benefits of SaO_2 monitoring are that it is non-invasive, it is accurate with a SaO_2 greater than 70% and can allow continuous monitoring. However, it has limitations. Inaccurate readings will be obtained in many situations; for example, excessive movement, known as motion artefact, will limit accuracy of monitoring. With conditions such as hypotension and shock, monitoring is affected by a poor pulsatile signal.

Balfour-Lynn et al. (2009) highlight the associated problems with monitoring, such as malpositioning of the probe which may let some of the light straight through to the photodetector and give falsely high readings. Outside light interference and nail varnish in dark colours can affect the readings through the nail bed. High bilirubin levels, such as in liver failure, also affect accurate monitoring.

There are many different systems in place for monitoring infants at home on oxygen. The controversy around the use of oxygen saturation monitoring at home is not a new phenomenon. For many years there has been widespread debate as to whether oxygen-dependent infants should go home with pulse oximeters in order for parents to monitor their child's oxygen saturation levels.

The provision of home saturation monitors should not be recommended as routine because there is no evidence of benefit or harm for their use. Some problems related to their use are increased

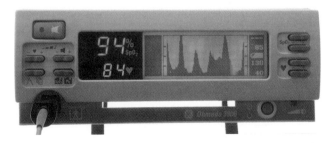

Figure 6.1 Oxygen saturation monitor. Reproduced with permission from Nottingham University Hospital.

Table 6.1   Pulse oximeter position/type of probes

Age	Site	Type of probe
Neonate/infant	Big toe, foot outer area	Adhesive single-patient use, size varies according to weight
Child	Across hand/finger	Adhesive single-patient use
	Big toe	
Adolescents	Finger index	Clip reusable

Table 6.2 SpO_2 and PaO_2 levels

SpO_2	PaO_2	mmHg	Status
98%	12–14 kPa	90–105	Normal
90%	8 kPa	60	Low
80%	6 kPa	45	Very low
75%	5 kPa	37.5	Very low

anxiety and undue parental reliance on the monitor, with some parents finding it difficult to accept the need to discontinue their use, when oxygen therapy is weaned. Other problems include unnecessary minor adjustments of flow rates, false reassurance of respiratory status, false alarms (less with newer motion-resistant technology) and cost. Nevertheless, some clinicians and parents may find this provision helpful in certain circumstances.

Home oxygen guidelines

In June 2003 the Department of Health announced plans to modernise the domiciliary oxygen service. The aim was to improve patient access to a wider range of modern technologies and to reduce the number of patients who receive oxygen therapy inappropriately (Godfrey 2004).

The home oxygen database and service commenced in October 2005 following new written guidelines issued by the Department of Health (2004) which have been updated in 2013. The new service ensures that oxygen is available on prescription as part of an integrated service (i.e. cylinder, concentrator and ambulatory oxygen) delivered directly to patients in their own homes. Oxygen equipment and servicing are all supplied and carried out by the oxygen provider.

The process involves obtaining consent from parents for their child's information to be stored on the database. Without a signed Home Oxygen Consent Form, the oxygen service is unable to supply the patient with the necessary equipment to administer supplementary oxygen. Once the consent form has been signed, a Home Oxygen Order Form (HOOF), updated in 2013, can be completed by any healthcare professional and faxed (not emailed) to the oxygen service.

Oxygen equipment can be delivered in three ways by the supplier. Emergency installation is within 4 h from acknowledgement of the faxed HOOF, next-day installation is available for hospital discharges and all other installations are standard delivery, which is within 3 working days. The cost of this service is funded by the patient's primary care trust. A nurse advisor from the oxygen company is available to assist with providing an individualised plan of care when initiating oxygen therapy.

How much oxygen should be given?

Balfour-Lynn et al. (2009) suggest that targets should be maintained for children's oxygen requirement which would be based on individual clinical symptoms.

In CNLD, oxygen therapy should be given to maintain a SpO_2 of 93% and above. The American Thoracic Society (ATS) guidelines recommend maintaining a saturation of 95% or more once past the age of oxygen-induced retinopathy (33 weeks postmenstrual or 4 weeks chronological age), as this provides a 'buffer' zone against oxygen desaturation that targets of 90% or more do not (ATS 2003). In other conditions, for example sickle cell disease, maintaining SpO_2 at 94–96% (to prevent painful crises and stroke) may be appropriate and for cystic fibrosis ≥90%. At present there are no data to guide target levels for SpO_2 in children with other respiratory conditions.

Generally practice is guided by studies which indicate that less than 5% of total study time should be spent below the saturation of 90%. It is not necessary to regularly assess CO_2 levels in infants with CNLD who are at home, but it may be useful in some neonates with other conditions and older children, especially when initiating home oxygen therapy. This would be carried out in hospital.

It is also good practice in infants with CNLD, prior to discharge, to perform an ECG or echocardiogram. This is useful to assess the right heart in order to exclude significant pulmonary hypertension, as previously discussed.

What equipment is required?

The home oxygen process will be discussed below. However, prescription requirements (examples in Table 6.3) may include oxygen concentrators that should be provided for LTOT, unless it is likely that the child will only require low-flow oxygen for a short while. Initially it is important to discuss and consider parent choice. Light-weight cylinders are easier to handle but they empty more quickly. Cylinders should be available for all children as part of the provision of home oxygen unless oxygen is only required at night.

When is it no longer necessary?

Discontinuing supplemental oxygen abruptly or gradually or weaning early or late does not seem to matter as long as weaning is done while maintaining the target oxygen saturations at the same level as when starting oxygen (Askie and Henderson-Smart 2001a,b).

Weaning of supplemental oxygen

This should be guided by overnight oxygen studies while maintaining the target oxygen saturations as previously discussed. Once the oxygen requirement is down to 0.1 L/min, the child may be ready to stop having supplemental oxygen.

Children can be weaned from continuous low-flow oxygen to night time and naps only, or remain in continuous oxygen throughout the 24 h until the child has no requirement at all. Oxygen equipment should be left in the home for at least 3 months after the child has stopped using it. If this is in a winter period, it is usually left until the end of winter. In CNLD, failure to reduce oxygen supplementation after 1 year warrants specialist review to rule out other conditions (see Chapter 11).

Discharge planning

Once it is deemed that the infant/child is ready for discharge and the need for oxygen is the only thing keeping the child in hospital, suitability for home oxygen therapy should be assessed. This should be carried out by a specialist with appropriate experience in the care of the relevant condition. This is usually either a respiratory paediatrician or a neonatologist (but may be a paediatric cardiologist, general paediatrician or palliative care specialist).

The family must also be assessed for their ability to manage home oxygen therapy and cope with all aspects of the child's care. The discharge planning should put in place a multidisciplinary follow-up to ensure a safe and smooth transition into the community. Parental education should include recognition of worsening clinical status and basic life support.

Before discharge, oxygen saturations must be measured continuously for at least 6–12 h to include periods of sleep, wakefulness and activity such as feeding; one-off measurements are insufficient. Feeding is quite a vigorous exertion for the infant and it is important to include a period of feeding as infants have an increased oxygen requirement during activity and infants with CNLD may develop feeding-related hypoxaemia. In addition, some children may only show evidence of nocturnal hypoxaemia without daytime hypoxaemia.

A period of sleep should also be included as clinically unsuspected sleep-related desaturations can occur in babies who are 'fully saturated' awake in air (Garg et al. 1998). Children can be discharged from the neonatal unit when their oxygen requirement is stable, with mean SpO_2 of $\geq 93\%$ and without frequent episodes of desaturation. The SpO_2 should not fall below 90% for more than 5% of the artefact-free recording period. There should be no other clinical conditions precluding discharge and the child must be medically stable.

Follow-up after discharge

The community children's nurse or nurse specialist should visit the child within 24 h of discharge. In particular, infants such as those with CNLD should have their SpO_2 monitored within a week of discharge, with subsequent recordings as clinically indicated (but not usually less often than 3–4 weekly); monitoring should include various activity states. Older children with other conditions who are clinically stable are likely to need home SpO_2 recordings performed less often than infants with CNLD.

Older children

For older children with other conditions previously mentioned, overnight oxygen studies inform the process of assessment and are useful in determining how well children will manage with the prescribed oxygen therapy at home. Circumstances will determine this; for example, children requiring oxygen for palliative care will have different physical demands that may be very short term. Children with uncorrected cardiac problems will also have needs that differ. For those with long-term conditions such as cystic fibrosis, oxygen may only be required at night. Therefore the nature of the assessment is very much individualised and disease specific.

Oxygen outside the home

Details surrounding the use of oxygen therapy in various situations outside the home environment will be discussed below. However, an appropriately trained individual should be present whilst the child is using the oxygen, but this does not necessarily have to be a school nurse or health professional. Other considerations include holidays where consideration needs to be given to high altitude, because during airline travel when rising there is a decreased inspired oxygen concentration. In a patient with marginal pulmonary reserves or who is maintained on supplemental oxygen, higher oxygen flows will be required which should be determined by a fitness-to-fly test.

Table 6.3 Equipment for home oxygen administration

Equipment	Use	Environment
Concentrator	LTOT	Home, school
Light-weight cylinder, low-flow regulator for some infants	Short term/LTOT	Outside home
Liquid oxygen	LTOT (>0.5 L/min only in most areas)	Outside home

LTOT, long-term oxygen therapy.

Potential disadvantages of home oxygen

It is rare for a child to be retained in hospital because the home environment is not conducive to carrying out the treatment. However, parent/carer smoking must be strongly discouraged. Parents/carers (and older children) must be made aware of the potential hazards of home oxygen, which will be addressed below. Equally, it is critical that parents and carers receive sufficient emotional support from their family, friends and healthcare services, including professionals such as community children's nurses.

Long-term oxygen therapy

When planning for discharge home, specific equipment is required to allow for low oxygen flow rates that some infants require. Almost all children receiving LTOT require ambulatory oxygen therapy, for example portable cylinders to use outside the home (see Table 6.3). Many children require LTOT overnight only, especially during the weaning stages. This is less than the 15 h that forms part of the adult LTOT definition. Ultimately all children will require supervision from a parent/carer with all this equipment. Another consideration is that provision of oxygen may be necessary at school for school-age children.

Equipment required

Parents have a number of oxygen delivery systems to become familiar with in order to care for their child safely (Allen and Kotecha 2002).

Oxygen concentrators are the most commonly used equipment for LTOT in the home environment (Figure 6.2). Concentrators work by drawing in room air through a series of filters to remove particulate matter (including bacteria) and nitrogen with the resultant oxygen stored in a reservoir before use (Dunbar and Kotecha 2000; McLauchlan 2002).

Two outlets are normally provided, one for the main living area and one for the bedroom (Balfour-Lynn et al. 2005). From these outlets, generous amounts of tubing are supplied to aid mobility to other rooms and if possible to the garden. The oxygen supplier maintains the concentrator as part of their contract. In the interim parents are taught how to change a simple external filter once weekly.

The concentrator runs off electricity and every quarter the cost of this is reimbursed to the family by the oxygen supplier (Barnett 2006). A large oxygen cylinder is supplied to parents as a back-up in case of machine or power failure.

Oxygen conservers are not indicated for young children but can be considered for older children capable of triggering the device. Humidification should be considered for high oxygen flows, when given by facemask. This is helpful especially for children with cystic fibrosis; a cold water bubble-through humidifier may be adequate for this purpose.

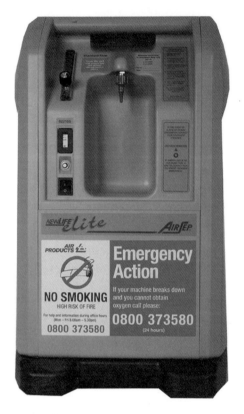

Figure 6.2   Oxygen concentrator. Courtesy of Air Products Healthcare.

When oxygen is given via a tracheostomy, heated humidification will generally be needed. A heat–moisture exchanger (Swedish nose) with an oxygen attachment may be an adequate alternative. Delivery methods such as nasal cannulae are preferable for infants and young children for flows ≤2 L/min (Figure 6.3). However, patient choice should be considered for older children (Figures 6.4, 6.5).

Ambulatory oxygen therapy

All children on LTOT (unless night time only) require portable cylinders for ambulatory use. Cylinders made of aluminium are now available and are much lighter than the original steel ones (Dunbar and Kotecha 2000). Although a priority for paediatric patients, these cylinders are not currently available to all infants as choice is dependent on safety, convenience and unfortunately cost. Low-flow meters are available for delivering small amounts of oxygen (0.1–1 L/min). Sized twin-pronged nasal cannulae, facemasks and extension tubing are all provided by the oxygen service (Balfour-Lynn et al. 2005).

Liquid oxygen therapy (Figure 6.6)

Other methods of oxygen delivery are also available for ambulatory use. Liquid oxygen has only been available on the NHS since the transformation of the oxygen service in 2006 but is rarely indicated for children. The equipment comes in two parts: the dewer and a refillable portable unit. A home

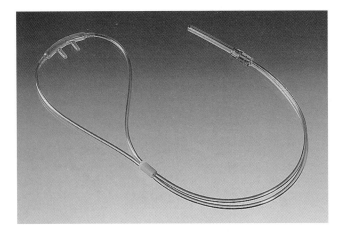

Figure 6.3 Nasal cannulae. Courtesy of Air Products Healthcare.

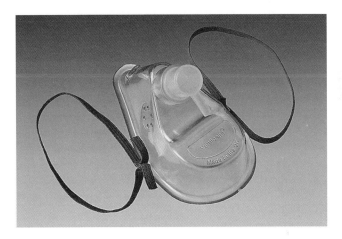

Figure 6.4 Basic oxygen mask. Courtesy of Air Products Healthcare.

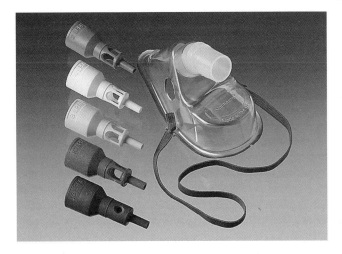

Figure 6.5 Venturi mask. Courtesy of Air Products Healthcare.

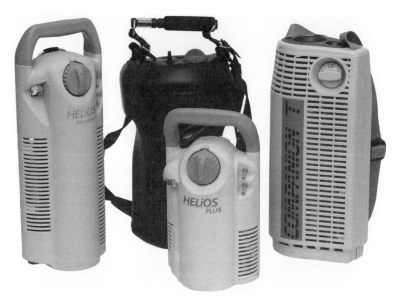

Figure 6.6   Liquid oxygen equipment. Courtesy of Air Products Healthcare.

assessment is required to ascertain suitability for the storage of the liquid oxygen dewer. Additional education and teaching on use and safety are provided by specialist liquid oxygen engineers.

The refillable unit should only be filled for use outside the home and a concentrator should be used in the home.

There are several oxygen providers in the UK. Each company will have different guidelines for the minimum oxygen requirement that can be delivered using liquid oxygen. Generally 0.5 L/min is the minimum in most areas (Air Products 2010). Therefore this mechanism is not suitable for infants who require quantities <0.5 L/min.

Liquid oxygen may be a more appropriate form of ambulatory oxygen if the child requires a larger prescription (more than 2 L/min) and spends a large proportion of their day out of the home (i.e. at school).

The lighter refillable unit lasts longer than a traditional oxygen cylinder. Care is essential as cold burns may result from accidental contact with the liquid oxygen (Dunbar and Kotecha 2000).

Oxygen in schools

Long-term oxygen therapy does not prevent children attending nursery or school (unless immune suppressed or prone to infection). Due to the growing number of children in the community on LTOT, there is an increasing demand for oxygen therapy to be available in nurseries and schools. Co-ordination is needed between the specialist nurse/children's community nurse and the school.

Within education, children with health needs often require a special educational needs statement (SEN), which is a local document often referred to as a 'statement' (DirectGov 2011). This process is currently under review, with proposed plans to replace the current system with a single assessment for health, social care needs and education (Department for Education 2011).

The school will apply for funding from the local education authority to support the health needs of the child in school, with the support of a learning support assistant (LSA). The LSA will support the child requiring LTOT, both physically and emotionally. This applies particularly to primary school children who will need adult supervision most of the time to ensure safety of the equipment.

Problems that can occur include other children turning the oxygen up, down or off. For adolescents, assistance is often required with navigating school corridors and class rooms at different levels.

Through closely working together, a healthcare plan can be devised for the individual child including all relevant contact numbers and a step-by-step emergency plan. A second HOOF must be completed for a separate oxygen source at school. If the child is to be carrying their oxygen cylinder themselves, lightweight equipment must be considered when ordering to make it easier for the child to handle (Balfour-Lynn et al. 2005). The school must ensure adequate insurance cover for staff and premises. Staff will require training on equipment use, storage and maintenance as well as the skills needed to identify any signs of respiratory distress (Balfour-Lynn et al. 2005; NHS 2010).

Holidays

It is possible to travel with a child dependent on LTOT but medical advice must be sought first. Currently, oxygen supplies are delivered free to most holiday destinations within the UK but there is a cost for this service when abroad. As from 2013 healthcare professionals will no longer need to complete a HOOF for a UK holiday order. For holidays abroad, the family must contact their oxygen supplier direct. On receipt of a separate HOOF, the oxygen company will communicate with the family to facilitate the process. If families are holidaying in the UK, the company will deliver and collect the equipment from the holiday address.

Families will need to give consideration to particular factors when planning their holidays.

- Is inflight oxygen required?
- Venue for holiday, i.e. cottage, holiday park.
- UK or abroad?
- Associated costs for holidays abroad.
- Electricity supply for privately rented accommodation.

Some companies will not provide oxygen supply at camp sites, because of the health and safety risks and lack of insurance cover when holidaying outdoors. The nurse has a responsibility to communicate this to families with assistance from the company, when families are considering their options for holidays. Therefore the nurse will work with the family to plan ahead. Ideally the companies require as much notice as possible, to ensure that the families' needs can be met safely.

Health and safety

Health and safety is paramount when oxygen is in the community setting, including the home environment; this will be addressed in more detail below. Oxygen is highly flammable, strongly supports combustion and increases the speed at which things burn once a fire starts. Nobody should smoke in the presence of oxygen (Balfour-Lynn et al. 2005). Therefore precautions must be taken and advice should be given about adopting a no smoking policy in the house. A child on oxygen should never be left in close proximity to gas cookers, open fires or birthday candles (Naylor 2003). The oxygen service engineers discuss this with parents as well as leaving comprehensive literature on installation, following a risk assessment of the home environment.

Care must also be taken with oil-based products. Grease, fat, oil or Vaseline-based products should never be used near the flow regulator, concentrator or cylinders. Oil-based products do not require a naked flame to combust in the presence of oxygen. The use of oil-based moisturising creams, massage oils and sun cream must also be avoided, using water-based products as an alternative.

Financial help

Every family caring for a child on LTOT is entitled to government help financially. Heath or social care professionals can assist families in accessing these funds. Disability Living Allowance (DLA) is a tax-free benefit for children and adults who need help with personal care or have walking difficulties because they are physically or mentally disabled. In addition, Carer's Allowance is a taxable benefit to help people who look after someone who is disabled. Health and social care professionals can also assist families who are struggling with applications to charitable funds, which all require support and co-ordination from nurses in the community.

Nursing management

Long-term oxygen therapy does not require a hospital environment (Allen and Kotecha 2002). However, the child's suitability for LTOT in the community should be assessed by a specialist paediatric respiratory consultant.

The family must also be carefully assessed as it is vital that parents understand the care they are expected to provide. Professionals also need to ascertain if the parents are able to cope with all aspects of the child's care (Balfour-Lynn et al. 2005; Fradd 1994). Family structure, patterns of daily living and family finances must all be scrutinised when considering discharge (Embon 1991). Equally important is the need to assess proximity to health services for the family and their responsiveness to the child's care needs.

The central role of discharge planning is to promote a seamless journey of care between hospital and home with the knowledgeable support of all involved (Moss and Bond 2002). Sending infants home while they are receiving oxygen therapy requires careful planning to ensure success (Allen and Kotecha 2002).

As soon as possible after deciding that the child should receive LTOT, a named nurse must be identified to co-ordinate the discharge planning. Following this, an education programme tailored to the individual child and family can commence. Through assigning the same nurse as a point of contact, the ongoing psychological and physical needs of the family can be comprehensively met (Broedsgaard and Wagner 2005).

A co-ordinated discharge planning meeting with parents, identified secondary carers, relevant staff and primary care clinicians should be organised a minimum of 2 weeks prior to discharge (Allen and Kotecha 2002; Balfour-Lynn et al. 2005; Dunbar and Kotecha 2000; Moss and Bond 2002). At these meetings parents' concerns can be discussed and addressed as well as medical history and future health needs. This meeting should also discuss the action plan to be followed if the infant/child becomes unwell once discharged home.

To successfully discharge a child home on LTOT, certain milestones must first be achieved. It is vital that the child is gaining adequate nutrition with or without the aid of a nasogastric tube, feeding supplements and/or high-calorie milk (Dunbar and Kotecha 2000). The treatment of gastro-oesophageal reflux, infection, cardiac dysfunction and, in neonates, retinopathy of prematurity (ROP) must be carried out whilst the child is an inpatient to avoid readmission to hospital. Immunisations should be up to date, including immunisation for influenza and respiratory syncytial virus (Dunbar and Kotecha 2000).

Respiratory effort should be stable. Oxygen saturation levels must be maintained above 94% in a consistent flow rate of supplementary oxygen when the child is awake, during feeding and whilst asleep (Naylor 2003). The most appropriate oxygen saturation level at which to maintain an infant has caused major controversy for many years. The clinical guidelines set out by Balfour-Lynn et al. (2005, 2009) can be followed.

The importance of empowering parents must be emphasised, helping them to build their confidence to provide an achievable degree of normality to family life through the use of appropriate information and teaching (Moss and Bond 2002). Teaching is normally commenced in the acute setting prior to discharge. This is then reinforced by the nurse specialist/children's community nurse (CCN) once at home and requires constant reassessment by all involved.

The nurse specialist/CCN therefore has considerable responsibility in ensuring that the family and other carers have the necessary instructions to enable the child to be cared for safely (Dimond 2005). Parents/carers need to be able to make a respiratory assessment of the infant and identify any changes from their normal respiratory pattern. They also need to assemble and safely use the equipment required for oxygen delivery, administer prescribed medication, initiate emergency treatment and basic resuscitation and be aware of pathways of help (Allen and Kotecha 2002; Balfour-Lynn et al. 2005; Dunbar and Kotecha 2000; Naylor 2003). In addition, health professionals should ensure that parents have easy contact for advice and support 24 h a day, 7 days a week (Dimond 2005; NHS 2010).

Maintaining a safe environment for these children once at home is also an essential part of the nurse specialist/CCN's role. Ensuring the family and infant maintain good health and wellbeing frequently requires input from all services, especially the county council and social services (Barnett 2006). Housing should be self-contained to facilitate adherence to safety issues for the safe storage and use of oxygen (Embon 1991). The family must always have access to a telephone in case of an emergency and it is vital that parents/carers and the child understand the potential hazards of oxygen therapy (Moss and Bond 2002). Therefore safety information is paramount prior to being discharged home on oxygen. It is the nurse specialist/CCN's responsibility to ensure that parents' skills are regularly updated and that their knowledge base continues to be at a level to safely care for their child's health needs.

None of this can be achieved without good communication with parents. Good communication is considered to be part of the duty of care owed to the child to ensure safety and support. To help parents follow their infant's oxygen therapy programme, it is advised that a care plan is written by the nurse specialist/CCN jointly with the family. This is kept in the home and can be used as a point of reference. The family must understand and be in agreement with the oxygen care plan if the programme is to be successful (Allen and Kotecha 2002; Naylor 2003).

It is essential to be aware that the nurse remains accountable for the actions of parents acting on their advice and teaching. If parents carry out a procedure that causes harm to the child, the nurse could be held responsible. This can be overcome by utilising a teaching checklist that parents sign to state they have been taught the skill (Dimond 2005). The CCN observes the parent/carer carrying out a taught procedure, a minimum of three times. Both the CCN and the parent/carer must be satisfied that the procedure has been done safely and confidently before the parent is signed as competent.

Measuring oxygen saturation levels using a pulse oximeter is a useful and non-invasive procedure (Allan and Kotecha 2002). The ATS has always supported the provision of oximeters to parents. However, their rationale seems to be mostly cost based in terms of reducing hospital and clinic/home visits (ATS 2003).

There is no question that non-invasive monitoring has revolutionised the ability to accurately track oxygenation status (Allen and Kotecha 2002). However, although pulse oximetry offers many benefits, it is only valuable if used correctly and in conjunction with a comprehensive respiratory assessment (Barnett 2006). An important aspect of nursing care when monitoring a child with a pulse oximeter is to ensure that the probe is rotated frequently to a different site. The skin also needs to be checked on a regular basis to prevent any damage from the infrared light that passes through the skin (Chandler 2000).

Parents already have a huge responsibility and steep learning curve when taking their oxygen-dependent child home without also taking on the responsibility of monitoring their child's oxygen saturation levels. Shielding them from continuous oxygen monitoring at home avoids parental dependence on these devices, which greatly increases anxiety especially when false readings occur due to artefacts (Dunbar and Kotecha 2000). Pulse oximeters all too often give false reassurance as oxygen saturation levels are only one aspect of the child's respiratory status.

Discontinuing parental use of pulse oximeters at home must therefore be considered. Each infant and unforeseen circumstance would have to be reviewed individually when making this decision. However, sense would suggest that if a child requires continuous monitoring then they are unlikely to be ready for hospital discharge (Balfour-Lynn et al. 2005).

To optimise oxygen delivery, it is recommended that formal overnight oxygen saturation studies (sleep studies) should be performed on all oxygen-dependent children prior to discharge. However, this very much depends on the circumstances; for example, this would not be appropriate in situations such as palliative care. Careful follow-up sleep studies, in particular for infants with CNLD, should take place in the community to ensure the child continues to receive the optimal amount of oxygen and is not discontinued too soon (Harrison et al. 2006; Primhak 2003).

Sleep studies can be carried out using saturation monitors with a data storage facility to record oxygen saturation levels overnight. The data can then be downloaded onto a computer and analysed (Naylor 2003). Results from regular formal sleep studies can then be medically and safely used with the input of the child's respiratory consultant and community nurse to wean an infant successfully off supplementary oxygen without putting the onus on parents. The child's oxygen flow rate can then be adjusted as appropriate (Naylor 2003).

Not having pulse oximeters in the home and health professionals regularly monitoring the infant mean that visits extend beyond a data collection exercise and start to generate feedback, prompt preventive care and support parent education (Balas and Lakovidis 1999). Most importantly, it gives parents more time to enjoy their child rather than merely nursing them.

Although this takes a degree of responsibility and control from parents, the risk of harm is reduced as weaning becomes medically based; ensuring oxygen saturation levels remain in the safety range removes the possibility of excessive adjustments of the flow rate by carers (Primhak 2003). Even after education, parents all too often think that keeping their child's oxygen saturation levels at 100% helps their child's recovery when in reality it can cause more harm than good.

When parents show concern that their child's oxygen needs increasing or decreasing (i.e. when the child has a cold), it is recommended that the child is seen in these circumstances, usually by the nurse specialist/CCN who can then make a full assessment (Balfour-Lynn et al. 2005). For children on LTOT, after viral infections, especially those requiring admission and increased oxygen requirements, they should be closely monitored and only discharged home when the oxygen requirement is stable.

The specialist nurse/CCN should evaluate the infant's and family's progress at each home visit. Parents' accounts/observation of their child's health should be discussed as additional information gained from the parents can prove useful in the evaluation.

Weaning from LTOT, as previously discussed, can also be carried out at home with the support of nurses and minimises the chance of nosocomial infection (Balfour-Lynn et al. 2005). This process will vary depending on each individual disease process. For example, chronic lung disease in children with CF or pulmonary fibrosis will not require frequent monitoring, as in an infant with CLD. Nurses caring for children in the community are reliant on guidelines such as those of the BTS. This places great emphasis on management of infants with CLD, which is essentially adapted to fit each specific disease profile.

Reassessment through regular sleep studies should be carried out monthly if the child is stable (Balfour-Lynn et al. 2005). Once the child is stable on 0.1 L/min of oxygen at night, a 2-h oximetry study in air can be carried out at home during the day (preferably including an oral feed if the child is able) (Simoes et al. 1997). If this is successful with no desaturations below 94%, the child can start having increasing periods of time in air during the day until fully weaned.

Infants are often successfully weaned in the day but still require oxygen at night. Once weaned in the day, a repeat study in air is carried out overnight. The aim is to achieve target saturation values similar to those used during oxygen therapy. Weaning is usually resisted during the winter periods since exacerbations with viral infection are likely (Dunbar and Kotecha 2000).

Once successfully weaned onto air, the oxygen equipment remains in the family home, after it is ensured that the infant can cope with at least one viral upper respiratory tract infection without problems (Balfour-Lynn et al. 2005).

This practice reflects current research when supported by excellent teaching and empowering of parents to take on the task at hand. The programme facilitates earlier discharge with benefits including improved feeding, growth and development, and enhanced parent–infant relationship (Naylor 2003). Parents are now being given back their status of being a parent, enabling them to enjoy their child rather than to nurse him/her.

Conclusion

Oxygen therapy has been revolutionised with the support of oxygen-providing companies, specialist clinicians and children's community nursing teams. The aim is to work with respiratory nurse specialists to support children and families in the community, in particular when children have worsening clinical symptoms; parents need advice and support to continue caring for their child at home.

Questions

1. What are the normal SpO_2 and PaO_2 levels?
2. What is ventilation/perfusion (V/Q) mismatch?
3. Causes of respiratory failure can be divided into three categories. What are they?
4. What are low SpO_2 and PaO_2 levels?
5. What other elements of oxygen therapy need consideration when prescribing equipment for home use?

References

Air Products (2010) A Guide to the Home Oxygen Service for Babies, Toddlers, Children and Teens. Available at www.airproducts.co.uk/homecare.

Allen J, Kotecha S. (2002) Oxygen therapy for infants with chronic lung disease. *Archives of Disease in Childhood Fetal and Neonatal* **87(1)**, F11–F14.

American Thoracic Society (ATS). (2003) Statement on the care of the child with chronic lung disease of infancy and childhood. *American Journal of Respiratory and Critical Care Medicine* **168(3)**, 356–96.

Askie LM, Henderson-Smart DJ. (2001a) Gradual versus abrupt discontinuation of oxygen in preterm or low birth weight infants. *Cochrane Database of Systematic Reviews* **4**, CD001075.

Askie LM, Henderson-Smart DJ. (2001b) Early versus late discontinuation of oxygen in preterm or low birth weight infants. *Cochrane Database of Systematic Reviews* **4**, CD001076.

Balas EA, Lakovidis I. (1999) Distance technologies for patient monitoring. *British Medical Journal* **319**, 1309.

Balfour-Lynn IM, Primhak RA, Shaw BNJ. (2005) Home oxygen for children: who, how and when? *Thorax* **60(1)**, 76–81.

Balfour-Lynn IM, Field DJ, Gringras P, *et al.*, on behalf of the Paediatric Section of the Home Oxygen Guideline Development Group of the BTS Standards of Care Committee. (2009) BTS guidelines for home oxygen in children. *Thorax* **64(Suppl II)**, ii1–ii26.

Barnett M. (2006) *Chronic Obstructive Pulmonary Disease in Primary Care*. London: John Wiley and Son Ltd.

Broedsgaard A, Wagner L. (2005) How to facilitate parents and their premature infants for the transition home. *International Nursing Review* **52(3)**, 196–203.

Chandler T. (2000) Oxygen saturation monitoring. *Paediatric Nursing* **12(8)**, 37–42.

Davies A, Carl M. (2003) *The Respiratory System. Basic science and clinical conditions.* London: Churchill Livingstone.

Department of Health. (2004) *A Modernised, Integrated Domiciliary Oxygen Service. Proposals for new guidelines for the use of domiciliary oxygen.* London: Stationery Office.

Department for Education. (2011) Government proposes biggest reforms to special education needs in 30 years. Available at: www.education.gov.uk.

Dimond B. (2005) Legal aspects of the community care of the sick child. In: Sidey A, Widdas D (eds) *Textbook of Community Children's Nursing*, 2nd edn. London: Harcourt, pp. 137–47.

DirectGov. Special education needs: statements (2011). Available at www.direct.gov.uk.

Dunbar H, Kotecha S. (2000) Domiciliary oxygen for infants with chronic lung disease of prematurity. *Care of the Critically Ill* **16(3)**, 90–3.

Embon CE. (1991) Discharge planning for infants with bronchopulmonary dysplasia. *Journal of Perinatal and Neonatal Nursing* **5(1)**, 54–63.

Fradd E. (1994) Whose responsibility? *Nursing Times* **90(6)**, 34–6.

Garg M, Kurzner S, Bautista D, Keens T. (1998) Clinically unsuspected hypoxia during sleep and feeding in infants with bronchopulmonary dysplasia. *Pediatrics* **81(5)**, 635–42.

Godfrey K. (2004) New guidance on long-term oxygen therapy management delivery. *Nursing Times* **100(38)**, 57.

Harrison G, Beresford M, Shaw N. (2006) Acute life threatening events among infants on home oxygen. *Paediatric Nursing* **18(1)**, 27–9.

McLauchlan L. (2002) Supplementary oxygen therapy in the community. *Nursing Times* **98(40)**, 50–2.

Moss D, Bond P. (2002) Home oxygen therapy for children. *Nursing Times* **98(30)**, 37–9.

Naylor H. (2003) O$_2$ go home – a home oxygen programme for neonatal graduates with bronchopulmonary dysplasia. *Nurse 2 Nurse* **3(3)**, 35–7.

National Health Service/Quality Improvement Scotland. (2010) *Best Practice Statement. Home oxygen therapy for children being cared for in the community.* Edinburgh: NHS Scotland.

Poets CF. (1998) When do infants need additional inspired oxygen? A review of the current literature. *Pediatric Pulmonology* **26**, 424–8.

Primhak RA. (2003) Discharge and aftercare in chronic lung disease of the newborn. *Seminars in Neonatology* **8(4)**, 117–26.

Simoes EA, Rosenberg AA, King SJ, Groothuis JR. (1997) Room air challenge: prediction for successful weaning of oxygen-dependent infants. *Journal of Perinatology* **17(2)**, 125–9.

Teague WG, Pian MS, Heldt GP, Tooley WH. (1998) An acute reduction in the fraction of inspired oxygen increases airway constriction in infants with chronic lung disease. *American Review of Respiratory Disease* **137**, 861–5.

Chapter 7

Long-term ventilation

David Thomas[1] and Beverley Waithe[2]

[1]*Paediatric Consultant*
[2]*Children's Community Matron, Nottingham Children's Hospital*

Learning objectives

In this chapter we will consider:

- the physiological basis of intervention
- prediction of long-term ventilation clinically
- outcomes of care
- different diseases
- practicalities of long-term ventilation
- ethical aspects
- the importance of competency assessment for parents/carers
- significance of continuing care packages in the community.

Introduction

Long-term ventilation (LTV) of children demands harmonious and well-orchestrated co-ordination of care between various health professionals and their families. Health professionals must lead, utilising the other agencies commonly involved, aiming to optimise care for children at home (Noyes 2006). One of the roles of the medical team is to identify situations when LTV may be indicated; nursing staff commonly lead on establishing care routines and become key workers in the journey home. Physiotherapists take the lead in optimising lung clearance. Carers, individuals without professional training who develop specific caring skills for LTV children, may be part of the team supporting transition home.

Normal respiration

Respiration in humans evolved to meet the continuous but variable demands of metabolism for gas exchange. Cyclical processes, breathing and heart contractions, lead to intimate and precise matching of two transport systems (blood and respired gases) in the respiratory zone of the lungs as

---

Children's Respiratory Nursing, First Edition. Edited by Janice Mighten.
© 2013 Blackwell Publishing Ltd. Published 2013 by Blackwell Publishing Ltd.

discussed in Chapter 1. The muscular pumps responsible for gas and blood flow share a common compartment, the chest. This has a symmetrical skeleton upon which the respiratory muscles act and within which the elastic properties of the lung exert an important influence. The circulation of blood is cyclical yet continuous within systemic and pulmonary circulations, there is marked elasticity on the arterial 'delivery' side and capacitance on the venous 'recovery' side. The timing of gas flow down the airways (conducting zone) into the airspaces (respiratory zone) is controlled by cyclical central nervous system pacemaker-like activity, itself influenced by chemoreceptors.

Chemoreceptor organs have generous blood flows that sense carbon dioxide and oxygen levels within the brain and the carotid body. Optimal airway calibre is ensured by phasic airway wall stiffening while inspiratory muscles draw gas into the respiratory zone. In health, at rest expiration then occurs passively as elastic recoil acts to expel gases back to air.

These processes are highly integrated and interdependent; they also lie at the centre of healthy metabolism. In the absence of disease there is considerable performance reserve to meet peaks in demand and allow recuperation during quieter periods.

The respiratory zone is free from contamination due to the combined effects of local immunity, the mucociliary escalator and cough. The normal cough reflex involves three well-co-ordinated phases: initial inspiration to 60–70% of total inspiratory capacity, then a brief but vital compressive period when forceful expiratory efforts are held by a closed glottis and finally the explosive expiratory period generating a plume of cleared respiratory secretions. Enhanced clearance aims to recreate the effects of coughing.

Pathophysiological aspects

Hypoxaemia, hypercarbia and lack of sleep are the three cardinal adverse effects that occur when the system fails. They may be ameliorated or reversed by breathing support as part of a package of care. A window of opportunity for intervention often presents, before and after which it may cause harm.

Inadequate gas exchange may be improved by LTV, particularly when there is relatively little parenchymal lung disease. The controlled gas flows of ventilation may straightforwardly overcome the ventilatory failure associated with disordered muscle function (low, high or variable tone) and the consequent restrictive pattern of lung function or moderate tracheobronchial or supraglottic obstruction.

This support is often effective in the long term. Children with advanced parenchymal disease may benefit temporarily during a period when time is precious. Sleep has a generally depressant effect on breathing and inadequate breathing commonly disturbs sleep. This vicious cycle may be interrupted by nocturnal LTV, enabling healthy daytime activities.

The restrictive pattern of lung disease commonly results from the compounded effects of muscular disease, skeletal deformity and paucity of lung growth and may be accompanied by cardiac elements. The metabolic consequences of sleep-disordered breathing (SDB), for example type 2 diabetes and ischaemic heart disease, emerge over a longer timescale. Intervention to support healthy gas exchange and avoid the increased work of breathing associated with most of these conditions may prevent or ameliorate these effects.

Lung development, growth and in particular healthy postnatal acquisition of increased numbers of alveoli are dependent upon chest movements. The normal excursions of tidal breathing and deeper breaths during increased demand (e.g. exercise) each play their part (Davies and Reid 1970). Without these growth-stimulating trophic effects, lung capacity is stunted and respiratory failure a natural consequence. Providing non-invasive ventilation (NIV) can promote healthier lung growth (Bach and Bianchi 2003).

Indications for long-term ventilation

Broadly, long-term ventilation may be of benefit in the circumstances listed in Box 7.1.

Predicting long-term ventilation

Ventilatory failure is the most common cause of death for all the patient groups in Box 7.1. Mechanical breathing support as part of a package of care can improve survival, quality of life or both. The timing and sequence of interventions require judgement, based upon measurements and intelligence about the individual patient in the context of knowledge about particular diseases and general principles.

Neuromuscular diseases

Our understanding of neuromuscular disorders has recently included descriptions of their molecular basis and improved characterization of the varied phenotypes.

Duchenne muscular dystrophy

Some diseases are relentlessly and predictably progressive; Duchenne muscular dystrophy is arguably the best described. It is rare in girls and mainly affects boys. Independent ambulation generally ceases around entry to secondary school and respiratory failure is highly probable by late

---

Box 7.1   Indications for LTV

Restrictive diseases

Neuromuscular diseases	Spinal muscular atrophy
	Duchenne muscular dystrophy
	Other muscular dystrophies
	Myopathies
	Myasthenia gravis
Chest deformities	Scoliosis
	Rigid spine syndrome

Airway obstruction

Congenital anomalies causing tracheobronchomalacia	Complex congenital heart disease
	Tracheo-oesophageal fistula
Congenital anomalies causing glottic or supraglottic airway obstruction	Pierre Robin sequence
	Vocal cord paresis
Low tone with anatomical vulnerability	Down's syndrome
	Achondroplasia

Lack of central drive to respiratory muscles

Congenital central alveolar hypoventilation
High spinal cord injury
Advanced parenchymal lung disease
Bronchiectasis
Cystic fibrosis

---

adolescence. These boys are capable of performing pulmonary function tests; longitudinal values reveal individual variation in decline that for forced vital capacity (FVC) averages 8% per annum (Phillips et al. 2001). A decline in FVC below 1 litre suggests survival of about 3 years (median value) without breathing support.

Short-term reversible decline in breathing performance occurs; for example, viral illnesses in this population cause a prolonged and disproportionate impairment in breathing (Noyes 2006; Poponick et al. 1997). An important predictive measurement is hypercarbia with the onset of sleep, REM related, after which a requirement for breathing support is expected within 2 years (Phillips et al. 1999; Ward et al. 2005). Peak cough flows (PCF) are measured when individuals cough, after a maximal inspiration, either through a peak flow meter or more sophisticated flow-sensitive device; normal values have been established from 5 years (Bianchi, Baiardi 2008). Their use for triggering interventions has not been established; in adult practice a value of less than 160L/s often triggers action (Weese-Mayer and Berry-Kravis 2004). When used to demonstrate the effectiveness of chest clearance techniques, the measurements provide encouragement.

Hypercarbia that persists around the clock – diurnal ventilatory failure – is, by consensus, an indication for offering non-invasive ventilation in Duchenne muscular dystrophy (Weese-Mayer and Berry-Kravis 2004) as it has been shown to prolong survival and improve quality of life (Simonds and Elliott 1995). Populations with Duchenne muscular dystrophy in which NIV is commonplace have witnessed increased survival (Jeppesen et al. 2003). Clear advantages of NIV described in this group include improved gas exchange (both CO_2 and O_2) (Simonds et al. 1998, 2000) and better sleep (Mellies et al. 2003). Similar benefits are observed in those presenting with acute decompensation with respiratory infection.

Spinal muscular atrophy

Children with spinal muscular atrophy (SMA) share a common genotype that varies greatly in expression – their phenotype. Natural outcomes range from death in the early years to survival into adulthood. By consensus, three types are recognised by their course: type 1 presenting in the first 6 months; type 2 between 6 and 18 months and others named type 3. Muscles particularly affected by the condition are the intercostal and bulbar groups. Breathing support for infants with type 1 SMA remains the exception and for those with type 2 the rule (Schroth 2009).

Other neuromuscular diseases

Disease progression cannot always be predicted with confidence. Neuromuscular disorders with a more variable overall course include myasthenia, spinal muscular atrophy with respiratory disease (SMARD) and other muscular dystrophies. Individuals with these conditions may experience a phase of weakness severe enough to require temporary breathing support, bridging to a healthier future and helping with lung growth or during a period of intense investigation for precise diagnosis.

Non-invasive ventilation: part of a package of care

Preparation for the possibility of NIV may occur in the phase before the onset of diurnal ventilatory failure. For the patient and their family, this is a further period of change during which much has to be accommodated. Patient surveys reveal that professionals and families usually underestimate their quality of life (Bach et al. 1991). Options for treatment should be presented in a clear-cut, non-directive fashion.

As the likelihood of respiratory infection is increased, protection should be implemented via immunization, having broad-spectrum antibiotics readily available and the learning of techniques enhancing lung clearance (Weese-Mayer and Berry-Kravis 2004). Lung clearance techniques should be tailored to the individual and their family. Mucociliary mechanisms are intact in neuromuscular disease while factors that can affect function include infection, mucous viscosity and exposure to cigarette smoke (Houtmeyers et al. 1999). Coughing is poor, leading to retained secretions. With effective glottic control, the inspiratory phase can be mimicked using breath-stacking techniques; air is delivered sequentially in supratidal volumes and held by glottal closure until a comfortable inspiratory capacity has been achieved. The final breath in the stack is followed by prompt external compression timed to coincide with release of the vocal cords.

When glottic control is poor chest clearance may be enhanced by mechanical insufflation-exsufflation (MIE). Active inspiratory and expiratory flows are switched rapidly in a time ratio of 2/1. The technique is well tolerated and maximal inspiratory and expiratory flows increase in proportion to the pressure utilised (Fauroux et al. 2008) with the effect of enhancing chest clearance; consensus agreement exists about its use (McCool and Rosen 2006; Miske et al. 2004).

Sleep-related hypercarbia would be expected during this phase, that varies in duration. As disease progression is generally slow patients may not describe symptoms, as the effects of respiratory failure may be tolerated. Specific symptom enquiry, with SDB in mind, may identify symptoms. In general, symptoms will prompt the introduction of NIV.

Many conditions requiring LTV allow that need to be anticipated. Skilful enquiry and the monitoring of breathing in children and young people with neuromuscular disease at outpatient clinics may allow the stepwise provision of support. As gas exchange and lung clearance deteriorate, support to optimise both may be required.

When coughing becomes inadequate, instructions in the techniques that enhance lung clearance generally precede the need for ventilation. The first experience of the child or young person with a ventilator may be when learning the techniques used to improve lung clearance.

Acute presentations

Alternatively, LTV requirements may be identified relatively acutely due to unpredictable events. These infants, children and young people will usually be resident on intensive care units. Failure to extubate and/or sustain breathing independently will prompt consideration of LTV, whether in the context of palliative or long-term support (Bach et al. 1991).

Neonatal care

In the neonatal intensive care unit, decisions regarding the aims of care may be particularly finely balanced and will require accurate diagnosis, allowing a discussion based on as high a degree of certainty as can be achieved at the beginning of independent life.

Infants with profound respiratory failure due to myopathy or congenital central alveolar hypoventilation require prompt diagnostic work-up but may not be easy to identify initially. Congenital central alveolar hypoventilation is diagnosed by identifying abnormalities in the gene (PHOX2B), that provides instructions for the production of protein in the early stages of development, with evidence of abnormal breathing responses to chemoreceptor stimulation. Autonomic nervous system instability, endocrine and other central nervous system-driven physiological anomalies may complicate management. Breathing support is generally required during sleep and may be required continuously, particularly during infective or other exacerbations (Maitra et al. 2004; Trang et al. 2005; Weese-Mayer et al. 1992).

Box 7.2   Conditions associated with obstruction of the upper airway that may require breathing support

Skeletal airway anomalies: craniofacial conditions	Treacher–Collins syndrome
	Crouzon's disease
	Pierre Robin sequence
	Stickler syndrome
	Achondroplasia
Low muscle tone – tongue and palate	Down's syndrome
Variable muscle tone	Cerebral palsies
Airway infiltrated	Mucopolysaccharidoses
Airway insufficiently rigid/compressed (often	Tracheomalacia
with other congenital abnormality, e.g.	Bronchomalacia
cardiac or tracheo-oesophageal fistula)	
Vocal cord function poor	Brainstem abnormalities
Adverse effects at many levels	Obesity
	Prader–Willi syndrome

   Home ventilation for neonatal chronic lung disease may become more commonplace but currently this is unusual.

Upper airway obstruction

Some populations with a high prevalence of SDB are listed in Box 7.2. In Down's syndrome up to two-thirds may have multichannel physiological recordings that define SDB (Dyken et al. 2003; Marcus et al. 1991) and the complexity of anatomical and functional factors contributing has been systematically described (Uong et al. 2001). Tonsillectomy may be effective in alleviating SDB (Bower 1995).

Outcomes of long-term ventilation

Long-term ventilation most commonly aims to enable children with ventilatory failure to live with their family at home, go to school and enjoy the best quality of life possible. LTV may be used as an aid for palliative care; respiratory failure is a common mode of death. As breathing becomes less effective and the effort required increases, the degree of comfort or distress and its timescale vary. Hypoxia and hypercarbia have sedative effects whereas dyspnoea, cough and secretions are unpleasant. Admission to hospital for nursing intervention may entrap the child and their family. LTV may enable comfort and care at home given appropriate support.

Long-term ventilation as a bridge to transplantation

Successful transplantation of lungs or heart and lungs may transform the lives of patients and their families with end-stage lung disease. LTV in combination with other intensive interventions increases the likelihood of successful transplantation for individuals. In advanced cystic fibrosis, advancing respiratory failure occurs with chronically infected bronchiectatic airways, impeding expiratory flow and causing airspace hyperinflation; consequently hypoxemia and hypoxic respiratory drive with nocturnal hypercarbia arise. Benefits from NIV might accrue from the resting of respiratory muscles, improved sleep and enhanced chest clearance, improving quality of life or allowing transplantation.

The optimal timing and regimen for patients with cystic fibrosis (CF) patients are unclear. Although benefits of NIV have been reported and gas exchange and dyspnoea improve in the short term, the acceptability of and adherence to positive pressure support strategies are poor and a substantial minority of potential users do not persist with the technique (Bower 1995; Fauroux et al. 1999; Gozal 1997; Moran et al. 2009).

Long-term ventilation considered and not commenced

Evidence that LTV prolongs life and improves the quality of life of some patient groups means that decisions to commence support may be straightforward on an outcomes basis, but this is not always the case.

From a day-to-day perspective, we consider the views of the individual and their family; potential benefit is balanced with possible harm in a rounded manner. Views vary amongst families according to their values, beliefs and other circumstances. The clinical team's job is to present a clear-cut description for the family to consider. Anticipation of future needs and exploration of what is acceptable at the outset help to negotiate the approach adopted. Views will often alter with circumstantial changes. The key outcome is that a personal resuscitation plan and escalation plan are agreed and disseminated between family and professionals (Wolff et al. 2011).

Where life is judged, either by the family or their child, as unbearable or of no purpose, if the child is in a permanent vegetative state or there is no chance of recovery and suffering is prolonged, life-sustaining treatment may be withheld or withdrawn (Royal College of Paediatrics 2004).

When disagreement between parties arises, the legal process may be involved. Often, in the background individuals or groups are advocating different plans of action, having considered the ethical and moral issues affecting the individual, their family and community. Where disagreement arises, the best framework for decision making is arguably one that involves experts in arbitration. More broadly, society's views must be considered and accounted for. Distributive justice requires that decisions made do not come into conflict with the needs of the many. When conflict exists or is foreseen, a second opinion and the views of the local clinical ethics committee may help (Larcher et al. 2010).

Technical aspects of long-term ventilation: equipment

Ventilation requires that gases for breathing are delivered down a circuit and via an interface to the patient's airway. Recent technical developments have improved the patient's experience and refinements to the options available are ongoing.

Ventilators (Figure 7.1)

Machines designed to support breathing entrain and accelerate gas flows to achieve targets set by the supervising medical team according to individual requirements. Components have improved in their performance, particularly size, quietness and responsiveness. Improvements are still required, particularly for our smallest and most profoundly affected patient groups.

As most breathing assistance is provided in the setting of considerable leakage of the gas flow produced, most ventilation is targeted to achieve a given pressure to the airway. (Ventilation

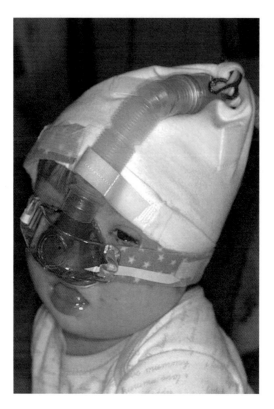

Figure 7.1   Ventilator.

to a given volume when measurement of that volume is inexact is difficult and may be dangerous.) The flow required to do this is preferably triggered by the earliest patient effort to optimise synchronised support. Flows to achieve the required pressure(s) are generated rapidly and are then sustained to maintain that pressure. Top pressures reached assist inspiration and give way to a lower setting, often still positive, that assists in sustaining airway calibre and thereby lung inflation.

This form of ventilation (pressure is set) is called pressure controlled; there are several terms for this form of breathing support. In pressure-controlled ventilation, the initial flows are generated rapidly for optimal inflation and then decelerate to avoid pressures overshooting. This optimises the inflation of the whole lung for gas exchange, maintaining open lung units and opening up ('recruiting') those that are not.

Volume-controlled modes require relatively little and constant gas leakage and are more commonly applied via a tracheostomy, sometimes with a cuffed tube. Achieving a known volume of inflation is attractive as the breathing support offered may adapt to ensure this target is achieved. Earlier volume-controlled techniques involved a constant flow of gas, which delivered a slow inflation; more recently, gas flows for volume-controlled ventilation can mimic those of pressure-controlled settings using rapid feedback from microprocessors.

The breathing actions of patient and machine should ideally be synchronous (the patient's effort should lead) at the start of both inspiratory and expiratory phases. Mismatch in the

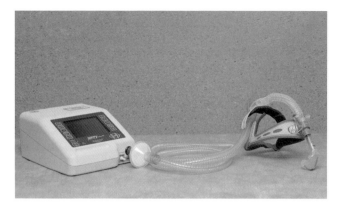

Figure 7.2   Facemask and circuit.

efforts of patient and machine is avoided by the machine's ability to detect or anticipate the terminal period of both phases.

Breathing circuits

Gases travel along tubing according to well-understood physical principles and a match between ventilator, tubing, interface and the patient is required bearing these in mind. Circuit calibre (radius) and to a lesser degree length and internal wall characteristics affect the resistance encountered. Humidification, normally achieved by the nasal passages, may be provided with suitable adaptation of the circuit. Gas flows are always delivered and monitored to the airway along an inspiratory limb; after the inflation, during the expiratory period, the gases may be returned to the ventilator for measurement or vented directly to the atmosphere. Single-limbed circuits are designed to work with large variation in leakage of gases. Double-limbed circuits require far less variation in leakage. Tubing should be lightweight, fairly rigid and available in lengths that encourage mobility locally when feasible. Oxygen flows may be added to the inspiratory circuit or directly into the ventilator; control of the inspired oxygen concentration is required.

Interfaces: masks

For non-invasive ventilation, adherence to treatment at home is the key aim, to allow realisation of the full benefits of this form of LTV. Early achievement of comfort with tangible benefits is an important outcome and encourages adherence. Mask designs have utilised materials that are soft, malleable, durable and amenable to cleaning; they form a gasket over the face spanning the nasal and/or mouth orifices without significantly impeding local skin blood flow (Figure 7.2). Masks are designed with a known resistance to airflow engineered in. They should be kept clean and are generally replaced every 6 months. Interfaces are held in place by a variety of headgear supplied with masks and in general not interchangeable.

Adaptation for the individual patient's comfort is sometimes required. Understanding that some leakage of gases is desirable is important otherwise families and professionals may overtighten masks, leading to painful and unsightly skin ulceration. A longer term effect of mask ventilation, particularly in infancy, is poor midfacial growth (Li et al. 2000).

Care of the child with long-term ventilation

Respiratory adjuncts

Ventilation to improve gas exchange is the most common primary objective. The clearance of secretions must also be addressed as this is commonly also impaired. Mucociliary clearance and coughing combine to keep the gas-exchanging zones of the lung in optimal condition for gas exchange. Mucociliary clearance in neuromuscular disease is unimpaired. The cough reflex is commonly impaired by the underlying diseases; the effects of neuromuscular weakness, deformity, poor brainstem function and vocal cord dysfunction may act individually or in combination to make coughing ineffective. Improvements can be taught for the everyday and step-up regimes agreed. Inspiratory volumes may be systematically enhanced to provide the additional volumes required to generate the high flows required to shear and expel secretions from the upper airways. These volumes may be generated through breath stacking (see above), cough assist machines and adjustments to the ventilator. During the expiratory phase external compression, carefully timed, can augment the native effort to accelerate gas flows.

Preparation for these manoeuvres should include consideration of the need for humidification, targeted positioning and vibration. The optimal length of treatment is assessed by a physiotherapist. Despite enhanced clearance, respiratory infection occurs. Preventive interventions include the primary course of immunisation augmented by protection from influenza. Nutrition should be optimised too, as effective defences depend upon healthy tissue and access to a variety of nutrients. In general, the early use of antibiotics is advocated; most will receive a broad-spectrum agent appropriate for community-acquired pneumonia; where microbiological intelligence is available, for example from sputum or cough swab cultures, a better targeted choice will be made. Some families will keep a course of treatment on standby at home.

Development of independence

Independence and self-esteem must be considered, as the child or young person dependent upon breathing support is commonly dependent in many other ways, with effects within the family. As individual cognitive abilities are generally little or not affected, the sophistication and complexity of psychological needs are greater than usual. The majority have grown up with a progressive condition while others become dependent unexpectedly; all have awareness of their environment and the abilities of their peers. Appreciation of the affected individual's quality of life by others, even family members, is usually impaired (Kohler et al. 2005).

A top priority is the development and maintenance of a dialogue with the affected individual in the broadest sense, the overall aim being an appreciation of their experience, views and wishes in an unhurried, confidential and increasingly individual manner. Control of the physical environment is another key priority for these young people who must master switches, joysticks and microprocessors, helping to achieve self-reliance with increasing sophistication. The activities of daily living to be considered may include sleeping posture, transfer to chair, wheelchair settings and direction, cough assist and ventilation devices, catering, personal toilet and communication aids.

Financial security is required for confidence and to sustain development. Various forms of family and individual breaks catering for such needs are available, which is important in allowing adventure, discovery and relaxation together or privately. Hospices in the UK are charitable organisations that cater in this way, having developed their scope of practice from end-of-life care. These communities have expertise and facilities for expert daily care for life-limiting conditions and some can support throughout childhood, adolescence and adult life (visit www.togetherforshortlives.org.uk).

Competence and self-determination are important principles for day-to-day life and in a court of law. Competence develops as reasoning, judgement and experience accrue until complete self-determination is realised. At all stages of development, the wishes of the individual should be taken into account and once competent, the individual's wishes are paramount within the ethical and legal framework.

Inclusion in mainstream education occurs for the majority, often with individual support from a teaching assistant for learning and personal care needs. Choices of career should be anticipated; roles and employment fulfilled by young people with neuromuscular disease become increasingly varied as life expectancy increases (see www.muscular-dystrophy.org).

Communication

Each representative professional's assessment of the needs of the child requiring LTV support should be shared and understood by the family and the LTV team. This allows the key aim of getting home with the family in a safe, sustainable fashion achievable in the shortest possible time. Once LTV is acknowledged to be required, relevant individuals from a range of agencies should be informed, with a request that they make their own assessments and action plans. It is good practice to identify the key workers from whom the core group will be established. Assessments are then shared both informally, such as during ward rounds, and formally in a multidisciplinary meeting.

Milestones of significance include diagnosis, agreement of a personal resuscitation plan, medical stability, first outing from ward, first day at home, first night at home, and last night in hospital. Within the hospital, once medical stability is attained, care should become nursing led and mimic general practice, ensuring that expectations are not overmedicalised; developmental needs should dominate. The daily routine, observations and record charts should be matched to those that are likely to prevail at home. The family-held record is commenced and will act as the focus of documentation and communication with the family for all professionals.

Long-term ventilation is offered in a variety of clinical situations and most hospitals will have a patient receiving this support in their catchment. Excellent team working should ensure that the best outcome and optimal independence at home are achieved.

Care in the community

The number of medically fragile children and young people has increased over the last 20 years and they have become part of a growing population of children surviving longer with life-limiting illnesses (Bush et al. 2005; Mentro 2003). Samuels (1996) suggested that advances in children's intensive care medicine have resulted in children surviving a critical illness or accident but failing to recover the ability to breathe without mechanical ventilation. Also children are surviving premature births and childhood illnesses as a result of earlier diagnosis, advances in technology and the ability to provide smaller portable medical equipment for home care (Kirk 1999). In 1999, Jardine et al. identified 141 children requiring LTV. Over the last 10 years this number has increased significantly and it is estimated that the number of children requiring LTV has in fact risen by 72%.

This increase brings new challenges for children's community nursing teams and, more recently, LTV support nurses. It also brings challenges to primary care trusts (PCT) that are responsible for commissioning appropriate services to meet the needs of these children. From 2002, it became the responsibility of strategic health authorities to lead on strategic planning within a defined population, including PCTs taking the lead on planning local children's services on behalf of the local health economy. PCTs , their commissioners and children's trusts now have a responsibility to review and develop services through joint commissioning that matches the needs of families. They also need to monitor these services to ensure they remain effective. However, from 2013, strategic health authorities and PCTs will be abolished under the government's new health service plan and replaced by consortia led by GPs who will commission services on behalf of the local community.

In its document *World Class Commissioning*, the Department of Health (2007) acknowledges that people are living longer and that aspirations and lifestyles are changing. Local PCTs will be at the forefront of the world-class commissioning vision, taking a strategic and long-term approach to commissioning services and designing services to meet the changing needs of their populations.

Healthy Lives, Brighter Futures (Department for Children, Schools and Families/Department of Health 2009) was produced in direct response for children, young people, parents and professionals. It is the first joint strategy to present the government's vision of how to improve outcomes for children. The aim of *Healthy Lives, Brighter Futures* is to build on the National Service Framework (Department of Health 2005), *Every Child Matters* (Department for Education and Skills 2003) and the *Children's Plan* (Department for Children, Schools and Families 2007) to enable teams to develop services that meet the needs of children and their families.

It has also been acknowledged that there is a need for increased support for disabled children and their families, including children requiring LTV, with an increase of £340 million in funding over the next 3 years. Funding has been pledged to improve palliative care services, improve equipment, produce high-quality short breaks and achieve world-class commissioning with evidence-based outcomes for disabled children.

Consequently, this poses the question of local strategic health authorities identifying children's services as a priority in local operational policies and implementation of the strategy. With no targets set against the outcomes, this may prove difficult. However, all PCT chief executives have been informed that the Department of Health and the Department for Children, Schools and Families will be mandating a local statement by the PCTs, setting out their actions specifically in four areas:

- short breaks
- community equipment
- wheelchair provision
- palliative care.

Nursing care

Nurses caring for children in the community have a responsibility to ensure that they are kept informed about changes in government policies and changes in practice. There is great emphasis on the need to be knowledgeable about current issues, ensuring that the children, young people and families nurses are caring for are always the centre of their activity.

The National Service Framework (NSF; Department of Health 2003) has been a driving force enabling change within the children's community setting. This 10-year plan set out goals, recommendations and guidance for best practice. One of the targets states that care for children with even the most complex disorders can be carried out away from hospital. Unlike many other government objectives, the NSF produced standards that appear workable in practice. Mountford and Widdas (2005) suggested that this framework was set to improve children's services using evidence-based knowledge and is aimed to improve inequalities and variations in care.

Children and young people on LTV often move from an intensive care environment, supported 24/7 by nursing staff, to home in the community, where the environment is very different. However, with support, the family can remain at home with a package of care. This will enable them to live ordinary lives (Department of Health 2004) and alleviate prolonged hospital admissions in an environment unsuitable for a child to develop and remain part of a family.

This care should be provided by children's community nursing teams. The UK Central Council for Nursing (1994), now superseded by the Nursing and Midwifery Council (NMC), defines a community children's nurse as a 'registered children's nurse who has completed a programme of education in community nursing, leading to registration with the United Kingdom Central Council for Nursing, Midwifery and Health Visiting and whose main focus of work is predominantly those children requiring treatment and care for acute and chronic ill health in a home setting'. Each child who requires LTV will have different needs and individual packages of care will have to be developed to meet them. With the huge variation of support needed, set rules and guidelines for a group of children with specific conditions would be difficult to use.

A recent study by Wilcock (2009) looked at 15 different trusts throughout the UK. The study looked at how much support and care families will receive at home and what factors nurses should consider when assessing packages of care. The study found that there was a disparity in service provision between NHS trusts and a current lack of national guidelines or standards.

The level of ventilation support a child/young person will need may vary significantly. Some children may also require non-invasive or invasive ventilation support for varying amounts of time throughout the day or night, as discussed earlier. There are children who need nasal or facial mask continuous positive airway pressure (CPAP) whilst they are asleep, and those who will require 24-hpositive pressure ventilation through a tracheostomy. There are also many different medical conditions that will result in paediatric LTV, as outlined earlier.

When considering the assessment process, the assessor should firstly take into consideration the needs of the child and their family, making sure that their views and thoughts are considered, and then plan how the services will meet these needs.

Jardine and Wallis (1998) produced guidelines for the discharge home of the child on LTV in the UK. They identified four goals of home mechanical ventilation:

- to enhance the quality of life
- to sustain and extend life without compromising quality
- to improve or sustain physical and psychological function and to enhance growth and development
- to provide cost-effective care.

Therefore discharge of the ventilator-dependent child must include a multidisciplinary approach. Jardine and Wallis (1998) suggest that this process should be co-ordinated by one person as the key worker, who will be responsible for liaising with all agencies. In addition, the PCT will need to start the planning process early, along with social care and any other party involved in the requirements for joint funding and the need to initiate the planning process.

Continuing care package

In addition to careful planning, there are many factors that need to be taken into consideration for the smooth transition of care from hospital to home. Noyes and Lewis (2005) have produced guidance for such planning and detail a care pathway for the discharge and ongoing management of a child requiring LTV. Factors they consider include:

- service costs: staff costs, recruitment and training, housing
- equipment: disposables, cost of ventilation at home, emergency procedures.

They also discuss the difficulties often encountered when obtaining agreement to fund packages of care. The main reason for these difficulties is cited as the lack of data concerning the costs associated with providing a package of care and different agencies agreeing who is responsible for specific areas of funding (Noyes and Lewis 2005).

The Lifetime Service in Bath (Lewis 2005) use a proforma, which is presented to commissioners to propose a package of care for a child with complex health needs. The principle of the information presented is the culmination of information from a multiagency assessment.

When considering recruitment of carers who may be employed to look after a ventilator-dependent child, again the needs of the family should be taken into consideration. Some families may prefer to care for their child themselves while others will request 24/7 service. Some parents feel their role as parents is taken away by having carers constantly in their home. The level of need should be assessed early in the discharge process through the multiagency assessment.

If a team of carers is needed, it should be led by a qualified paediatric nurse. Jardine and Wallis (1998) suggest that carers other than the team leader do not necessarily need a nursing qualification, as long as a well-designed comprehensive training programme is in place for the daily management of the child. This appears to be the case in most areas utilising clinical support workers in practice. A patient-specific training package should be completed and carers should be assessed as competent at the hospital prior to the child leaving this setting. These carers could be part funded by social care, but health will remain responsible for the training and ongoing competency assessment of the carers and the ongoing medical care.

Discharge of this group of children should not be rushed but approached gradually, with possibly an interim time in a transitional unit. The family as well as the carers should spend time providing care to the child in a hospital setting, as this time may be crucial in highlighting any problems and can allow the parents to be trained to proficiently care for the child. This should then be followed by a trial run at home.

Conclusion

There is no reason why children requiring LTV cannot be cared for safely at home. Intensive care is an inappropriate setting for a child both developmentally and psychologically. It is acknowledged that the discharge process is complex and expensive and may take a long period of time. However, a high-quality service can be provided to this group of children in the community to sustain care at home, with the right personnel and appropriate training for all.

Questions

1. Name four respiratory disease categories that may lead to non-invasive ventilation.
2. What are the three adverse consequences when respiratory systems fail overnight?
3. How do nocturnal and diurnal respiratory hypercarbia differ?
4. What preparation is required for children and families requiring LTV support, prior to discharge home?
5. What consideration needs to be given to care in the community?
6. In what circumstances might it be legal to withhold life-saving support?
7. Describe in your own words what a home ventilator does.
8. How do invasive and non-invasive ventilation differ?

References

Bach JR, Bianchi C. (2003) Prevention of pectus excavatum for children with spinal muscular atrophy type 1. *American Journal of Physical Medicine and Rehabilitation* **82(10)**, 815–19.

Bach JR, Campagnolo DI, Hoeman S. (1991) Life satisfaction of individuals with Duchenne muscular dystrophy using long-term mechanical ventilatory support. *American Journal of Physical Medicine and Rehabilitation* **70(3)**, 129–35.

Bianchi C, Baiardi P. (2008) Cough peak flows: standard values for children and adolescents. *American Journal of Physical Medicine and* **87(6)**, 461–7.

Bower C. (1995) Tonsillectomy and adenoidectomy in patients with Down syndrome. *International Journal of Pediatric Otorhinolaryngology* **33**, 141–8.

Bush A, Fraser J, Jardine E, Paton J, Simmonds A, Wallis C. (2005) Respiratory management of the infant with type 1 spinal muscular atrophy. *Archives of Disease in Childhood* **9**, 709–11.

Davies G, Reid L. (1970) Growth of the alveoli and pulmonary arteries in childhood. *Thorax* **25**, 669–81.

Department for Children, Schools and Families. (2007) *The Children's Plan; building brighter futures*. London: Stationery Office.

Department for Children, Schools and Families/Department of Health (2009) *Healthy Lives, Brighter Futures: the strategy for children and young people's health*. London: Stationery Office.

Department for Education and Skills. (2003) *Every Child Matters*. London: Stationery Office.

Department of Health. (2003) *Getting the Right Start. National Service Framework for Children, Young People and Maternity Services*. London: Stationery Office.

Department of Health. (2004) *The Children Act*. London: Stationery Office.

Department of Health. (2005) *Commissioning Children's and Young Peoples Palliative Care Service. National Service Framework for Children, Young People and Maternity Services*. London: Stationery Office.

Department of Health. (2007) *World Class Commissioning: vision summary*. London: Stationery Office.

Dyken ME, Lin-Dyken DC, Poulton S, Zimmerman MB, Sedars E. (2003) Prospective polysomnographic analysis of obstructive sleep apnea in Down syndrome. *Archives of Pediatric and Adolescent Medicine* **157(7)**, 655–60.

Fauroux B, Boule M, Lofaso F, *et al.* (1999) Chest physiotherapy in cystic fibrosis: improved tolerance with nasal pressure support ventilation. *Pediatrics* **103(3)**, e32.

Fauroux B, Guillemot N, Aubertin G, *et al.* (2008) Physiologic benefits of mechanical insufflation-exsufflation in children with neuromuscular diseases. *Chest* **133(1)**, 161–8.

Gozal D. (1997) Nocturnal ventilatory support in patients with cystic fibrosis: comparison with supplemental oxygen. *European Respiratory Journal* **10(9)**, 1999–2003.

Houtmeyers E, Gosselink R, Gayan-Ramirez G, Decramer M. (1999) Regulation of mucociliary clearance in health and disease. *European Respiratory Journal* **13(5)**, 1177–88.

Jardine E, Wallis C. (1998) Core guidelines for the discharge home of the child on long term assisted ventilation in the United Kingdom. *Thorax* **53**, 762–7.

Jardine E, O'Toole M, Paton J, Wallis C. (1999) Current status of long term ventilation of children in the United Kingdom: questionnaire survey. *British Medical Journal* **318**, 295.

Jeppesen J, Green A, Steffensen BF, Rahbek J. (2003) The Duchenne muscular dystrophy population in Denmark, 1977: prevalence, incidence and survival in relation to the introduction of ventilator use. *Neuromuscular Disorders* **13(10)**, 804–12.

Kirk S. (1999) Caring for children with specialised health care needs in the community, the challenges for primary care. *Health and Social Care in the Community* **7(5)**, 350–7.

Kohler M, Clarenbach CF, Boni L, Brack T, Russi EW, Bloch KE. (2005) Quality of life, physical disability, and respiratory impairment in Duchenne muscular dystrophy. *American Journal of Respiratory and Critical Care Medicine* **172(8)**, 1032–6.

Larcher V, Slowther AM, Watson AR. (2010) Network UKCE. Core competencies for clinical ethics committees. *Clinical Medicine* **10(1)**, 30–3.

Lewis M. (2005) *Life Time Service*. Bath: Child Health Department.

Li KK, Riley RW, Guilleminault C. (2000) An unreported risk in the use of home nasal continuous positive airway pressure and home nasal ventilation in children. *Chest* **117(3)**, 916–18.

Maitra A, Shine J, Henderson J, Fleming P. (2004) The investigation and care of children with congenital central hypoventilation syndrome. *Current Paediatrics* **14(4)**, 354–60.

Marcus CL, Keens TG, Bautista DB, von Pechmann WS, Ward SLD. (1991) Obstructive sleep apnea in children with Down syndrome. *Pediatrics* **88(1)**, 132–9.

McCool FD, Rosen MJ. (2006) Nonpharmacologic airway clearance therapies. *Chest* **129(1 suppl)**, 250S–9S.

Mellies U, Ragette R, Dohna Schwake C, Boehm H, Voit T, Teschler H. (2003) Long-term noninvasive ventilation in children and adolescents with neuromuscular disorders. *European Respiratory Journal* **22(4)**, 631–6.

Mentro AM. (2003) Nursing care of children and families. *Journal of Paediatric Nursing* **18(4)**, 225–32.

Miske LJ, Hickey EM, Kolb SM, Weiner DJ, Panitch HB. (2004) Use of the mechanical in-exsufflator in pediatric patients with neuromuscular disease and impaired cough. *Chest* **125(4)**, 1406–12.

Mountford S, Widdas D. (2005) A new national health service. In: Sidey A, Widdas D (eds) *Textbook of Community Children's Nursing*. London: Elsevier.

Moran F, Bradley JM, Piper AJ. (2009) Non-invasive ventilation for cystic fibrosis. *Cochrane Database of Systematic Reviews* **1**, CD002769.

Noyes J. (2006) The key to success: managing children's complex packages of community support. *Archives of Disease in Childhood – Education & Practice Edition* **91**, 106–10.

Noyes J, Lewis M. (2005) *From Hospital to Home: guidance on discharge management and community support for children using long-term ventilation*. London: Barnardo's.

Phillips MF, Smith PEM, Carroll N, Edwards RHT, Calverley PMA. (1999) Nocturnal oxygenation and prognosis in Duchenne muscular dystrophy. *American Journal of Respiratory and Critical Care Medicine* **160(1)**, 198–202.

Phillips MF, Quinlivan RCM, Edwards RHT, Calverley PMA. (2001) Changes in spirometry over time as a prognostic marker in patients with Duchenne muscular dystrophy. *American Journal of Respiratory and Critical Care Medicine* **164(12)**, 2191–4.

Poponick JM, Jacobs I, Supinski G, Dimarco AF. (1997) Effect of upper respiratory tract infection in patients with neuromuscular disease. *American Journal of Respiratory and Critical Care Medicine* **156(2)**, 659–64.

Royal College of Paediatrics. (2004) *Withdrawing or Withholding Life Sustaining Treatment in Children: a framework for practice*. London: Royal College of Paediatrics.

Samuels M. (1996) Long-term ventilation. *Paediatric Respiratory Medicine* **2**, 24–31.

Schroth MK. (2009) Special considerations in the respiratory management of spinal muscular atrophy. *Pediatrics* **123**(suppl 4), S245–9.

Simonds AK, Elliott MW. (1995) Outcome of domiciliary nasal intermittent positive pressure ventilation in restrictive and obstructive disorders. *Thorax* **50(6)**, 604–9.

Simonds AK, Muntoni F, Heather S, Fielding S. (1998) Impact of nasal ventilation on survival in hypercapnic Duchenne muscular dystrophy. *Thorax* **53(11)**, 949–52.

Simonds AK, Ward S, Heather S, Bush A, Muntoni F. (2000) Outcome of paediatric domiciliary mask ventilation in neuromuscular and skeletal disease. *European Respiratory Journal* **16(3)**, 476–81.

Trang H, Dehan M, Beaufils Fo, Zaccaria I, Amiel J, Gaultier C. (2005) The French Congenital Central Hypoventilation Syndrome Registry. *Chest* **127(1)**, 72–9.

UKCC (1994) *The Future of Professional Practice. The Council's standards for education and practice following registration: programmes of education leading to the qualification of specialist practitioner*. London: UKCC.

Uong EC, Mcdonough JM, Tay-Kier CE, *et al.* (2001) Magnetic resonance imaging of the upper airway in children with Down syndrome. *American Journal of Respiratory and Critical Care Medicine* **163(3)**, 731–6.

Ward S, Chatwin M, Heather S, Simonds AK. (2005). Randomised controlled trial of non-invasive ventilation (NIV) for nocturnal hypoventilation in neuromuscular and chest wall disease patients with daytime normocapnia. *Thorax* **60(12)**, 1019–24.

Weese-Mayer DE, Berry-Kravis EM. (2004) Respiratory care of the patient with Duchenne muscular dystrophy: ATS consensus statement. Genetics of congenital central hypoventilation syndrome: lessons from a seemingly orphan disease. *American Journal of Respiratory and Critical Care Medicine* **170(4)**, 456–65.

Weese-Mayer D, Silvestri J, Menzies L, Morrow-Kenny A, Hunt C, Hauptman S. (1992) Congenital central hypoventilation syndrome: diagnosis, management, and long-term outcome in thirty-two children. *Journal of Pediatrics* **120(3)**, 381–7.

Wilcock S. (2009) An investigation into the factors that nurses consider when assessing parental participation in caring for their child/young person with complex health needs at home. University of Nottingham, unpublished.

Wolff A, Browne J, Whitehouse WP. (2011) Personal resuscitation plans and end of life planning for children with disability and life-limiting/life-threatening conditions. *Archives of Disease in Childhood – Education & Practice Edition* **96(2)**, 42–8.

Section III

Respiratory conditions

Chapter 8

Management of lung infection in children

Alan R. Smyth

Professor of Child Health, School of Clinical Sciences, University of Nottingham; Honorary Consultant in Paediatric Respiratory Medicine, Nottingham Children's Hospital

---

Learning objectives

After studying this chapter, the reader will:

- understand the range of pathogens causing lung infection in children
- be aware of strategies to prevent serious lung infection in children and to prevent cross-infection in the hospital setting
- understand the diagnostic difficulties which may arise
- be familiar with the emergency management of paediatric lung infection
- be familiar with the specific antimicrobial therapies available and ways of improving effectiveness through increased adherence.

Introduction

Respiratory infections in children are common. One-third of all preschool children will be seen in primary care at least once a year because they are coughing (Hay et al. 2005). Respiratory infections are one of the most common reasons for children to be admitted to hospital; respiratory syncytial virus (RSV) infection alone is estimated to account for 20% of hospital admissions in preschool children in the US (Hall et al. 2009). The cost to the UK National Health Service of treating acute cough in preschool children has been estimated at over £30 million per year (Hollinghurst et al. 2008).

Respiratory symptoms (such as poor feeding, cough and difficulty breathing) may indicate a self-limiting upper respiratory infection or the early stages of a severe lower respiratory infection (such as bronchiolitis, croup or pneumonia). Careful nursing observations will ensure effective triage and assessment, as well as guiding the supportive treatment which is the cornerstone of care.

Children's Respiratory Nursing, First Edition. Edited by Janice Mighten.
© 2013 Blackwell Publishing Ltd. Published 2013 by Blackwell Publishing Ltd.

Bronchiolitis

Acute bronchiolitis is one of the most common causes of hospital admission in children in the UK, during the months of November through to the end of February. In other parts of the world, different seasonal peaks occur and, in many tropical countries, the peak in admissions corresponds with the rainy season.

Bronchiolitis is most commonly caused by RSV but other important causes are human metapneumovirus, parainfluenza virus type 3, influenza and adenovirus. The clinical syndrome is the same, irrespective of the virus responsible, with the exception of some forms of adenovirus which have the capacity to cause severe pneumonia and a form of permanent lung damage known as obliterative bronchiolitis. Infants have smaller airways than older children and these are more likely to become blocked (leading to air trapping) when inflammation, due to virus infection, produces inflammatory secretions and oedema. A 1 mm rim of oedema in an airway of 4 mm in diameter will increase airways resistance 16-fold. Much of the inflammation in bronchiolitis is caused by neutrophils and an excessive response by the infant's immune system (McNamara and Smyth 2002).

Bronchiolitis is primarily a condition of the first year of life. It is a clinical syndrome, character-ised by coryza, cough and a chest which appears hyperinflated (air 'trapped' in the chest). When a stethoscope is applied, crackles are heard at the lung bases. In North America, the term bronchiolitis may be applied to young children with episodic (viral) wheeze.

In most cases the infant's mother will report poor feeding. In the early stages of infection, this may be due to coryza, causing nasal obstruction. As infection progresses over several days, poor feeding may be related to tachypnoea. Where this is severe, infants are at risk of aspiration. Infants under 6 weeks of age with RSV infection are at risk of central apnoea.

There is no active immunisation against RSV infection. Infants with chronic lung disease of prematurity who are receiving home oxygen, those with some forms of congenital heart disease and severe immune deficiency are at greater risk of severe bronchiolitis. Passive immunisation with palivi-sumab (a monoclonal antibody against RSV) should be offered to these children (JCVI 2004). This is expensive and needs to be administered at monthly intervals usually in five doses over the winter period.

Viral diagnostic tests may help with measures to prevent cross-infection in hospital, e.g. nurs-ing infants with RSV infection in cubicles or cohorting larger groups with RSV infection in 'bronchiolitis bays' (SIGN 2006). Each institution will have its own infection control policy, which should be followed. Nasopharyngeal aspirates can be analysed by direct immunofluorescence but increasingly polymerase chain reaction (PCR, see Glossary) methods are used. A chest x-ray is rarely helpful, unless a complication such as aspiration is suspected.

The treatment of viral bronchiolitis is supportive. Babies who are feeding poorly should have nasogastric feeds (SIGN 2006). However, if the infant is very tachypnoeic (>60 breaths per minute), consider nil by mouth and intravenous fluids for a short period to avoid aspiration of feeds. Supplementary oxygen should be administered if the oxygen saturation is consistently <92%. This is best given through nasal cannulae. A small proportion of infants, often those with a known risk factor for severe disease (see above), may require ventilatory support. There is as yet no evidence that the use of nasal continuous positive airway pressure (nasal CPAP), in a deteriorating infant, will avoid intubation and mechanical ventilation (Palanivel and Anjay 2009). Many infants require a 'trickle' of oxygen to maintain normal oxygen saturations levels for several days after their respiratory symptoms have settled.

A borderline saturation in air, in an otherwise well baby, is not a reason to keep them in hospital. Simple nursing measures, such as gentle suction of nasal secretions, may also be helpful. One specific therapy has been shown to be of benefit in recent years – nebulised hypertonic saline (Zhang et al. 2008). This is administered as a 3% solution (usually 4 mL nebulised very 8 h) and in randomised controlled trials has improved clinical score and shortened hospital stay by approximately 24 h.

Ribavirin is an antiviral agent which is effective against RSV and may be given in nebulised form. It can cause genetic abnormalities in pregnancy, it is also difficult to administer and there is little evidence of benefit (Ventre and Randolph 2007). Bronchodilators, steroids and antibiotics are of no benefit in most infants with bronchiolitis and should not be used (although they frequently are) (Calogero, Sly 2007; Gadomski, Bhasale 2006; Spurling et al. 2007). Young children who are admitted with acute bronchiolitis may go on to have recurrent episodes of wheezing in the coming months. There is no effective preventive treatment for this complication (Blom et al. 2007). Even at 10 years of age, children who were admitted with bronchiolitis in infancy will wheeze more frequently than matched controls (Noble et al. 1997).

Pneumonia

Pneumonia is the most common cause of death in children under 5 years worldwide, accounting for 2 million deaths (19% of all deaths) (Bryce et al. 2005). In 2000, 42 countries accounted for 90% of deaths from pneumonia and over half the children in these countries failed to get the antibiotic they needed (WHO 2005). In the developed world there are few deaths and the incidence of pneumonia in children under 5 is around 36 cases per 1000 children per year, just under half requiring admission to hospital (Jokinen et al. 1993).

In the UK, infection with some of the organisms which can cause pneumonia may be prevented through the primary immunisation schedule. These include pneumococcus and pertussis (UK Immunisation Schedule 2010). Children in at-risk groups should also be given specific immunisations, e.g. influenza immunisation for children with chronic respiratory disease, such as cystic fibrosis, and 25-valent pneumococcal vaccine for children with sickle cell disease (Department of Health 2010).

Infants with pneumonia may present with non-specific symptoms such as poor feeding, lethargy and fever. There may be specific respiratory signs such as grunting and tachypnoea. However, in children under a year, the presentation may be one of 'sepsis' with a respiratory cause only apparent once an infection 'screen' has been undertaken and antibiotics started. Even in older children, symptoms may be misleading – abdominal pain is seen as well as chest pain and cough may be a late feature. In young infants, respiratory examination may reveal tachypnoea and chest indrawing. In older children classic physical signs such as a dull sound when the chest is percussed (tapped) and bronchial (harsh) breathing are more likely to be present and may allow the affected lung (and lobe) to be determined (Smyth 2001).

In younger children, viral infection (such as RSV) is the most common cause of pneumonia. Bacterial organisms are more common in older children, most commonly *Streptococcus pneumoniae* ('the pneumococcus'), followed by *Haemophilus influenzae, Mycoplasma pneumoniae* and *Chlamydia pneumoniae*. The pneumococcus is transmitted through droplet spread (close prolonged contact) and some forms can live in the nasopharynx without causing symptoms. Young children are at greater risk of pneumococcal infection than adults, particularly children with poor splenic function (e.g. sickle cell disease) or immune deficiency. *Staphylococcus aureus* is an uncommon cause of pneumonia. Children appear much sicker, and may develop complications such as pneumatocoele (thin-walled cavities on chest x-ray). If *Staph. aureus* is suspected, intravenous flucloxacillin should be given. As with bronchiolitis, a nasopharyngeal aspirate may help to identify the causative virus in infants.

Diagnosis of bacterial infection is more difficult. Children admitted to hospital should have blood sent for culture (though the test is insensitive), and serum sent immediately and at 6-week follow-up looking for antibodies to atypical organisms such as *Mycoplasma* and *Chlamydia*. Where a firm clinical diagnosis has been made, a chest x-ray is not necessary (Figure 8.1) (BTS 2002).

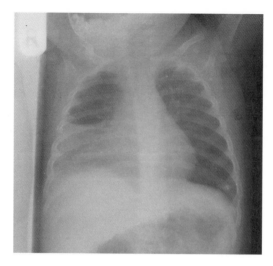

Figure 8.1   Chest x-ray showing right middle lobe and right lower lobe pneumonia.

Oxygen should be administered to all children with an oxygen saturation <92%. Some children will have become dehydrated and will need nasogastric or intravenous fluids. Most children with pneumonia can be treated with oral antibiotics (Atkinson et al. 2007). Exceptions include those with very low oxygen saturation (<85%), children who are shocked and those who are immune deficient (Atkinson et al. 2007). Oral amoxicillin is a good first-line treatment (or intravenous benzylpenicillin if oral antibiotics are contraindicated). If infection with *Mycoplasma* or *Chlamydia* is suspected, then a macrolide antibiotic such as clarithromycin should be given. Children who are drinking adequately and who no longer require oxygen can complete their treatment at home.

Empyema

Uncommonly, children with pneumonia develop a persisting fever and worsening dyspnoea. Percussion of the chest reveals dullness on one side, there may be a small patch of bronchial breathing above the dull area and the spine may curve to avoid expanding the chest on the affected side (scoliosis). A chest x-ray will reveal a dense white shadow on the affected side indicating fluid between the lung (which is lined by the visceral pleura) and the chest wall (parietal pleura). This is called a pleural effusion and it occurs when inflammation of the lung spreads to involve the pleura and fibrin 'gums up' the pleural lymphatics. Initially the fluid may be clear (uncomplicated parapneumonic effusion) but in many cases the pleural effusion itself becomes infected (complicated parapneumonic effusion or empyema). In some cases the effusion develops without evidence of prior pneumonia and a child with pneumonia can develop a large pleural effusion over the space of a few days. Empyema has become more common in the UK in recent years (Rees et al. 1997).

Mycoplasma and *Chlamydia* usually cause only small effusions and the most common organism in empyema is the pneumococcus, though *Staph. aureus*, other streptococci and gram-negative organisms can be responsible. Children with suspected empyema should have a chest x-ray and ultrasound scan of the chest (Balfour-Lynn et al. 2005). The latter will show if pleural thickening

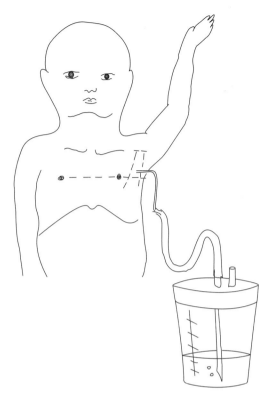

Figure 8.2 Diagram of a chest drain showing the 'triangle of safety' and the underwater seal.

and fibrinous loculations (pockets) are present, which may make it difficult for fluid to drain and antibiotics to penetrate.

All children should have pleural fluid sent for culture. Prolonged antibiotic treatment (often for several weeks) may be needed. Initially, intravenous benzylpenicillin (with flucloxacillin if *Staph. aureus* is suspected) should be given and antibiotics amended if and when culture results become available (Balfour-Lynn et al. 2005).

In most cases empyema can be effectively treated with a small (10–12 Fr) chest drain (inserted using the Seldinger technique), though occasionally a larger drain may be inserted under anaesthesia. The drain is connected to an underwater seal (Figure 8.2) and low-grade suction (-20 cm water) may be applied (see below). The site of insertion is determined by chest ultrasound, though larger drains should be inserted in the 'triangle of safety' bounded by pectoralis major medially, latissimus dorsi laterally and the internipple line below (see Figure 8.2).

A large volume of purulent fluid may drain initially. Once rapid drainage has ceased, urokinase should be instilled into the drain. A commonly used approach cited by Thomson et al. (2002) is to instil 40,000 units of urokinase in 40 mL of saline which is left to dwell for 4 h with the drain clamped and then placed under low-grade suction for 8 h. Six × 12-hcycles are given over 3 days. If ultrasound shows thick pleural 'peel' or fibrous loculations, or initial management is unsuccessful, then surgical decortication may be necessary (Eastham et al. 2004). Following discharge, a repeat chest x-ray should be performed after at least 6 weeks have elapsed. Figure 8.3 shows a sequence of x-rays in a child with empyema, showing the effects of drain insertion and appearance at follow-up.

(a)   (b)   (c)

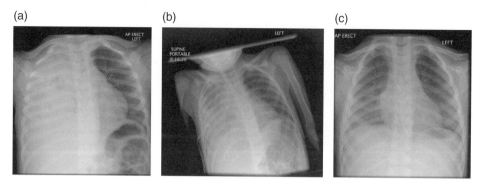

Figure 8.3   A series of chest x-rays of a 5-year-old boy who presented with a 1-week history of fever and shortness of breath, caused by right-sided empyema. Note the scoliosis with the thoracic spine flexed to the patient's right in (a) and (b). After drain placement, the patient received 3 days of urokinase instillation as described in the text. (a) Initial presentation. (b) After placement of a right-sided narrow-gauge chest drain. (c) At follow-up 6 weeks later.

Infectious and non-infectious causes of acute stridor in children

The most common cause of acute stridor in children is viral croup. Box 8.1 shows the differential diagnosis of acute stridor in children. For the sake of completeness, two non-infectious causes (inhaled foreign body and anaphylaxis) are also included.

Croup

Viral croup or laryngotracheobronchitis occurs most frequently in spring and autumn and affects preschool children. The most common organisms are parainfluenza virus types 1 and 2, though other viruses may be responsible – RSV, rhinovirus and (in the unimmunised) measles. Partial airways obstruction is caused by inflammation of the vocal cords and trachea. Clinical features include a characteristic barking cough, hoarse voice and inspiratory stridor. There is often a prodromal viral illness. The diagnosis is clinical – blood tests and x-rays are unhelpful.

Management depends on the severity of respiratory distress and any hypoxaemia but should initially follow the airway, breathing, circulation (ABC) approach. Toddlers with croup are best left sitting on their mother's lap and will automatically adopt the best position to maintain their own airway. Oxygen should be held gently to the face, if the oxygen saturation is <92%. Croup scores are frequently used in clinical trials but not in routine clinical practice. The Westley score is reliable and has been validated (Westley et al. 1978). The essential components of this describe the severity of croup using a scoring system, which enables an assessment of the presenting symptoms for a child with croup, which is summarized in Table 8.1.

Steroid treatment is proven to be effective and can be administered as nebulised budesonide (relatively expensive) or oral dexamethasone (Russell et al. 2004). Both treatments work quickly (within 6 h) and last for up to 12 h. Steroid treatment reduces the duration of hospital stay by an average of 12 h and reduces readmissions. There is no difference in the (small) number of children needing intubation and intensive care, with steroid use. Budesonide is administered as a fixed dose of 2 mg and dexamethasone at a dose of 0.3 mg/kg. In either case, a single dose should be administered and the effect reviewed after several hours. Nebulised adrenaline (1–5 mL of 1/1000)

Box 8.1   Causes of acute stridor in children

Common

Viral croup

Less common but usually mild

Spasmodic croup

Less common but severe

- Epiglottitis
- Bacterial tracheitis
- Inhaled foreign body (non-infectious)
- Anaphylaxis (non-infectious)

Rare

- Epstein–Barr virus ('glandular fever')
- Severe bacterial tonsillitis
- Peritonsillar abscess

Table 8.1   The Westley croup score

Symptoms	Severity of croup	Score
Stridor	Mild	<4
Conscious levels		
Air entry	Moderate	4–6
Cyanosis		
Intercostal recession	Severe	>6

may be used as a temporising measure in children with croup, while waiting for expert anaesthetic support to arrive.

Spasmodic croup

Some children with a background of atopic disease (such as eczema and asthma) may develop barking cough and stridor in the absence of viral infection – 'spasmodic croup'. This is generally unresponsive to any of the therapies used for viral croup but is usually self-limiting.

Epiglottitis

Epiglottitis due to *Haemophilus influenzae* is now rarely seen in the UK and other developed countries due to immunisation with *Haemophilus influenzae* group B vaccine (HiB) (UK Immunisation Schedule 2010). Children with epiglottitis present with high temperature and signs of bacteraemia which may include shock (cool peripheries, prolonged capillary refill and tachycardia). There is no prodrome. They may drool because of inability to swallow saliva.

Urgent assessment by an experienced anaesthetist and ear, nose and throat (ENT) surgeon is needed as complete airway obstruction may occur rapidly. Once the airway has been secured, intravenous antibiotic treatment (guided by local antibiotic protocols) is needed.

Bacterial tracheitis

Children with bacterial tracheitis present in a similar manner to epiglottitis. The most common organism is *Staph. aureus* and pus may sometimes be seen, welling from beneath the cords during intubation. Airway management is the same as for epiglottitis and intravenous antibiotics (including flucloxacillin) should be started immediately.

Inhaled foreign body

Inhalation of a foreign body, which lodges in the hypopharynx, larynx or trachea, may be life threatening and back blows and chest thrusts should be commenced immediately, if the episode is witnessed (Mackway-Jones et al. 2005). The foreign body may be coughed out or the rescuer may be able to remove the foreign body from the mouth. The management of inhaled foreign body in the lower airway is discussed in Chapter 4, under bronchoscopy.

Anaphylaxis

Acute stridor due to anaphylaxis may be suspected if the child has known allergies and has been in an environment where exposure is likely (e.g. a birthday party). Stridor may be accompanied by urticarial rash and facial swelling. The ABC approach to management should be followed. Definitive treatment is intramuscular adrenaline 10 μg/kg or 0.1 mL/kg. Alternatively, the dose can be chosen according to age band outlined in Table 8.2 (Advanced Life Support Group 2011). This should be combined with antihistamine and a short course of prednisolone.

Rare causes of acute stridor

Epstein–Barr virus

Epstein–Barr virus (EBV), which causes glandular fever, may cause massive tonsillar enlargement with upper airways obstruction and intubation may be needed. A positive monospot test suggests the diagnosis and this can be confirmed by testing for EBV viral capsid antigen IgM. There is no effective antiviral agent. Treatment is supportive.

Bacterial tonsillitis

Bacterial tonsillitis may rarely cause severe tonsillar enlargement with airways obstruction. The cause is usually group A β-haemolytic streptococci and this can be diagnosed with a tonsillar

Table 8.2 Dose of adrenaline for anaphylaxis

Age	Dose of adrenaline in micrograms	Dose of adrenaline in mL
Below 6 years	150	0.15
Between 6–12	300	0.3
Between 12–18	500	0.5

swab. Airway management is as described above and specific treatment is penicillin. Occasionally, tonsillitis is followed by severe unilateral pain and swelling in the throat with spasm of the jaw muscles (trismus). This indicates a peritonsillar abscess. Intravenous antibiotics should be started and an urgent ENT opinion requested.

Tuberculosis in children

In many cases tuberculosis (TB) infection will be contained by the child's immune system and will not cause TB disease. The only manifestation may be a small area of infection in the lung, often just beneath the pleura (the Ghon focus), and enlarged mediastinal lymph nodes. This combination is called the 'primary complex'. Bloodstream spread may occur at this stage and the TB may lodge in the lung or in other parts of the body such as the spine, the central nervous system or the joints. Here the organism may remain inactive indefinitely or may reactivate later to cause pulmonary or extrapulmonary TB.

Most children who develop infection with *Mycobacterium tuberculosis* are free of symptoms (TB infection) but a small proportion may develop disease in the chest (pulmonary TB) or spread of disease outside the chest (extrapulmonary TB). Box 8.2 summarises the different forms of pulmonary and extrapulmonary TB which may be seen.

Primary tuberculosis

Tuberculosis remains prevalent in the developing world and may be associated with HIV infection. In the UK the incidence varies greatly in different parts of the country, with the highest incidence seen in Greater London (>40/100,000 per annum). Effective tuberculosis control requires close working relationship between public health, primary care and hospital teams. Specialist nurses play a crucial role in contact tracing, tuberculin skin testing, immunisation and supporting adherence to treatment.

Immunisation with bacillus Calmette Guérin (BCG) vaccine is indicated in the newborn period, for babies who come from an area of the UK where the incidence of TB is >40/100,000 per

---

Box 8.2   Pulmonary and extrapulmonary tuberculosis

Pulmonary tuberculosis

Primary complex (focal pulmonary lesion and mediastinal lymph node enlargement) – seen in young children
Cavity formation (often upper lobes) – seen in adolescents
Mediastinal lymph node enlargement with lobar collapse
TB pleural effusion
Miliary tuberculosis

Extrapulmonary tuberculosis

Cervical lymph node enlargement
Spinal TB
TB meningitis
TB arthritis – usually a small number of large joints affected
Less commonly seen in children – abdominal TB and genitourinary TB

annum – currently only London, Birmingham and Leicester. It is also indicated for infants (and unvaccinated preschool children) whose parents or grandparents come from a high-prevalence country (Department of Health 2010). School-age children who have not had BCG should have a tuberculin skin test in the following circumstances:

- they have a parent or grandparent from a high-prevalence country
- they were born in or have lived in a high-prevalence country
- they are a household contact of pulmonary TB.

If the skin test is negative they should receive BCG immunisation. BCG does not prevent TB infection completely but moderates the severity of disease and reduces the risk of serious complications such as TB meningitis.

Children with primary TB are not infectious to others and are often identified through the screening of a member of the household who is smear positive, i.e. sputum shows acid- and alcohol-fast bacilli on Ziehl Neelson (ZN) staining (see Glossary). Screening is best done using the Mantoux test (tuberculin skin test) (see Glossary) (Coulter 2008). An intradermal injection of 0.1 mL of 20 units per mL tuberculin purified protein derivative is given and the result read after 48–72 h. A positive Mantoux test is defined as >6 mm in those who have not had BCG and >15 mm in those who have had the immunisation. If the test is positive in a child (over 2 years) exposed to TB, an interferon-γ release assay (IGRA) should be performed (e.g. Elispot™, Quantiferon™ or Tspot™) (for definitions see Glossary). This is negative if the positive skin test is due to BCG alone but positive in the case of TB infection (NICE 2011). If both the skin test and the IGRA are positive, then the child should be investigated for TB (Health Protection Agency 2008). This should include careful questioning to elicit any constitutional symptoms, e.g. weight loss, lethargy and night sweats. Young children should have 3×gastric aspirates for ZN staining and TB culture. This usually requires hospital admission, as a gastric aspirate sample must be taken from the child on first waking and before they have sat up or eaten (Pomputius et al. 1997). Older children may be able to expectorate sputum or sputum may be induced with hypertonic saline. All children should have a chest x-ray at this stage (Figure 8.4).

Other forms of pulmonary tuberculosis

Older children and adolescents may present with a picture similar to adult pulmonary TB with a cavity in the upper lobes or upper segments of the lower lobes on chest x-ray. These children may be smear positive and hence infectious to others. As with primary TB, Mantoux and IGRA testing may be helpful. However, sputum should be sent were possible (for ZN staining and TB culture) and treatment should not be delayed, where x-ray appearances are characteristic.

In some cases, young children with primary TB may develop very enlarged mediastinal lymph nodes which can compress an adjacent bronchus, leading to collapse of a lobe. In these circumstances oral prednisolone should be prescribed (in addition to the anti-TB treatment listed above) (Toppet et al. 1990). Prednisolone has the effect of shrinking the mediastinal nodes, allowing re-expansion of the affected lobe.

Just as the child with pneumonia may develop a pleural effusion, a pleural effusion may occur in pulmonary TB. A TB pleural effusion may be composed of a large volume of fluid, causing shortness of breath (Figure 8.5). In this case, the diagnosis of TB is best made by pleural biopsy (see Figure 8.5). Drainage should be performed to relieve dyspnoea only, as chest drains can introduce secondary bacterial infection into the pleural space. Treatment is the same as for uncomplicated pulmonary TB and will lead to the resolution of the effusion. In addition, a short course of prednisolone may allow the effusion to resolve more quickly.

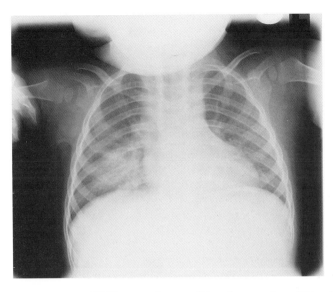

Figure 8.4 The x-ray in primary TB. There are two possible outcomes when children have a positive Mantoux and IGRA test. 1. The gastric aspirates or induced sputum are positive or the chest x-ray suggests TB. Give 6 months of TB treatment. Standard treatment is rifampicin, isoniazid, pyrazinamide and ethambutol for 2 months followed by rifampicin and isoniazid for a further 4 months. 2. All tests for clinical TB are negative. Treat as TB infection, not TB disease. Give 3 months of rifampicin and isoniazid alone.

(a)   (b)

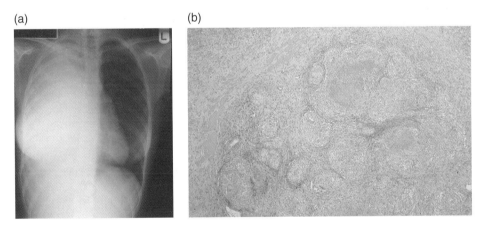

Figure 8.5 (a) Right-sided TB and pleural effusion with (b) histology from pleural biopsy.

Miliary TB (so called because of the appearance of many tiny white dots on the chest x-ray which look like millet seeds) affects mainly younger children and the immunosuppressed (Coulter 2008). Infection may spread in the bloodstream and investigations should include a lumbar puncture to look for TB meningitis. Standard anti-TB treatment should be given, with prednisolone added if there is TB meningitis as well as miliary TB.

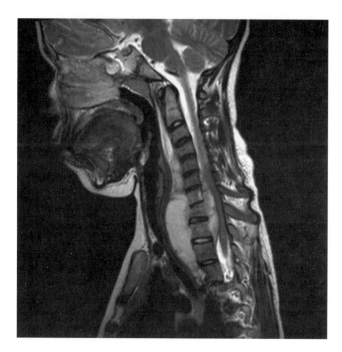

Figure 8.6   Spinal TB in an 11-year-old girl.

Extrapulmonary tuberculosis

Tuberculosis may affect not just the lungs but other systems as well (see Box 8.2). TB infection in children, outside the lungs, includes enlargement of lymph nodes in the neck, involvement of the vertebral bodies (spinal TB), TB meningitis and infection of a joint. Rarely, there may be infection of the abdominal cavity or the kidneys but this is beyond the scope of this book.

In children who have significantly enlarged lymph nodes in the neck for weeks or months, a number of diagnoses should be considered, including recurrent tonsillitis (tonsilar nodes only), infection similar to TB but with a different organism (non-tuberculous mycobacteria), TB and lymphoma. In children with recurrent tonsillitis, the diagnosis is usually obvious. If the node is small and does not enlarge further over some weeks then parents can be reassured. However, large nodes, particularly if there is a lymph node 'mass', should be biopsied and the tissue sent for culture and histology. If culture shows non-tuberculous mycobacteria, then removal of the node is curative. If histology suggests TB (or TB is cultured), then 6 months of standard therapy (see above under pulmonary TB) should be given.

Children with TB of the spine usually present with difficulty in walking and may have the constitutional symptoms of TB mentioned above (Coulter 2008). Infection starts in the anterior part of the vertebral body and leads to collapse of one or more vertebrae, causing a sharp angulation of the spine ('gibbus'). Necrotic (caseous) material may form an abscess and press on the spinal cord, leading to weakness in the arms or legs. A Mantoux test should be performed and tissue sent for TB culture or histology, if the child has surgery. Magnetic resonance imaging (MRI; Figure 8.6) should be performed and advice sought from a spinal surgeon and paediatric neurologist. Most paediatricians would give 12 months of TB treatment and in the early stages prednisolone may help to relieve symptoms of cord compression.

(a)   (b)

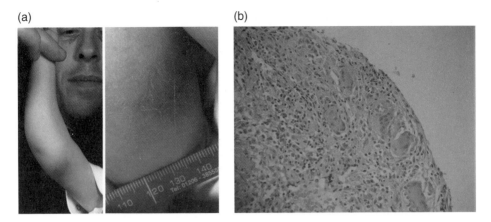

Figure 8.7   (a) TB arthritis affecting the right elbow in a 2-year-old girl. (b) Synovial biopsy.

Tuberculosis of a large joint may be confused with septic arthritis (most commonly due to *Staph. aureus*) or juvenile chronic arthritis. The large joints, such as knees and elbows, are more commonly affected. A careful history should be taken, asking about contact with TB and constitutional symptoms. A Mantoux test should be performed. Confirmation of the diagnosis is with synovial biopsy (Figure 8.7). Treatment is with standard TB drugs for 6 months (see above).

Conclusion

Pulmonary infection, particularly pneumonia, is the leading cause of death in the under-5s worldwide. Bronchiolitis is an important cause of hospital admissions in the developed world, though children with this condition rarely die. Children may present with signs of acute upper airway obstruction from infective causes (such as croup) or non-infectious causes (such as anaphylaxis). In all these acute conditions, timely supportive care with airway management, oxygen and fluids is crucial, before specific therapy is commenced. TB can cause infection in many body systems and often has an insidious onset. Careful history taking, combined with appropriate use of the Mantoux and IGRA tests, imaging and biopsy (where appropriate), is the key to early diagnosis and treatment.

Questions

Answer true or false.

1. The following are causes of acute bronchiolitis.
   a. *Haemophilus influenzae*
   b. Influenza virus
   c. Respiratory syncytial virus (RSV)
   d. Human papillomavirus
   e. Human metapneumovirus

2. The following are effective treatments for acute bronchiolitis.
   a. Intravenous fluids
   b. Oxygen

   c. Antibiotics

   d. Oral dexamethasone

   e. Hypertonic saline

3. Which of the following statements about immunisation are true?

   a. BCG prevents almost all TB infection in children

   b. Palivisumab may prevent RSV in high-risk children

   c. Pneumococcal immunisation is 99% effective in preventing pneumonia

   d. Immunisation is effective in preventing croup

   e. HiB immunisation has helped reduce the incidence of epiglottitis

4. The following are causes of upper airways obstruction.

   a. Croup

   b. Bacterial tracheitis

   c. Pneumococcal infection

   d. Bronchiolitis

   e. EBV infection

5. Empyema:

   a. Should be managed without drainage once loculations have formed

   b. Should be managed without antibiotic treatment

   c. May be managed with decortication

   d. May be managed with chest drainage plus urokinase

   e. Is almost never seen since the introduction of pneumococcal vaccine

6. The following are possible sites of TB infection.

   a. Lung

   b. Pleura

   c. Meninges

   d. Vertebral body

   e. Lymph node

7. The following can be useful in the diagnosis of TB.

   a. Careful history taking

   b. Mantoux test

   c. Hypertonic saline

   d. IGRA test

   e. Urokinase

8. The following drugs are useful in the treatment of TB.

   a. Rifampicin

   b. Penicillin

   c. Prednisolone

   d. Isoniazid

   e. Budesonide

9. Which of the following statements about the Mantoux test are true?

   a. The Mantoux test requires intramuscular administration of tuberculin

   b. The Mantoux test is not affected by previous BCG immunisation

   c. IGRA tests should not be performed where BCG has been given previously

   d. The Mantoux test is read at 12 h

   e. The Mantoux test is useful in TB contact screening

10. In childhood pneumonia:

   a. Most children will respond to oral antibiotics

   b. A chest x-ray should be performed in every case

   c. Most children can produce sputum which should be sent for culture

   d. Respiratory viruses are often responsible in young children

   e. Pneumococcus is the most common cause of bacterial pneumonia

References

Advanced Life Support Group. (2011) *Advanced Paediatric Life Support: the practical approach*, 5th edn. Chichester: Wiley Blackwell.

Atkinson M, Lakhanpaul M, Smyth A, *et al.* (2007) Comparison of oral amoxicillin and intravenous benzyl penicillin for community acquired pneumonia in children (PIVOT trial): a multicentre pragmatic randomised controlled equivalence trial. *Thorax* **62**, 1102–6.

Balfour-Lynn IM, Abrahamson E, Cohen G, *et al.* (2005) BTS guidelines for the management of pleural infection in children. *Thorax* **60(suppl I)**, i1–i21.

Blom DJM, Ermers M, Bont L, van Woensel JBM, van Aalderen WMC. (2007) Inhaled corticosteroids during acute bronchiolitis in the prevention of post-bronchiolitic wheezing. *Cochrane Database of Systematic Reviews* **1**, CD004881.

British Thoracic Society. (2002) *Guidelines for Treatment of Community Acquired Pneumonia in Children*. London: British Thoracic Society.

Bryce J, Boschi-Pinto C, Shibuya K, Black RE. (2005) WHO Child Health Epidemiology Reference Group. WHO estimates of the causes of death in children. *Lancet* **365**, 1147–52.

Calogero C, Sly PD. (2007) Acute viral bronchiolitis: to treat or not to treat – that is the question. *Journal of Pediatrics* **151**, 235–7.

Coulter JBS. (2008) Bacterial infections: Mycobacterium tuberculosis. In: McIntosh N, Helms P, Smyth R, Logan S (eds) *Forfar and Arneil's Textbook of Paediatrics*, 7th edn. Edinburgh: Churchill Livingstone, pp.1227–39.

Department of Health. (2010) Immunisation against infectious disease. *The Green Book*. London: Stationery Office. Available at: www.dh.gov.uk/prod_consum_dh/groups/dh_digitalassets/documents/digitalasset/dh_113539.pdf.

Eastham KM, Freeman R, Kearns AM, *et al.* (2004) Clinical features, aetiology and outcome of empyema in children in the north east of England. *Thorax* **59**, 522–5.

Gadomski AM, Bhasale AL. (2006) Bronchodilators for bronchiolitis. *Cochrane Database of Systematic Reviews* **3**, CD001266.

Hall CB, Weinberg GA, Iwane MK, *et al.* (2009) The burden of respiratory syncytial virus infection in young children. *New England Journal of Medicine* **360(6)**, 588–98.

Hay AD, Heron J, Ness A. (2005) ALSPAC study team. The prevalence of symptoms and consultations in pre-school children in the Avon Longitudinal Study of Parents and Children (ALSPAC): a prospective cohort study. *Family Practice* **22(4)**, 367–74.

Health Protection Agency. (2008) Position statement on the use of Interferon Gamma Release Assay (IGRA) tests for tuberculosis (TB). Interim guidance. London: Health Protection Agency.

Hollinghurst S, Gorst C, Fahey T, Hay AD. (2008) Measuring the financial burden of acute cough in pre-school children: a cost of illness study. *BMC Family Practice* **9**, 10.

Jokinen C, Heiskanen L, Juvonen H, *et al.* (1993) Incidence of community-acquired pneumonia in the population of four municipalities in eastern Finland. *American Journal of Epidemiology* **137**, 977–88.

Joint Committee on Vaccination and Immunisation (JCVI). (2004) Minutes of the JCVI RSV Subgroup 11th November 2004. Available at: www.advisorybodies.doh.gov.uk/jcvi/mins111104rvi.htm.

Mackway-Jones K, Molyneux E, Phillips B, Wieteska S. (2005) *Advanced Paediatric Life Support*, 4th edn. Oxford: Blackwell.

McNamara PS, Smyth RL. (2002) The pathogenesis of respiratory syncytial virus disease in childhood. *British Medical Bulletin* **61**, 13–28.

National Institute for Health and Clinical Excellence (NICE). (2011) *Clinical Diagnosis and Management of Tuberculosis and Measures for Its Prevention and Control*. London: Stationery Office. Available at: www.nice.org.uk/nicemedia/pdf/CG033FullGuideline.pdf.

Noble V, Murray M, Webb MSC, Alexander J, Swarbrick AS, Milner AD. (1997) Respiratory status and allergy nine to 10 years after acute bronchiolitis. *Archives of Disease in Childhood* **76(4)**, 315–19.

Palanivel V, Anjay M. (2009) Question 3. Is continuous positive airway pressure effective in bronchiolitis? *Archives of Disease in Childhood* **94(4)**, 324–6.

Pomputius WF III, Rost J, Dennehy PH, Carter EJ. (1997) Standardization of gastric aspirate technique improves yield in the diagnosis of tuberculosis in children. *Pediatric Infectious Disease Journal* **16**, 222–6.

Rees M, Spencer D, Parikh D, Weller P. (1997) Increase in incidence of childhood empyema in West Midlands,UK. *Lancet* **349**, 402.

Russell KF, Wiebe N, Saenz A, *et al.* (2004) Glucocorticoids for croup. *Cochrane Database of Systematic Reviews* **1**, CD001955.

Scottish Intercollegiate Network (SIGN). (2006) *Bronchiolitis in Children: a national clinical guideline.* Available at: www.sign.ac.uk.

Smyth A. (2001) Physical examination: signs. In: Silverman M, O'Callaghan CL (eds) *Practical Paediatric Respiratory Medicine*. London: Arnold.

Spurling GKP, Foneska K, Doust J, del Mar C. (2007) Antibiotics for bronchiolitis in children. *Cochrane Database of Systematic Reviews* **1**, CD005189.

Thomson AH, Hull J, Kumar MR, Wallis C, Balfour-Lynn IM, on behalf of the British Paediatric Respiratory Society Empyema Study. (2002) Randomised trial of intrapleural urokinase in the treatment of childhood empyema. *Thorax* **57**, 343–7.

Toppet M, Malfroot A, Derde MP, *et al.* (1990) Corticosteroids in primary tuberculosis with bronchial obstruction. *Archives of Disease in Childhood* **65**, 1222–6.

UK Immunisation Schedule. (2010) Available at: www.immunisation.nhs.uk/Immunisation_Schedule.

Ventre K, Randolph A. (2007) Ribavirin for respiratory syncytial virus infection of the lower respiratory tract in infants and young children. *Cochrane Database of Systematic Reviews* **1**, CD000181.

Westley CR, Cotton EK, Brooks JG. (1978) Nebulized racemic epinephrine by IPPB for the treatment of croup: a double-blind study. *American Journal of Diseases of Childhood* **132(5)**, 484–7.

World Health Organization. (2005) *Make Every Mother and Child Count*. Geneva: World Health Organization. Available at: www.who.int/whr/2005/whr2005_en.pdf

Zhang L, Mendoza-Sassi RA, Wainright C, Klassen TP. (2008) Nebulized hypertonic saline solution for acute bronchiolitis in infants. *Cochrane Database of Systematic Reviews* **4**, CD006458.

Chapter 9

Pharmacology and the respiratory system

Andrew Prayle[1] and Janice Mighten[2]

[1]*Research Fellow, School of Clinical Sciences*
[2]*Children's Respiratory/Community Nurse Specialist, Nottingham Children's Hospital*

Learning objectives

After studying this chapter, the reader will have an understanding of:

- pharmacodynamics
- respiratory drug therapy
- the importance of monitoring patients for unwanted effects
- the nurse's role in drug administration.

Introduction

Safe, effective prescribing and administration of medications is a cornerstone of good practice. There are several important references with which all practitioners should be familiar. The *British National Formulary for Children* (BNFc; Royal Pharmaceutical Society 2011) is the single most important reference in the UK at present. Additional guidance is also available from the National Institute for Health and Clinical Excellence (NICE). Locally, most institutions have their own guidelines, usually for specific groups of patients such as those with cystic fibrosis or those on intensive care.

Prescribing and administration guidelines allow for the safe administration of medicines. There is increased risk with prescribing for children, because many medications are relatively understudied in children, and also doses require adjustment for each child (usually according to their age or weight). Pharmacology is the study of the modes of action, effects and side-effects and uses of drugs (Neal 2005). An understanding of pharmacology is essential to the safe prescription and administration of drugs.

How drugs work

The ideal drug is usually one which has a specific action on a specific organ to do a specific job with minimal side-effects or toxicity. So, after administration of the drug, it has to be transported through the body to the target organ (or, in the case of some respiratory medicines, it is administered directly

---

Children's Respiratory Nursing, First Edition. Edited by Janice Mighten.

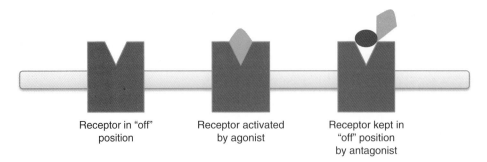

Receptor in "off"
position

Receptor activated
by agonist

Receptor kept in
"off" position
by antagonist

Figure 9.1   Schematic of agonist and antagonist action. Receptors can be located on the cell surface or within the cell. An agonist binds to the receptor and activates it, turning on a process within the cell. An antagonist binds to the receptor and prevents the body's natural agonists from activating the receptor.

to the lungs). At the target organ, the drug binds with a component of the organ's cellular machinery (often a specific protein or cell surface receptor). This binding causes the drug's effect. A receptor can be thought of as a kind of biological switch which turns a process in a cell on or off. A drug which turns a receptor on is an agonist, and one which blocks a receptor, stopping it from being turned on, is an antagonist (Figure 9.1). After binding, the drug is often metabolised into breakdown products, and following this the drug is excreted from the body.

Absorption

Absorption is the process by which a drug passes from the site of administration (often the gastro-intestinal tract after being taken orally) into the bloodstream. For orally administered drugs, the small intestine is usually the site of absorption. Intravenous drugs are administered directly into the bloodstream and do not require absorption.

A key feature of absorption is that not all the drug administered by the oral route will be absorbed – some will pass directly through the gut without interacting with the body. The fraction of the drug which is absorbed is termed its bioavailability. Many intravenous drugs are given via the intravenous route because their oral bioavailability is low. Aminoglycoside antibiotics are an example of these. Oral absorption is slow and so the onset of action of oral drugs occurs after an equivalent dose of an intravenous drug. So if rapid analgesia is required, intravenous preparations of morphine are preferred over oral morphine.

Oral drugs are generally absorbed over 1–3 h but gut absorption is affected by foods given at the same time as the drugs, largely due to the effect of food on gut motility (the speed at which things pass through the gut) and the acid content of the stomach.

Distribution

After passing into the blood, a drug is then distributed through the various tissues of the body. Drugs are rarely evenly distributed between body tissues – for example, some antibiotic drugs do not penetrate into the brain, and some antibiotics such as gentamicin are actively taken up into the kidneys.

Metabolism

Metabolism occurs when the body chemically alters a drug into metabolites. These metabolites are often easier to excrete from the body. The process of metabolism changes the chemical structure of the drug, and often this means that the metabolites do not have the same properties as the original drug. The liver is usually the site of metabolism.

Some metabolism of a drug can occur before it gets into the body's circulation for orally administered drugs. After being absorbed in the gastrointestinal tract, the drug enters the portal veins which drain into the liver. Some drug is metabolised in the liver as the drug passes through it, reducing the amount of blood which gets into the systemic circulation. This is termed 'first-pass metabolism' and it reduces the bioavailability of orally administered drugs (Rang et al. 2007).

Elimination

Most drugs are removed from the body by the kidneys. Some drugs can be excreted by the lungs, for example gaseous anaesthetic agents administered during a general anaesthetic. Drugs can be removed in the urine in their original form, such as gentamicin, which has an increased risk of toxicity and has been shown to cause damage to the kidneys (Bertenshaw et al. 2007; Detlef et al. 2009). However, often only their metabolites are removed by the kidneys.

The kidneys and liver are important for drug metabolism and elimination

As most drugs are metabolised by the liver and most are excreted by the kidneys, decreased kidney and liver function can lead to accumulation of drugs in the body. For this reason, dosages of drugs are often adjusted for patients with kidney damage or liver failure.

At different ages, children's kidney and liver function varies. For example, preterm neonates have low kidney function compared to term infants. For this reason drug doses are adjusted not just for weight but also for the age of the child.

The inhaled route of drug administration

Many therapies given in respiratory practice need to get to the lungs to effect their action. For example, salbutamol is given in asthma to dilate the airways, improving airflow and gas exchange in the lung. The site of action of salbutamol is a cell surface receptor called the β2-receptor. In the lungs, activation of the β2-receptor causes bronchodilation. β-Receptors are also present in the heart, where activation of the receptor causes the heart rate to increase. Salbutamol is usually given by the inhaled route, as it gets directly to the site where it is needed in the lungs. This allows low doses to be used. Some drug does get absorbed via the lungs into the bloodstream but because the dose given is low, very little gets to the heart, so tachycardia (a side-effect) is minimised. In contrast, if inhaled salbutamol is not effective for an asthma attack, a salbutamol infusion is often given. This requires a higher dose (as not all the drug will be distributed to the lungs) and so more drug gets to the heart, and the tachycardia is greater with the intravenous route.

Because many children cannot co-ordinate their breathing, inhaled drugs from an inhaler are usually given with a spacer. Nebulised therapies are usually delivered in hospital, although some patients such as those with cystic fibrosis receive nebulised therapies at home.

Frequently administered respiratory drugs

A comprehensive discussion of respiratory drugs prescribed for children is beyond the scope of this chapter. However, an outline of several respiratory drugs may be helpful.

In asthma, therapy is geared towards minimising inflammation and bronchoconstriction (narrowing of the airways). Patients are usually prescribed a bronchodilator such as salbutamol or ipratropium bromide, which temporarily dilates the airways. Longer acting bronchodilators are also given, such as salmeterol. Oral therapies can also be given such as theophylline and montelukast. Montelukast is a leucotriene receptor antagonist (an antagonist turns off a receptor). It prevents leucotrienes from interacting with their receptor. Their normal job seems to be to turn on inflammation, so by inhibiting their receptor, montelukast reduces inflammation.

Inhaled corticosteroids are frequently used in asthma, to reduce the symptoms between an asthma attack and the risk of an asthma attack. They reduce inflammation in the lung. Frequently prescribed inhaled steroids are beclomethasone, budesonide and fluticasone. There are many side-effects of inhaled steroids and for this reason, the dose is often adjusted up or down when the patient is seen in clinic to get the best response with the smallest dose. Oral steroids are used with some caution as their side-effect profile is much more severe than that of inhaled steroids (Sharek and Bergman 2000). However, oral steroids are highly effective when given as a short course for an asthma attack.

Oral antibiotics are frequently administered for pneumonia. Intravenous antibiotics are usually reserved for patients who require oxygen or those who are not tolerating oral antibiotics, for example due to vomiting. Paracetamol is frequently given for fever associated with chest infections but this is to relieve symptoms rather than to treat the underlying infection.

Patients with cystic fibrosis (CF) receive numerous medications, including nebulised antibiotics, nebulised sputum mucolytics (such as dornase), nebulised hypertonic saline, oral antibiotics and intravenous antibiotics. They are frequently admitted to hospital for a period of intensive antibiotic therapy, physiotherapy and dietetic and specialist nursing care. Due to the polypharmacy involved (numerous drugs given at the same time), extra care needs to be taken with their prescriptions. Children with CF often require different dosages of drugs compared to other patient groups. Many units will have their own guidelines.

Some of these drugs need careful monitoring of drug levels; in particular, aminoglycosides such as tobramycin and gentamicin (which is less frequently used in CF) require blood level monitoring. If levels are too high, kidney damage (nephrotoxicity) is a risk, and even with careful monitoring nephrotoxicity can still occur.

The nurse's role in drug administration

The Nursing and Midwifery Council (NMC 2010) clearly outlines the professional responsibility and accountability of practitioners when administering medicines; it is 'not solely a mechanistic task. It requires thought and professional judgement' (p. 1). Although training provides the basis for safe drug administration, it is ultimately the responsibility of each professional to adhere to their local policy.

Human factors will no doubt contribute to errors with drug administration so the Department of Health (Department of Health 2004) suggests that practitioners should take into account the 'five rights' of safe drug administration (Box 9.1). Adopting this approach ensures that practitioners provide safe and accurate care. Local policy also supports and incorporates the principle of the 'five rights' in order to carry out all the necessary checks of the drug administration process listed in Table 9.1.

When administering medicines to children, it is important to get co-operation from the child but equally important is the need to involve the family (Trounce et al. 2004). It is also important to acknowledge other considerations such as the significance of correct doses in children and the need to adhere to local medicines administration policy. These points are outlined in Table 9.1. It is also good practice to question prescribers and clarify the correct dose to be given before administration to children (Trounce et al. 2004).

Pharmacology training for nurses is now an integral part of the modern health service. This enables nurse prescribers to work closely with other healthcare professionals locally in support of their extended role, such as specialist pharmacists when appropriate (Trounce et al. 2004). It is also

---

Box 9.1   The 'five rights' for drug administration (adapted from Department of Health 2004)

The right …
Patient
Time
Route
Dose
Drug

Table 9.1   Checks required during all stages of drug administration (adapted from Nottingham University Hospital 2011)

Patient	Day	Route	Formulation/dose	Record
Identification, e.g. hospital number, date of birth	Correct date, day and time	Correct route, e.g. IV/oral	Tablets/liquid/ capsules IV/IM	Check drug chart is signed and legible Second checker
Right drug chart Any allergies Recheck identity before administration	Date and time last dose was given	Administer one drug per route at a time to minimise the risk of wrong route	Knowledge of drug Calculation Check BNFc	Sign for drugs when given Document if drugs not given Document/report any problems

BNFc, *British National Formulary for Children*; IM, intramuscular; IV, intravenous.

good practice for all nurses, irrespective of their level of knowledge, to acknowledge the need to check drug doses with the BNFc on every occasion before administration, as a safety mechanism.

Conclusion

There is widespread availability of medicines within all specialties. It is important for healthcare professionals to understand not only the significance of how medicines work but also the impact of such drugs on the respiratory system. Nurses should also have the ability to discuss with families the significance of monitoring for unwanted effects. The overall objective of this is to ensure that side-effects can be treated sooner rather than later.

Questions

1. Following oral administration, what factors affect absorption?
2. What is the cause of some side-effects such as tremor when using salbutamol?
3. Where does drug distribution take place in the body?
4. What is nephrotoxicity?
5. What is montelukast?

References

Bertenshaw C, Watson A, Lewis S, Smyth A. (2007) Survey of acute renal failure in patients with cystic fibrosis in the UK. *Thorax* **62**, 541–5.

Department of Health. (2004) *Building a Safer NHS for Patients: improving medication safety*. London: Department of Health.

Detlef B, Martin JH, Robert K. (2009) Cystic fibrosis, amino glycoside treatment and renal acute renal failure: the not so gentamicin. *Pediatric Nephrology* **24**, 925–8.

Neal MJ. (2005) *Medical Pharmacology at a Glance*, 5th edn. London: Blackwell.

Nottingham University Hospital. (2011) *Medicines Code of Practice: administration of medicines*. Nottingham: Nottingham University Hospital.

Nursing and Midwifery Council. (2010) *Standards for Medicines Management*. London: Nursing and Midwifery Council.

Rang HP, Dale MM, Ritter JM, Flower RJ. (2007) *Rang and Dale's Pharmacology*, 6th edn. London: Churchill Livingstone.

Royal Pharmaceutical Society of Great Britain. (2011) *British National Formulary for Children*. London: BMJ Group.

Sharek P, Bergman D. (2000) Beclomethasone for asthma in children: effects on linear growth. *Cochrane Database of Systematic Reviews* **2**, CD001282.

Trounce J, Greenstein B, Gould D. (2004) *Trounce's Clinical Pharmacology for Nurses*, 17th edn. London: Churchill Livingstone.

Chapter 10

Management of asthma and allergy

Jayesh Bhatt,[1] Harish Vyas[2] and Debra Forster[3]

[1]*Consultant Respiratory Paediatrician*
[2]*Consultant in Paediatric Respiratory Medicine*
[3]*Specialist Practitioner in Children's Community Nursing, Nottingham Children's Hospital*

Learning objectives

After studying this chapter the reader will have an understanding of:

- the pathophysiology of asthma
- the treatment and management of asthma in children
- the management of severe asthma
- the importance of nursing support
- the need for education and monitoring.

Introduction

Asthma is one of the most common chronic conditions and 10–15% of children in western society suffer from it (Pearce et al. 1993), with boys twice as likely as girls to be affected. Asthma UK estimates (2009) that:

- 5.4 million people in the UK are currently receiving treatment for asthma
- 1.1 million children in the UK are currently receiving treatment for asthma
- there is a person with asthma in one in five households in the UK.

The International Study of Asthma and Allergies in Childhood (ISAAC) has shown the rising prevalence of self-reported asthma symptoms and has allowed worldwide comparisons of the prevalence of asthma symptoms and changes over time (ISAAC 1998; Pearce et al. 2007). Despite the rise in overall prevalence, the number of acute asthma episodes in the community has shown a recent decline (Sunderland and Fleming 2004).

There is a significant cost burden to the NHS due to asthma. The Office of Health Economics (2004) estimated that the costs to the NHS in 2001 totalled £889 million.

Children's Respiratory Nursing, First Edition. Edited by Janice Mighten.
© 2013 Blackwell Publishing Ltd. Published 2013 by Blackwell Publishing Ltd.

Definition of asthma

The word asthma derives from Greek *aazein*, 'to breath with open mouth or to pant'.

'This disorder starts with a common cold, & the patient is forced to gasp for breath day & night, until the phlegm is expelled, the flow completed & the lung well cleared', from *Treatise on Asthma* by Moses Maimonides (AD 1135–1204).

The Global Initiative for Asthma (GINA) is an organisation which works to increase awareness of asthma among health professionals, public health authorities and the general public, with the objective of improving prevention and management through a concerted worldwide effort. The GINA (2008) definition of asthma is as follows.

> Asthma is a chronic inflammatory disorder of the airway in which many cells play a role, in particular mast cells, eosinophils, and T-lymphocytes. In susceptible individuals this inflammation causes recurrent episodes of wheezing, breathlessness, chest tightness and cough particularly at night and/or in the early morning. These symptoms are usually associated with widespread but variable airflow limitation that is at least partly reversible either spontaneously or with treatment. The inflammation also causes an associated increase in airway responsiveness to a variety of stimuli.

This descriptive definition highlights the three underlying cardinal pathophysiological factors in asthma.

- *Reversible bronchoconstriction*: this is mainly caused by contraction of the airway smooth muscle in response to various triggers. Airway inflammation also contributes to airway narrowing and airflow limitation. Wheeze on auscultation is indicative of airflow limitation; this can be reversed either on its own or with treatment. Bronchoconstriction can be assessed by performing lung function measurements including peak expiratory flow rates (PEFR), spirometry or other measures of airway resistance, as discussed in Chapter 5.
- *Chronic airway inflammation*: this is the result of a variety of inflammatory mediators and chronic cellular infiltrates. Oral or inhaled corticosteroids, which form the mainstay of asthma treatment, control inflammation. Methods of assessing airway inflammation are generally invasive (bronchial biopsy) or require significant co-operation (induced sputum to assess cellular type and inflammatory mediators) and are generally not routinely performed in children. Fraction of exhaled nitric oxide is a measure of underlying eosinophilic inflammation and is now being increasingly used in clinical practice.
- *Airway hyper-responsiveness (AHR)*: 'twitchy breathing tubes' is a tendency of the airways to narrow excessively in response to a variety of stimuli which normally would have little or no effect in individuals without asthma. The AHR can be assessed in the respiratory function laboratory and can be objectively measured. Some of the classic symptoms of asthma, including episodic breathlessness, cough, wheeze and chest tightness on exertion, at night, exposure to inhaled allergens or temperature changes, are due to underlying AHR which can lead to bronchoconstriction and airway inflammation.

Godfrey (2000) classifies the AHR challenges as allergen mediated, direct and indirect. Challenges with an inhaled allergen to which the susceptible individual has become sensitised could be potentially dangerous because of severe reactions; they are rarely used except for research.

Chemicals such as methacholine or histamine will act directly on the airway smooth muscle. This test of AHR is commonly used as an endpoint in asthma clinical trials to determine the effectiveness of an intervention (Liem et al. 2008). These chemicals act directly on airway smooth muscle (ASM) to cause narrowing of the ASM in all individuals. In normal individuals, a much higher dose is required to do this while in those with AHR, this happens at a much lower dose. The difference in the asthmatic child is quantitative and not qualitative.

With indirect challenges, the stimulus causes changes in the bronchial environment which are similar to what happens during an attack of asthma. The most common indirect challenge is the exercise test which under standardized environmental conditions in the laboratory assesses whether there is (greater than 12–15%) decline in lung function after a standardized level of exercise.

Treatment of asthma

Diagnosis

When considering treatment, it is important to acknowledge that a diagnosis of asthma is not made on a single symptom. History taking is just as important as clinical features, investigations or tests and the whole process is often like putting several pieces of a jigsaw together to get the whole picture. The episodic nature of symptoms including breathlessness, cough, chest tightness and wheeze should raise the possibility of an asthma diagnosis.

Parents often use the term 'wheeze' to describe any abnormal respiratory noise which on further investigation turns out to be a different respiratory noise (rattle or stridor) and not wheeze; therefore parents are often better at locating sounds than describing them (Elphick et al. 2001; Cane and McKenzie 2001). It is sometimes helpful to imitate various respiratory noses and clarify the wheeze as a whistling noise on breathing out (expiration). Wheeze on auscultation is a continuous, high-pitched musical sound coming from the chest.

While taking the history, one should clarify that the child indeed has wheeze and not any other cause of noisy breathing. Once it is established that the child has a wheeze, one should try and ascertain if this is episodic or persistent as there are many different causes of wheeze in childhood and different clinical patterns of wheezing can be recognised in children. When wheezing is persistent or frequent and associated with symptoms in between episodes, the likelihood of these symptoms being due to asthma is greater. Children who have persisting or interval symptoms are most likely to benefit from therapeutic interventions.

Enquiry should also be made about the presence or absence of atopy (inherited predisposition to produce IgE antibodies to various allergens). A personal history of atopic disorder (eczema, intermittent or persistent allergic rhinitis) or a family history of atopic disorder and/or asthma increases the probability of a diagnosis of asthma (BTS 2011). Atopic status can be established by performing skin rick tests or measuring blood-specific IgE to various inhaled or food allergens. A positive test is only indicative of sensitisation (the production of specific IgE antibody to the relevant allergen). Assessing atopy is also helpful in identifying triggers and in an individual may be related to the severity of current asthma and persistence through childhood.

Presence of certain clinical features lowers the probability of an asthma diagnosis and alternative or additional diagnoses need to be considered. These features include symptoms associated with a cold only, with no interval symptoms. Others include isolated cough in the absence of wheeze or difficulty breathing, history of moist cough, prominent dizziness, light-headedness and peripheral tingling.

Other elements would include repeatedly normal physical examination of chest when symptomatic, measurements such as normal peak expiratory flow (PEF) or spirometry when symptomatic, and medication provided for a trial period can demonstrate no response to a trial of asthma therapy when taken correctly through an appropriate inhaler device. Therefore the clinical features point to an alternative diagnosis, for example cystic fibrosis or vocal cord dysfunction. Normal oxygen saturation levels in association with sudden onset of wheezing, without any clear trigger, may indicate the presence of other conditions such as vocal cord dysfunction or hyperventilation.

The BTS guidelines recommend that in children with a high probability of asthma, a trial of treatment should be started and the response reviewed within 2–3 months. In those children with a low probability of asthma and an additional or an alternative diagnosis, further investigations or specialist assessment would be appropriate.

Goals for treatment

The GINA report (2008), based on a global strategy for asthma management, recommends specific goals for asthma treatment: minimal, and ideally no, symptoms during the day or at night; minimal, and ideally no, asthma episodes (exacerbations), including minimal use (less than daily) of a reliever medication (short-acting β2-agonist (SABA) such as salbutamol). Other variables include normal activities, normal lung function (PEFR/forced expiratory volume in 1 second (FEV1) $\geq 80\%$ of the child's personal best) and minimal, or ideally no, adverse effects from medications.

In children and young adults, often it is better to set personal goals as well, for example the ability to complete a game of football without the need to take the reliever medication frequently. Treatment should be commenced at the appropriate level of severity for the individual patient. The BTS guidelines recommend a stepwise approach as described later in this chapter.

When commencing inhaled treatment, an appropriate inhaler device should be prescribed after reviewing the technique and a spacer device should be prescribed for children for use with a pressurised metered dose inhaler. Children over 6 may be able to use a dry powder inhaler, and the device that the child demonstrates that they can use best and prefers should be prescribed. Regular review of inhaler technique should be carried out at each clinic as reinforcing the training is required to continue to maintain correct inhaler technique (Kamps et al. 2002). A more detailed discussion on use of inhaled devices is presented later in this chapter.

Monitoring of treatment response and asthma control will be clinical and symptom based in the majority of patients. A structured symptomatic assessment is required to correctly assess the severity of asthma as unstructured assessments lead to underestimating the severity and could adversely influence the treatment decisions (Halterman et al. 2006). Several patient-based validated tools are available, including the Asthma Control Test (ACT) (Schatz et al. 2006) and are also included as recommendations by the BTS guidelines.

The ACT helps to identify patients with poorly controlled asthma (Schatz et al. 2006). This tool consists of five pertinent questions, shown in Box 10.1, relating to symptoms and quality of life over a 4-week period. Essentially, the higher the ACT scores, the better the control. A score of 20 or more indicates good control and the goal should be an ideal score of 25 for complete control.

Other things that need to be included in assessing control are lung function, number and severity of exacerbations requiring use of healthcare resources, oral corticosteroid use and time off school or work since last assessment. Treatment concordance should also be assessed, especially if the response to correctly prescribed treatment is not as expected. Adverse environmental influences,

---

Box 10.1   ACT test questions (adapted from Schatz et al. 2006)

1. In the past 4 weeks, how often did your asthma stop you from doing daily activities like going to school?
2. How frequently were you breathless?
3. How many times did you wake with your asthma at night or in the morning before you were due to get up?
4. How frequently did you use your reliever medication such as a salbutamol inhaler?
5. At the moment, how well would you say that your asthma is controlled?

including exposure to environmental tobacco smoke, ongoing allergen exposure and psychosocial factors need to be reviewed in those with 'difficult' asthma (Ranganathan et al. 2001).

Allergen avoidance

Even though it has been shown that increased allergen exposure in sensitised individuals is associated with an increase in asthma symptoms, bronchial hyper-responsiveness and deterioration in lung function, the research evidence supporting reduction in allergen exposure to reduce morbidity and/or mortality in asthma is tenuous (BTS 2009, 2011).

House dust mite

Measures to decrease house dust mites have been shown to reduce their numbers but have not been shown to have an effect on asthma severity. Cochrane reviews on house dust mite control measures in a normal domestic environment have concluded that chemical and physical methods aimed at reducing exposure to house dust mite allergens cannot be recommended (Gøtzsche et al. 2004).

Some very committed families with evidence of house dust mite sensitisation may wish to try mite avoidance by considering the following:

- complete barrier bed-covering systems
- removal of carpets
- removal of soft toys from beds
- high-temperature washing of bedlinen
- applying acaricides to soft furnishings
- good ventilation with or without dehumidification.

Other allergens

The literature on pet avoidance is very confusing and generally speaking, individual aeroallergen avoidance strategies have limited or no benefit. A multifaceted approach is more likely to be effective if it addresses all the indoor asthma triggers.

Treatment and management need the co-operation of the child and parents. Advances in medicines and proficient guidelines have facilitated care based on best practice.

British Thoracic Society guidelines for the management of asthma

The 2008 BTS *Guideline on the Management of Asthma* was based on review of the literature published up to March 2007. The 2011 revision includes updates on monitoring asthma, a whole new section on asthma in adolescents and pharmacological management. These revisions are clearly highlighted as 2011 changes and stress the importance of using closed questions when asking about asthma control and being aware that the best predictor for future exacerbations is level of current control. On an annual basis at least, the following should be monitored:

- symptom score/exacerbations
- oral corticosteroid use
- time off school/nursery due to asthma since last assessment
- inhaler technique
- adherence
- possession/use of self-management and personalised asthma action plan

- exposure to tobacco smoke
- growth (height and weight centile).

It should be recognised that doses of inhaled steroids are referenced against beclomethasone dipropionate (BDP) with hydrofluroalkane (HFA) propellants and that these products are more potent and all should be prescribed by brand.

In children (5–12 years) on inhaled corticosteroids (ICS) at a dose of 400 μg/day of BDP equivalent, addition of an inhaled long-acting β2-agonist (LABA) is the first choice. These agents improve lung function AND symptoms, and decrease exacerbations. This should be done before doubling the dose of ICS as the dose–response curve with ICS is flat beyond a certain dose so the likelihood of systemic side-effects increases. A flat dose–response curve means that increasing the dose is unlikely to give additional benefit and more likely to produce side-effects. LABAs should never be used on their own without ICS. A review by the Medicines and Healthcare products Regulatory Agency (MHRA) has concluded that the benefits of these medicines used in conjunction with ICS in the control of asthma symptoms outweigh any apparent risks. Leukotriene receptor antagonists may provide improvement in lung function, a decrease in exacerbations, and an improvement in symptoms.

Omalizumab (humanised monoclonal antibody which binds to circulating IgE) has NICE approval for use in patients >12 years old. The criteria for its use in this age group include the use of high-dose ICS and LABA, impaired lung function, symptomatic with frequent exacerbations and IgE levels 30–1300 kilounits (KU)/L. Omalizumab is given as a subcutaneous injection every 2–4 weeks and should only be initiated in specialist centres with experience of evaluation and management of patients with severe and difficult asthma. It is also licensed for use but not NICE approved for children 6–12 years of age and the IgE levels in this age range should be lower than 1500 KU/L.

The guidelines recommend a stepwise approach to management and initial treatment should be at the step most appropriate to the initial severity of the patient's asthma. The goals should be individualised (see GINA above) but with a stepwise approach, the aim should be to abolish symptoms as soon as possible and to optimise lung function.

The aim is to achieve early control and to maintain control by stepping up treatment as necessary and stepping down when control is good. For paediatric patients, there are different recommendations for stepwise management across three age ranges including children >12 years old (similar to adults), children 5–12 years, and children under 5 years. The evidence to support treatment recommendations is less clear in children under 2 and the threshold for seeking an expert opinion should be lowest in these children.

Step 1: mild intermittent asthma

An inhaled SABA (salbutamol or terbutaline) as short-term reliever therapy should be prescribed for all patients with symptomatic asthma. SABAs work more quickly and/or with fewer side-effects than the alternatives (inhaled ipratropium bromide, β2-agonist or theophylline tablets). This should be on an as-required basis and ideally there should be little or no need for SABA use. Patients who require inhaled SABA three times a week or more or are symptomatic three times a week or more or waking one night a week should move to step 2.

Step 2: introduction of regular preventer therapy

Inhaled corticosteroids

Inhaled corticosteroids such as beclomethasone, used in recommended doses, are the most effective and safe preventer drugs for achieving symptom control, improvement in lung function, and prevention/reduction of exacerbations. ICS should be considered for children aged 5–12 and children under the age of 5 if they:

- are using inhaled β2-agonists three times a week or more
- are symptomatic three times a week or more or waking one night a week
- have had an exacerbation of asthma requiring oral corticosteroids in the last 2 years.

Reasonable starting doses are, in children > 12 years old (similar to adults), 400 µg per day, and in children 5–12 years, 200 µg per day. In children less than 5 years of age, higher doses may be required if there are problems in obtaining consistent drug delivery. The dose should be titrated to the lowest dose at which effective control of asthma is maintained. Leukotriene receptor antagonists can be used as monotherapy in this age group if ICS cannot be used.

Safety and side-effects of inhaled corticosteroids

Inhaled corticosteroids have been in use since the 1970s and are safe drugs when taken in recommended doses as discussed above. However, systemic side-effects secondary to ICS have come to light since the late 1990s and every clinician prescribing ICS should be vigilant to the possibility of side-effects, especially if there is additional steroid burden in the form of frequent courses of oral steroids for exacerbations as well as cumulative steroid burden, for example an atopic child also receiving steroid creams for eczema and nasal steroids for significant allergic rhinitis.

Patients on higher dose ICS could be issued steroid warning cards but this may have an impact on compliance and the benefits of this suggestion are not clearly defined.

Administration of ICS at or above 400 µg a day of BDP or equivalent may be associated with systemic side-effects, including growth failure and adrenal suppression. It has been known for some years that suppression of the hypothalamic-pituitary-adrenal (HPA) axis occurs in children exposed to ICS (Broide et al. 1995; Fitzgerald et al. 1998; Kannisto et al. 2000). More recently, clinical adrenal insufficiency at the time of intercurrent illness has been identified in a small number of children who have become acutely unwell (Patel et al. 2001). Most of these children had been treated with high doses of ICS, such as budesonide, fluticasone and beclomethasone, outside the recommended doses (Todd et al. 2002).

The dose or duration of ICS treatment required to place a child at risk of clinical adrenal insufficiency is unknown but is likely to occur at ≥ 800 µg per day of BDP or equivalent. The low-dose ACTH test (short synacthen) is considered to provide a physiological stimulation of adrenal responsiveness but it is not known how useful such a sensitive test is at predicting clinically relevant adrenal insufficiency and also how often it should be repeated if abnormal.

Regular review of ICS doses should be undertaken, stepping down on dose with good control, being vigilant about cumulative steroid exposure and prescribing the lowest dose of ICS required for disease control. Systemic side-effects of ICS should be kept in mind and specific written advice about steroid replacement in the event of a severe intercurrent illness should be part of the management plan.

Although recommended in previous guidelines and as part of asthma action plans, doubling the dose at the time of an exacerbation is of unproven value.

Step 3: initial add-on therapy

At each clinical review and when asthma control is not achieved, inhaler technique should be checked and reinforced. Treatment adherence needs to be explored, checked and encouraged and trigger factors eliminated as far as possible.

Stepping up and using a trial of add-on therapy should be considered if control is not good.
The options for add-on therapy are as follows.

- In children (5–12 years) on ICS at a dose of 400 µg/day, addition of an inhaled LABA is the first choice. These agents improve lung function and symptoms, and decrease exacerbations. This should be done before doubling the dose of ICS as the dose–response curve with ICS is flat beyond a certain dose and the likelihood of systemic side-effects increases. A flat dose–response curve means that increasing the dose is unlikely to give additional benefit and more likely to produce side-effects. LABAs should never be used on their own without ICS.
- Leukotriene receptor antagonists may provide improvement in lung function, a decrease in exacerbations, and an improvement in symptoms.
- Increasing the dose of ICS.
- Theophyllines may improve lung function and symptoms but side-effects occur more commonly and blood levels need to be measured because of the narrow therapeutic window.

Long-acting β2-agonists are not licensed for use in children under 5 years old and step 3 for these children should be as follows.

- On ICS >200–400 µg/day, consider addition of a leukotriene receptor antagonist (LTRA).
- In those children taking a LTRA alone, consider addition of an ICS 200–400 µg/day.
- In children under 2 years, consider referring to a specialist respiratory paediatrician.

Combination inhalers

Guidance from NICE recommends that in children with chronic asthma in whom treatment with an ICS and LABA is considered appropriate, the following apply.

- The use of a combination device within its marketing authorisation is recommended as an option.
- The decision to use a combination device or the two agents in separate devices should be made on an individual basis, taking into consideration therapeutic need and the likelihood of treatment adherence.

There is no difference in efficacy in giving ICS and LABA in combination or in separate inhalers. However, once a patient is on stable therapy, combination inhalers have the advantage of guaranteeing that the LABA is not taken without ICS.

Step 4: poor control on moderate dose of inhaled steroid plus add-on therapy: addition of fourth drug

In children under 5 years of age, if control is not achieved on step 3, indicating persistently poor control, early referral to a respiratory paediatrician should be made.

If control remains inadequate on 800 µg daily (>12 years) or 400 µg daily (children) of an ICS plus a LABA, consider the following interventions.

- Increase ICS.
- Leukotriene receptor antagonists.
- Theophyllines.

However, remember that this should be as a trial and if it is ineffective, stop the drug or reduce the dose back.

Step 5: continuous or frequent use of oral steroids

Use daily steroid tablets at the lowest dose providing adequate control and refer to a respiratory paediatrician. Regular monitoring of systemic side-effects should be undertaken, including measuring blood pressure, growth, urine sugar, adrenal insufficiency, cataracts and bone health.

Steroid tablet-sparing medication

The aim of treatment is to control the asthma using the lowest possible dose or, if possible, to stop long-term steroid tablets completely (BTS 2009). Treatment trials of steroid-sparing agents such as immunosuppressants (methotrexate, ciclosporin and oral gold), intravenous immunoglobulin and continuous subcutaneous terbutaline should only be undertaken in centres with relevant experience and facilities.

Omalizumab (humanised monoclonal antibody which binds to circulating IgE) has NICE approval for use in patients > 12 years old on high-dose ICS and LABA who have impaired lung function, are symptomatic with frequent exacerbations, and have IgE levels 30–700 KU/L. It is given as a subcutaneous injection every 2–4 weeks and should only be initiated in specialist centres with experience of evaluation and management of patients with severe and difficult asthma (Kulis et al. 2010).

Stepping down

Patients should be maintained at the lowest possible dose of ICS and the dose reduction should be slow and individualised but can be considered every 3 months, decreasing the dose by approximately 25–50% each time.

Once asthma control is achieved, stepping down therapy should be undertaken. This should be done at regular clinical reviews and the lowest dose of ICS that achieves asthma control should be used as maintenance treatment.

For those admitted to hospital with severe asthma, a different approach is required.

Acute severe asthma

Acute severe asthma is a major reason for admission to hospital and remains the most common medical emergency in children. Prevalence of asthma has increased by 50% since 1980. Severe asthma still remains a cause of death; it is tragic that one-third of these patients would have been previously diagnosed as being mild. The last few years have seen a steady increase in the number of patients admitted to paediatric intensive care units (PICU), although the majority of them stay for a relatively short period.

Pathophysiology

Elements of respiratory system development have been discussed in Chapter 1. During an acute attack of asthma there is marked airway inflammation producing excessive mucus, leading to airway plugging. In addition, bronchospasm produces severe airflow limitation, leading to progressive respiratory failure. In a small group of children acute anaphylaxis will lead to intense bronchospasm without significant mucus plugging. In the majority of children there are no specific identifiable precipitating factors although occasionally a history of anaphylaxis may be present.

History

A detailed history is essential for rapid and appropriate management. The following details are required.

- Past history of asthma, prematurity, chronic lung disease, surgery for congenital lung anomalies such as tracheo-oesophageal fistula.
- Family history of atopy.
- Previous hospital admission.
- Frequency of attacks and details of precipitating factors.
- Current medical therapy and history of compliance.
- Duration of current attack and precipitating factor.

The most common precipitating factors are viral infections, allergens such as exposure to cats or grass pollen, and food such as eggs and peanuts. Occasionally emotional and social factors may bring on a severe attack (Halterman et al. 2006).

Differential diagnosis

It is always necessary to exclude other diagnoses such as lower respiratory tract infection, bronchiolitis and pneumonia. As well as infection, there could also be lower respiratory tract obstruction. Therefore in a child with no previous history, there is the need to rule out foreign body inhalation or mediastinal tumour, e.g. lymphoma. Another area to consider is upper airway obstruction (usually inspiratory stridor would be obvious). A variety of conditions such as epiglottitis, croup or bacterial tracheitis, foreign body, polyps/tumour, vascular ring or tracheomalacia can contribute towards upper airway obstruction. Other possibilities include:

- obliterative bronchiolitis
- cystic fibrosis
- aspiration
- psychogenic hyperventilation
- metabolic acidosis, e.g. diabetic ketoacidosis
- salicylate poisoning.

Risk factors for severe asthma

Some of the risks associated with a severe attack of asthma include a history of sudden and rapid deterioration, possibly due to acute anaphylaxis. With poor compliance in clinical practice, it is noted that these children will often have a severe attack. If there is evidence of previous attacks of severe asthma requiring PICU admission and mechanical ventilation, this can also be a contributing factor to the increased risk associated with severe asthma attacks. Again, the evidence suggests that excessive use of β-agonists also increases the risk, including a reluctance to recognise severity and poor perception of hypoxia.

General management

General points for all asthmatics referred

- Administer high-flow oxygen via a facemask with a rebreathing bag with the aim of maintaining $SaO_2 > 94\%$. (SaO_2 = the percentage of available haemoglobin saturated with oxygen).

Table 10.1   Assessment of severity

	Age 0–5 years	Age 5–15 years
Moderate-severe	Too breathless to talk Too breathless to feed Respiratory rate >50 Pulse >130 bpm Significant respiratory distress	Too breathless to talk PEFR <50% predicted Respiratory rate >30 Pulse >120 bpm Use of accessory muscles
Life-threatening (any of these features)	• Cyanosis • Silent chest • Poor respiratory effort • Fatigue or exhaustion • Agitation or reduced level of consciousness • (PEFR <33% – monitoring unlikely to be tolerated)	

bpm, beats per minute; PEFR, peak expiratory flow rate.

- Provide a calm and reassuring environment and allow the child to assume the most comfortable position – often sitting upright reduces distress and improves chest wall movement. This position reduces ventilation/perfusion mismatch when β-agonists are administered.
- Monitor:
  - continuous pulse oximetry and electrocardiogram (ECG)
  - non-invasive blood pressure (BP)
  - serum electrolytes and blood glucose; watch carefully for hypokalaemia.

Note: PEFR measurement is not tolerated by acutely distressed or young children.

Assessment of severity of the attack is shown in Table 10.1 and the initial management in the emergency department is summarised in Figure 10.1.

Management of acute asthma in the emergency department

Initial management as always involves emergency treatment to maintain the airway, such as providing high oxygen concentration using a reservoir bag. Nebulised salbutamol continuously with oxygen also assists in the process, giving consideration to the fact that poor response may be due to inadequate gaseous exchange. In such cases intravenous salbutamol should be administered.

We have already established that the process involved in asthma includes inflammation so early steroid, either orally if tolerated or intravenously, is essential. Sitting the child up will minimise ventilation/perfusion mismatch but failure to improve with the initial treatment necessitates admission to the PICU.

Clinical evaluation and monitoring

Regular medical and nursing observations are essential. It is important to assess, evaluate and monitor clinical signs regularly, for example an increasing heart rate is a sign of worsening asthma. Respiratory rate and the degree of breathlessness, including the use of accessory muscles, should be assessed and evidence of air entry on auscultation is significant. In relation to this element, wheezing may be biphasic and may disappear on worsening airway obstruction. Following regular

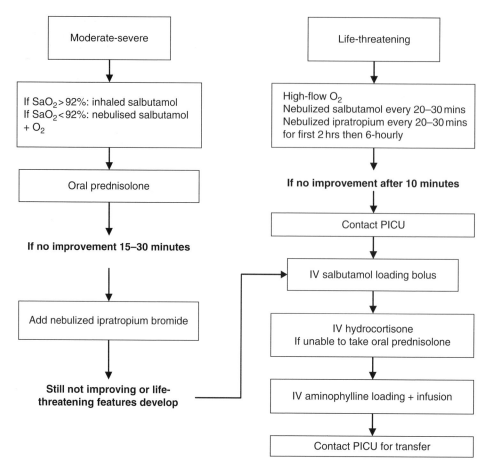

Figure 10.1   Initial medical treatment. IV, intravenous; PICU, paediatric intensive care unit.

checks and observation, any signs of progressive agitation or obtundation indicate end-stage respiratory failure and require urgent intubation.

Monitoring should include the following.

• Continuous pulse oximetry.
• ECG and BP.
• Blood electrolytes and glucose. Hypokalaemia should be treated.
• Blood gases (usually capillary). A rising $PaCO_2$ indicates imminent respiratory collapse.

Peak flow measurements are not normally undertaken in an acutely distressed or very young child.

Treatment prior to admission to high-dependency or paediatric intensive care unit

Initial treatment is similar to the management of acute asthma in the emergency department but if there is a poor response to continuous nebulised medication, intravenous salbutamol is indicated. This may be due to poor air entry as a result of progressive airway obstruction. A loading dose followed by continuous infusion helps aeration and improves work of breathing. Failure of this therapy mandates an intravenous aminophylline bolus followed by continuous infusion. Aminophylline has a narrow therapeutic range and significant adverse effects such as tachycardia, arrhythmias, nausea, vomiting, convulsions and hyperglycaemia, and therefore requires monitoring.

Magnesium sulphate should be administered upon arrival to the PICU and may help with improved oxygenation.

Other possible options include the use of non-invasive ventilation (NIV) which may help while waiting for the medical therapy to work. It may also help in children who are getting tired and drifting into respiratory failure. However, it requires a co-operative child and should be discontinued if there is worsening of hypoxia or blood gases or the child looks tired and is drifting into coma.

Risks of intubation and ventilation

Presenting symptoms such as worsening bronchospasm which could include additional factors, for example laryngospasm, worsening hypoxia, hypotension due to induction agents, antecedent dehydration and worsened by positive pressure ventilation and cardiac arrest. Another significant factor is that barotrauma in an overinflated chest may produce pneumothorax and surgical emphysema.

Criteria for intubation

- Respiratory arrest.
- Hypoxia and rising hypercarbia despite maximum oxygen and medical treatment and NIV.
- Exhaustion and inability to vocalise.
- Altered mental status.

Worsening blood gases should not be used alone to initiate intubation. Fifty percent of complications occur during or immediately after intubation, so an experienced senior physician must be present when intubation is planned and it must be carried out by a very experienced clinician.

Issues during ventilation

Sedation and paralysis

Adequate sedation is essential to allow permissive hypercapnia and prevent patient–ventilator dysynchrony which can worsen dynamic hyperinflation. Paralysis in conjunction with steroids may lead to myopathy/neuropathy and should be avoided or restricted to less than 48 h.

Delivery of bronchodilators

Either metered dose inhalers or nebulisers can be inserted into the ventilatory circuit to deliver salbutamol + ipratropium, when a child is ventilated. Following extubation, there is usually a rapid improvement in oxygenation. Steroids and nebulised bronchodilators should be continued. Transfer to the ward should be determined by the improvement in oxygen requirement and clinical air entry. Before discharge, plans should be made for long-term follow-up in a specialist respiratory clinic. Inhaler technique that is carried out correctly will help but requires good support from nursing input.

Nursing management

This section will discuss nursing management including inhaler technique, education and support for children with asthma and their families.

The role of the asthma nurse

The respiratory nurse specialist provides an important role in facilitating care delivery for children with asthma. With specialist skills and knowledge, such care delivery is evident in both primary and secondary care, with treatment regimes that can be complex at times (Wooler 2001). McKean and Furness (2009) emphasise the importance of a respiratory nurse within secondary care to support nursing colleagues with the delivery of education for asthma patients. Therefore the nurse specialist is at the forefront of planning a suitable care pathway for the child and family, through education and continual support.

Education

The aim of management for children with asthma is to reduce the number of acute exacerbations and hospital admissions. This can be achieved through education, providing the parents with the correct information and continued monitoring and support. Without correct inhaler technique and a management plan for reference, an assessment of clinical outcome can be difficult.

However, the role of the respiratory nurse caring for children with asthma is not simply about checking inhaler technique, although this is vital. Increasingly, professionals agree that patient education is crucial to achieving good control of asthma symptoms (McPherson et al. 2002). The philosophy of participation and family-centred care in children's nursing is well established and provides the child and family with the opportunity to gain greater control over the management of their health (Rowen 2002).

The nurse with a high level of expertise and knowledge of asthma, together with effective communication skills, is in an ideal position to aid in the management of asthma in children. Indeed, the role of the specialist asthma nurse is promoted in the BTS guidelines (2011). Effective management is not achieved by simply giving advice and explanation (McPherson et al. 2002). It takes time, effort and commitment from all parties. A multidisciplinary approach is also advocated (Wesseldine et al. 1999).

We have already established that written information is beneficial in supporting the care management plan set by the primary care team. Equally important is the provision of patient information leaflets. Asthma UK has produced a wealth of literature for the management of asthma in children. Therefore professionals can signpost parents and young people to their website (www.asthmauk.org) in order to support their knowledge and understanding.

A leaflet for parents of children under 5 with wheeziness or asthma has recently been produced in collaboration between the hospital and community services (Forster 2010). This aims to provide comprehensive written information for parents of this client group by healthcare professionals in either the community or hospital. Giving consideration to quality standards, this leaflet has been produced using evidence-based practice from NICE (2000) and BTS guidelines (2011).

Parents will always have questions surrounding the management of their child's asthma, in particular drug therapy. Chapter 9 provided a comprehensive overview of respiratory pharmacology. However, frequently asked questions about the side-effects of steroids and the overuse of bronchodilators need to be answered appropriately and reinforced to parents.

Inhaler technique

Correct inhaler technique is a cornerstone of effective asthma management. Overall, it is perceived to be a waste of time and prescription if individuals do not use inhalers correctly. A well-conducted study by Brocklebank et al. (2001) has shown that the ability to use inhalers correctly does indeed vary. Teaching the correct method does definitely improve technique and therefore the amount of drug actually deposited in the lungs (NICE 2000).

The BTS *Guideline on the Management of Asthma* (2011) strongly recommends that practitioners should 'prescribe inhalers only after patients have received training in the use of the device and have demonstrated satisfactory technique' (p.48). However, it also states that there is little or no available evidence on which to base recommendations for choice of inhaler device.

Therefore it is imperative that a practitioner with experience of working with children and asthma management decides on which inhaler is most effective for each individual patient. Factors such as age, physical ability, lifestyle, attitude and the influence of peers should not be underestimated in inhaler choice. This is because a child may not want to take an inhaler in the class, in front of their peers. Therefore peer pressure may have an influence on their attitude towards the inhaler (Education for Health 2006).

As previously stated, the child's age and development will have an impact on choosing and using an inhaler device. Children may have also had previous experience of using or seeing others using devices. Naturally, older children can be involved in choosing the device. The younger child can be given the impression that they are involved in choosing the device and practitioners experienced in child development will have no problem achieving this task.

Encouraging parents to use the inhaler devices with the child's favourite doll or cuddly toy is a frequent suggestion. Another suggestion is to decorate the spacer devices to make them more attractive and child friendly. Using plenty of praise and encouragement when the child uses the device with less fuss is always recommended too.

In addition, it is vital that inhaler technique is checked regularly, for example whenever the child is reviewed by a nurse or doctor. This should certainly take place during a routine clinic visit, so that small discrepancies can be rectified quickly and easily. On a practical note, teaching and supporting a child to use an inhaler correctly take time, patience and innovation.

A recent study has shown that 50% of children have assumed responsibility for the use of their daily preventive medications by the age of 11 (Orrell-Valente et al. 2008). If parents are not observing their child using their inhalers, the child's technique may actually be suboptimal and poor symptom control may be the result. Poor inhaler technique is often a problem in a severe episode of asthma (Chandler 2001), because the medication would not get to where it is needed to improve symptoms.

Inhalers used in asthma management can be grouped into three broad categories (Figure 10.2):

- pressurised metered dose inhalers (MDI)
- breath actuated
- dry powder devices.

Within these categories there are several different types of inhalers. Each of these devices has different mechanical characteristics, which, when combined with factors such as the child's/carer's thoughts, perceptions and behaviour, will lead to variation in both the quantity of drug delivered by the device and the amount actually deposited in the lungs (NICE 2000).

This section will not discuss in detail the technique for each device. However, there are some important factors that should be mentioned. When using an MDI or breath-actuated inhaler, the device must be shaken before each dose. Problems when using the MDI alone usually occur due to the difficulties with co-ordinating device actuation and inhalation at the same time.

Brocklebank et al. (2001) found that 57–77% of people did not demonstrate correct MDI technique. This team also showed that 41–47% did not demonstrate correct technique using dry powder devices and 41–47% had difficulty using a spacer with an MDI. This study clearly highlights the huge variations in inhaler technique. Further, much is known about the pharmacokinetics, importance of particle size and deposition site in the respiratory system of inhaled medications. Therefore, the importance of correct technique when using an inhaler cannot be overestimated. The Asthma UK website illustrates how to use many types of inhalers (www.asthma.org.uk/using_your_inhaler.html).

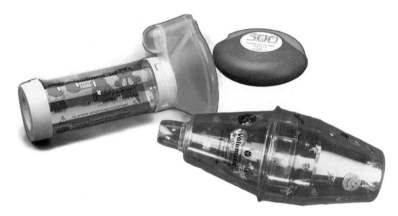

Figure 10.2   Inhalers and spacers.

Asthma action plans

A written, personalised asthma action plan should be included in best practice, especially for those with moderate to severe disease, and does lead to good outcomes, in particular in relation to health-care resource use (BTS 2011). The education provided as part of the asthma action plan empowers patients and/or carers to undertake self-management more appropriately and effectively. The discussion points should include:

• nature of the disease
• nature of the treatment
• identifying areas where patient most wants treatment to have effect
• how to use the treatment
• development of self-monitoring/self-assessment skills
• negotiation of the personalised action plan in light of identified patient goals
• recognition and management of acute exacerbations
• appropriate allergen or trigger avoidance.

Examples of asthma action plans

Asthma action plan for children who do not do peak flow measurements

Name
Date

When well: not really coughing, wheezing or breathless. Give usual doses of inhalers, for example if coughing/wheezing and a little breathless but not distressed, give usual dose of reliever (blue inhaler). Your child should <u>not</u> need their reliever every 4 hours at this point.

Not so well: coughing/wheezing and breathless or has a cold, which usually triggers the asthma. Your child is distressed by the symptoms of cough/breathlessness/wheeze.

• Give usual dose of reliever (blue inhaler), but every 4 hours up to 6 times in 24 hours.
• Continue to give preventer (brown/orange/lilac inhaler), but still give only morning and evening.
• Do not forget to reduce dose of inhalers (usually after about a week).

<u>Not very well</u>: very distressed, coughing, wheezing and breathlessness. Usual doses of reliever are not lasting 4 hours.

- Give at least 5 (maximum 10) puffs of reliever slowly through spacer every 4 hours up to 6 times in 24 hours, i.e. during the night too.
- Continue to give preventer.
- If increased puffs of reliever are not lasting 4 hours then the child will need to see the GP **AS SOON AS POSSIBLE**.

If your child's breathing becomes worse and the reliever inhaler is not working or they are blue and gasping, they must see a doctor immediately or you must call for an ambulance.

Asthma action plan (for those measuring peak flow)

<u>Name</u>
<u>Date</u>

Best peak flow when well ......
If peak flow is above ..... and you feel fine, continue usual treatment.

CAUTION
If peak flow falls below ..... and/or you have been coughing/wheezing more than usual:

- give reliever (*blue* inhaler)
- check peak flow again at least 5 minutes after giving inhaler.

If you do not feel any better and peak flow is not improved much, you should:

- give reliever every 4 hours
- continue to give preventer inhaler (**brown/orange/purple**).

Continue to check peak flow twice a day until it remains above ..... or 2 days, then reduce treatment to usual doses.

DANGER
If peak flow falls below .... and you are very distressed by coughing/wheezing/ breathlessness:

- give up to 10 puffs of your reliever slowly through a spacer
- check peak flow again at least 5 minutes after giving reliever
- if you feel better and peak flow is above ..... continue to give up to 10 puffs of your reliever through a spacer every 4 hours
- continue to give preventer inhaler.
- **You must see your GP**.

BUT

- If you do not feel better and peak flow is not improved, give a further 10 puffs of your reliever.
- **See a doctor immediately**.
- Start steroids as instructed by doctor. You are aiming at a peak flow above .....
- If response to treatment is slow or poor, call doctor, come to hospital or casualty, especially if you are gasping or looking blue.

Asthma action plan for school

Name
Date

When well: not really coughing, wheezing or breathless. Give usual doses of inhalers; for example, if coughing/wheezing and a little breathless but not distressed, give usual dose of reliever (blue inhaler). The child should not need their reliever every 4 hours at this point.

Not so well: coughing/wheezing and breathless or has a cold, which usually triggers the asthma. The child is distressed by the symptoms of cough/breathlessness/wheeze.

- Give usual dose of reliever (blue inhaler), but every 4 hours.
- Inform parents/carers of need for inhalers.

Not very well: very distressed by coughing, wheezing and breathlessness. Usual doses of reliever are not lasting 4 hours.

- Give at least 5 (maximum 10) puffs of reliever slowly through spacer.
- Contact NHS Direct or parents for advice.
- The child must see their GP.
- If increased puffs of reliever are not lasting 4 hours, the child's breathing becomes worse and the reliever inhaler is not working, or they are blue and gasping, dial 999 and ask for an ambulance. You may be asked to repeat the increased puffs of reliever through a spacer.

Audit

Audit is a tool used to compare current practice to existing models of best practice, in order to identify areas for change and development (NICE 2002a). The BTS *Guideline on the Management of Asthma* (2011) offers a summary of recommended audits for the care of people with asthma. One such audit is recording the percentage of patients with satisfactory inhaler technique and their use of a spacer device. The completion of a form used by both the nurses and doctors in the clinic for patients with asthma as a follow-up appointment allows for an easier audit process.

On each visit the child and parent are asked which inhalers (usually by the colour, then name) they are currently using and which device. Inhaler technique is then checked and this information is all recorded. The information can then be assessed against national recommendations, such as the BTS *Guideline on the Management of Asthma* (2011) and NICE guidance (2000, 2002b) on the use of inhaler devices with children.

Care in the community

The majority of children with asthma are managed in the community. Therefore it is also important to provide training for professionals from both primary and secondary care settings. The respiratory nurse must also have systems in place to work closely with community colleagues such as GPs, practice nurses and school nurses. Equally, the same principles apply to many children with asthma and allergy, where the ethos now is to educate community children's nurses.

The National Service Framework for Children, Young People and Maternity Services (Department of Health 2004) highlights the need for health services to be created around the needs of the child through high-quality, child-centred services and pathways. This concept has become a reality in the joint working of the hospital-based children's respiratory nurse, school nurses and children's community nurses within the East Midlands. The process has enabled identified asthma link school nurses to complete a recognised asthma course, thus providing a first-line resource for their colleagues in school nursing teams. This service has also enabled these nurses to work alongside the hospital-based respiratory team in the clinic on a regular basis (Forster and Winser 2007).

The respiratory nurse is pivotal to the success of managing children with allergy. Therefore it is also good practice to create a partnership, in order to work with parents effectively with treatment and management. Following skinprick testing, the respiratory nurse will provide education for parents on future management such as the use of an Epipen and food avoidance. This ongoing management can also include other professionals who support the family in the community, such as health visitors or school nurses.

Conclusion

Multidisciplinary working is paramount in the management of children with asthma. This requires regular training, contact and communication with colleagues across all boundaries. Projects that involve working in partnership with colleagues across boundaries, also promotes the aim of delivering a high quality seamless service for the benefit of children with asthma.

Questions

Answer true or false.

1. Asthma is an inflammatory disease involving various cells such as mast cells, eosinophils and T-lymphocytes.
2. Fraction of exhaled nitric oxide is not a measure of eosinophilic inflammation.
3. Patients with severe persistent allergic asthma and IgE levels of less than 1300 KU/L (age 6–12) are treated with omalizumab subcutaneous injection.
4. Excessive use of β-agonists increases the risk of a severe asthma attack.
5. There is no benefit from IV salbutamol during an acute attack of asthma, when there is little response to nebulised salbutamol.
6. The criteria for intubation following a severe attack of asthma include hypoxia, hypercarbia and altered levels of consciousness.
7. BTS guidelines state that inhalers can be prescribed before any training is given to patients.
8. According to NICE guidance, teaching correct inhaler technique improves lung deposition.
9. The lower the ACT scores, the better the control.
10. A written, personalised asthma action plan for those with moderate to severe disease leads to good outcomes.

References

Asthma UK. (2009) *All About Asthma*. Available at: www.asthma.org.uk.

British Thoracic Society (BTS). (2009) *Guideline on the Management of Asthma: a national clinical guideline*. London: British Thoracic Society.

British Thoracic Society (BTS). (2011) *Guideline on the Management of Asthma: a national clinical guideline (revised)*. London: British Thoracic Society.

Brocklebank D, Ram F, Barry P, *et al.* (2001) Comparison of the effectiveness of inhaler devices in asthma and chronic obstructive airways disease: a systematic review of the literature. *Health Technology Assessment* **5(26)**, 1–149.

Broide J, Soferman R, Kivity S, *et al.* (1995) Low-dose adrenocorticotropin test reveals impaired adrenal function in patients taking inhaled corticosteroids. *Journal of Clinical Endocrinology and Metabolism* **80**, 1243–46.

Cane RS, McKenzie S. (2001) Parents' interpretations of children's respiratory symptoms on video. *Archives of Disease in Childhood* **1(84)**, 31–4.

Chandler T. (2001) Reducing re-admission for asthma: impact of a nurse-led service. *Paediatric Nursing* **19(10)**, 19–21.

Department of Health. (2004) *National Framework for Children, Young People and Maternity Services.* London: Department of Health.

Education for Health. (2006) *Simply Devices: a practical pocket book.* Leamington Spa: Salvo.

Elphick H, Sherlock P, Foxall G, *et al.* (2001) Survey of respiratory sounds in infants. *Archives of Disease in Childhood* **1(84)**, 35–9.

Fitzgerald D, van Asperen P, Mellis C, Honner M, Smith L, Ambler G. (1998) Fluticasone propionate 750 micrograms/day versus beclomethasone dipropionate 1500 micrograms/day: comparison of efficacy and adrenal function in paediatric asthma. *Thorax* **53(8)**, 656–61.

Forster D. (2010) Wheeziness at home for under fives: in association with Nottingham Community Health. Unpublished.

Forster D, Winser C. (2007) The role of asthma link nurses for schools. *Nursing Times* **103(45)**, 52–3.

Global Initiative for Asthma (GINA). (2008) *Global Strategy for Asthma Management and Prevention.* Global Initiative for Asthma. Available at: www.ginasthma.org.

Godfrey S. (2000) Bronchial hyper-responsiveness in children. *Paediatric Respiratory Review* **1(2)**, 148–55.

Gøtzsche PC, Johansen HK, Schmidt LM, Burr ML. (2004) House dust mite control measures for asthma. *Cochrane Database of Systematic Reviews* **4**, CD001187.

Halterman JS, Yoos H, Kitzman H, *et al.* (2006) Symptom reporting in childhood asthma: a comparison of assessment methods. *Archives of Disease in Childhood* **91(9)**, 766–70.

International Study of Asthma and Allergies in Childhood (ISAAC) Steering Committee (1998) Worldwide variations in the prevalence of asthma symptoms: the International Study of Asthma and Allergies in Childhood (ISAAC). *European Respiratory Journal* **12**, 315–35.

Kamps AW, Brand P, Roorda R. (2002) Determinants of correct inhalation technique in children attending a hospital-based asthma clinic. *Acta Paediatrica* **91(2)**, 159–63.

Kannisto S, Korppi M, Remes M, Voutilainen R. (2000) Adrenal suppression, evaluated by a low dose adrenocorticotropin test, and growth in asthmatic children treated with inhaled steroids. *Journal of Clinical Endocrinology and Metabolism* **85**, 652–7.

Kulis M, Herbert J, Garcia E, Fowler-Taylor A, Fernandez C, Blogg M. (2010) Omalizumab in children with inadequately controlled severe allergic (IGE-mediated) asthma. *Current Medical Research and Opinion* **26(6)**, 1285–93.

Liem JJ, Kozyrskyj AL, Donald W, Cockcroft D, Allan B, Becker MD. (2008) Diagnosing asthma in children: what is the role of methacholine bronchoprovocation testing? *Pediatric Pulmonology* **43(5)**, 481–9.

McKean M, Furness J. (2009) Paediatric respiratory nursing posts in secondary care reduce asthma morbidity, but provision is variable. *Archives of Disease in Childhood* **94(8)**, 644.

McPherson A Glazebrook C, Forster D, Smyth A. (2002) The Asthma Files: evaluation of a multimedia package for children's asthma education. *Paediatric Nursing* **14(2)**, 32–5.

National Institute For Clinical Excellence. (2000) *Guidance on the Use of Inhaler Systems (Devices) in Children under the Age of 5 Years with Chronic Asthma.* Technology Appraisal Guidance No. 10. London: National Institute For Clinical Excellence.

National Institute For Clinical Excellence. (2002a) *Principles for Best Practice in Clinical Audit.* Abingdon: Radcliffe Medical Press.

National Institute for Clinical Excellence. (2002b) *Inhaler Devices for Routine Treatment of Chronic Asthma in Older Children (Aged 5–15 Years).* Technology Appraisal Guidance No. 38. NICE London.

Office for Health Economics. (2004) *Compendium of Health Statistics*, 15th edn. London: Office for Health Economics.

Orrell-Valente JK, Jarlsberg LG, Hill LG, Cabana MD. (2008) At what age do children start taking daily medicines on their own? *Pediatrics* **122(6)**, 1186–92.

Patel L, Wales JK, Kibirige MS, Massarano AA, Couriel JM, Clayton PE. (2001) Symptomatic adrenal insufficiency during inhaled corticosteroid treatment. *Archives of Disease in Childhood* **85(4)**, 330–4.

Pearce N, Welland S, Keil U, *et al.* (1993) Self reported prevalence of asthma symptoms in children in Australia, England, Germany and New Zealand: an international comparison using the ISAAC protocol. *European Respiratory Journal* **6**, 1455–61.

Pearce N, Ait Khaled N, Beasley R, *et al.* (2007) Worldwide trends in the prevalence of asthma symptoms: phase III of the International Study of Asthma and Allergies in Childhood (ISAAC). *Thorac* **62(9)**, 758–66.

Ranganathan SC, Payne D, Jaffe A, McKenzie S. (2001) Difficult asthma: defining the problems. *Pediatric Pulmonology* **31(2)**, 114–20.

Rowen J. (2002) *Nursing Care of Children: principles and practice*, 2nd edn. Philadelphia: Elsevier.

Schatz M, Sorkness C, Pharm D, *et al.* (2006) Asthma Control Test: reliability, validity, and responsiveness in patients not previously followed by asthma specialists. *Journal of Allergy and Clinical Immunology* **117(3)**, 549–56.

Sunderland RS, Fleming DM. (2004) Continuing decline in acute asthma episodes in the community. *Archives of Disease in Childhood* **89**, 282–5.

Todd GR, Acerini CL, Ross-Russell R, Zahra S, Warner JT, McCance D. (2002) Survey of adrenal crisis associated with inhaled corticosteroids in the United Kingdom. *Archives of Disease in Childhood* **87(6)**, 457–61.

Wesseldine L, McCarthy P, Silverman M. (1999) Structured discharge procedure for children admitted to hospital with acute asthma: a randomised trial of nursing practice. *Archives of Disease in Childhood* **80**, 110–14.

Wooler E. (2001) The role of the nurse in paediatric asthma management. *Paediatric Respiratory Reviews* **2(1)**, 76–81.

Useful websites

Asthma in children – corticosteroid guidance, available at: http://guidance.nice.org.uk/TA131.

Asthma in adults – understanding NICE guidance, available www.asthma.org.uk.

Chapter 11

Complications with lung development and progressive airway injury

Jayesh Bhatt,[1] Chhavi Goel[2] and Sarah Spencer[3]

[1] *Consultant Respiratory Paediatrician*
[2] *Consultant Paediatrician*
[3] *Specialist Practitioner in Children's Community Nursing, Nottingham Children's Hospital*

Learning objectives

After studying this chapter the reader will have an understanding of:

- complications with lung development
- common congenital anomalies of lungs
- the causes of bronchial wall destruction
- the significance of nursing support.

Chronic lung disease of prematurity

Chronic lung disease of prematurity (CLD) (synonyms: chronic neonatal lung disease (CNLD), chronic lung disease of infancy (CLDI), bronchopulmonary dysplasia (BPD)) was first described by Northway and colleagues more than 40 years ago and included clinical and radiological features in preterm infants who had severe respiratory distress syndrome (RDS), who had been treated with high inspired oxygen (O_2) concentrations and prolonged mechanical ventilation with high positive airway pressures, resulting in inflammation, fibrosis and smooth muscle hypertrophy in the airways ('classic or old BPD') (Northway et al. 1967). Neonatal intensive care has advanced beyond recognition since this early description but despite advances in the prevention and management of RDS such as the use of antenatal steroids, surfactant treatment, better nutritional interventions, careful monitoring of oxygen therapy, better ventilators and ventilation strategies, CLD is still one of the major complications in mechanically ventilated neonates.

Any disorder that produces an acute lung injury and/or requires treatment with positive pressure mechanical ventilation and high concentrations of inspired oxygen during the initial weeks of life predisposes the infant to the development of CLD.

With the survival of extremely premature infants (23–24 weeks' gestation), a different type of CLD has emerged. This type of CLD ('new BPD') represents a disorder of intrauterine inflammation and premature extrauterine lung development characterised by alveolar simplification, in contrast

---

Children's Respiratory Nursing, First Edition. Edited by Janice Mighten.
© 2013 Blackwell Publishing Ltd. Published 2013 by Blackwell Publishing Ltd.

to the early descriptions of BPD, in which postnatal inflammation and fibrosis due to barotrauma and oxygen toxicity played more of a role (American Thoracic Society 2003).

Definition

Bancalari et al. (1979) maintain that there are three basic criteria required to define BPD:

- supplemental oxygen requirement at 28 days of postnatal life
- persistent abnormalities of the chest radiograph
- tachypnoea in the presence of crackles, which are the crackling noises heard on auscultation during inhalation.

However, some researchers feel that as 'new BPD' occurs in very low-birthweight infants with gestational ages of 30 weeks or less, the cut-off for supplemental oxygen should be 36 weeks postconceptional rather than beyond 28 days of age in 'old or classic BPD' (Shennan et al. 1988).

The BTS guidelines (2009) define CNLD as an infant requiring supplemental oxygen at a corrected age of 36 weeks' gestation who is at least 28 days old.

It is difficult to estimate the true prevalence of BPD due to changing definitions but it is felt that as neonatal care has changed and more premature babies are surviving, the prevalence seems to have gone up but it is less severe now. CLD (oxygen requirement at 36 weeks after conception) developed in 19% of the very low-birthweight babies born during the period of 1993–1994 in an American study (Stevenson et al. 1998). In a more recent prospective follow-up study of extreme premature babies born at ≤25 weeks' gestation in 1995 in the UK, 74% of this population received supplementary oxygen at 36 weeks' postmenstrual age and 36% were discharged with supplementary oxygen, i.e. more than one-third of the babies born at ≤25 weeks' gestation have CLD (Hennessy et al. 2008).

Pathophysiology

The cause of BPD is multifactorial. The immature lung is most vulnerable to disruption of alveolar development in the stage before alveolar formation begins (23–26 weeks' gestation). Factors that increase inflammation in the lung – such as oxygen toxicity, mechanical ventilation-induced trauma from volume and pressure changes, and infection – are associated with the development of BPD. Exposure to inflammation of fetal membranes, such as chorion caused by bacterial infection, known as chorioamnionitis, with resultant foetal inflammatory syndrome and high levels of circulating proinflammatory cytokines, also places preterm infants at increased risk of BPD.

Foetal inflammatory syndrome, including high levels of circulating proinflammatory cytokines, which are inflammatory mediators, also places preterm infants at increased risk of BPD. Inflammation has an important role in the pathogenesis of BPD and the pharmacological modulation of the inflammatory response may be protective (Eichenwald and Stark 2007). The 'new BPD' is believed to represent less the effects of severe lung injury and its repair and more a disruption or arrest of lung development. Changes in the pulmonary vasculature structure ('dysmorphic circulation') are increasingly being recognised as contributory to the pathogenesis of CLD (Jobe and Bancalari 2001). A pulmonary score to define the severity of CLD has also been developed, which is useful to guide practice (Coalson 2000).

Treatment

Nutrition

Infants with CLD have higher energy needs compared to healthy age-matched infants. Some may have feeding difficulties secondary to oral aversion related to the lengthy neonatal intensive care unit (NICU) interventions and are more likely to have gastro-oesophageal reflux. This may also lead to difficulties with sucking and swallowing co-ordination due to evolving neurodevelopmental problems. It is important to optimise nutrition in these infants but this can be very challenging due to the above reasons. Feeding with calorie-dense formulae does result in 'catch-up' weight gain but height velocity often remains subnormal even up to school age (Madan et al. 2005).

Bronchodilators

The response in babies with CLD is variable and in symptomatic babies with definite wheeze, a trial of salbutamol or ipratropium via spacer may be given. If there is definite clinical improvement, these agents can be used on an as-required basis at times when the babies are symptomatic. An appropriate drug delivery device and facemask should be chosen.

Corticosteroids

Postnatal oral corticosteroids have been widely used in evolving or established CLD but their use still remains controversial. Early, moderately early and delayed use (Giacoia et al. 1997; Halliday et al. 2003a–c) are associated with significant side-effects including hyperglycaemia, hypertension, gastrointestinal bleeding, intestinal perforation, decreased growth, adrenal suppression, cardiomyopathy and interventricular septal hypertrophy and nosocomial infection. Delayed side-effects include abnormal neurological examinations, cerebral palsy and developmental delay. There are also concerns regarding decreased alveolar number (American Thoracic Society 2003).

In infants with severe BPD who are ventilator dependent, use of corticosteroids might improve survival without increasing adverse neurological outcome (Halliday et al. 2003a). More research is required to establish the optimal steroid as well as dosing regimen.

Inhaled corticosteroids (ICS) can facilitate extubation in ventilator-dependent infants when used over 1–4 weeks but the onset of action is slower compared to systemic steroids and no firm conclusions can be drawn about efficacy in non-ventilated infants (Doyle et al. 2005). Regular ICS reduce symptoms, improve lung function and lessen the need for bronchodilator therapy in those infants with CLD who are symptomatic at follow-up (Lister et al. 2000).

Oxygen therapy

This is covered in more detail in Chapter 6 but some of the aspects of oxygen therapy specific to babies with CLD are discussed in this section.

The duration of supplemental oxygen therapy is generally less than 6 months as shown in the studies listed in Table 11.1. In a child who is not weaning as expected from supplemental oxygen therapy, it is necessary to consider whether the child is not getting the oxygen because the supply has run out or if there is a problem with non-adherence. Other issues include unnoticed dislodgement of cannula and blocked tube or valve, all of which can be assessed by the nurse during home visits. This will be covered below.

Consequently, in CLD, failure to reduce oxygen supplementation after 1 year warrants specialist review to rule out other conditions such as:

- another or an additional medical diagnosis (unsuspected congenital cardiac defects, upper airway obstruction from enlarged tonsils and adenoids or subglottic cyst, and chronic aspiration with gastro-oesophageal reflux)
- condition increasing in severity, frequently after a respiratory illness
- pulmonary hypertension.

Table 11.1 Infants discharged home on supplemental oxygen

No. of babies	Gestation	Duration	Reference
18	Mean gestation 28 weeks	Mean 7.9 months	Yuksel and Greenough 1992
30	2 weeks to 17 months	Mean 4.5 months	Abman et al. 1984
35	26 weeks	Mean 14.1 weeks (0.5–36 weeks)	Hudak et al. 1989
21	24–37 weeks	Mean 97 days (15–320 days)	Campbell et al. 1983
146	<25 weeks	Median 2.5 months (75th percentile: 8.5 months)	Hennessy et al. 2008

Very occasionally, long-term ventilation (LTV) at home may be required in infants with severe CLD who have never been able to be weaned from the ventilator in the NICU, or in those who have been weaned from the ventilator but have suffered a setback severe enough to warrant reinstitution of mechanical ventilation (American Thoracic Society 2003).

Diuretics

Despite the widespread use of different diuretics, little is known about the effects of long-term diuretic therapy in infants with developing or established CLDI with regard to survival, duration of ventilator support or oxygen administration, potential complications and long-term outcome (American Thoracic Society 2003).

Discharge planning

The importance of discharge planning cannot be overestimated. This involves prior preparation of the home environment, competent parents, equipment and the appropriate professional support. This will be discussed in more detail below.

Immunisation

Passive immunisation with humanised monoclonal antibody (palivizumab) against the respiratory syncytial virus should be offered according to the Joint Committee on Vaccination and Immunization criteria. The JCVI considers palivizumab cost-effective when used as recommended for preterm infants with CLD (defined as oxygen dependency for at least 28 days from birth) at the chronological ages at the start of the RSV season and gestational ages at birth covered within the shaded area in Table 11.2.

Consider palivizumab for the prevention of RSV in the following categories:

- children with chronic lung disease (in other words, oxygen dependency for at least 28 days from birth) who have specific risk factors
- infants who have haemodynamically significant, acyanotic congenital heart disease and are less than 6 months old
- children who have severe combined immunodeficiency syndrome until they are immune reconstituted.

Other immunisations include influenza vaccine for the child after 6 months of age and for the close family contacts.

Table 11.2   Cost-effective use of palivizumab (shaded area) for preterm infants with CLD by chronological age (months) at the start of the RSV season (beginning of October) and gestational age at birth (weeks) (reproduced from Department of Health 2010)

Chronological age (months)	Gestational age at birth (weeks)						
	≤24	24–26	26–28	28–30	30–32	32–34	≥35
1.0 to <1.5	▓	▓	▓	▓	▓	▓	
1.5–3	▓	▓	▓	▓	▓		
3–6	▓	▓	▓				
6–9	▓						
>9							

Other issues

Parents and carers should be counselled about environmental tobacco smoke exposure, avoidance of viral exposures as far as possible and the importance of hand washing to prevent spread of infections.

Parents should also be counselled that infants with CLD are likely to require significant escalation of care including oxygen requirement and paediatric intensive care unit (PICU) care may be required in some infants, especially in the winter season.

Long-term complications can include lung transplantation. This may be indicated, although very rarely, in a small number of infants with very severe CLD when all other treatment has failed.

Modern medicine has assisted in the process of better clinical outcome and prognosis for infants with CLD. With companies providing home oxygen and children's community nursing support as discussed in Chapter 3, children with this congenital abnormality of the lungs can be cared for in their homes successfully with the ultimate aim of weaning from oxygen therapy.

Interstitial lung disease

The pulmonary interstitium is the tissue in between the air sacs (alveoli) and the capillaries. Gas exchange occurs by diffusion across the epithelium of the capillaries across the interstitial space, and across the alveolar epithelium.

Definition

Interstitial lung disease(s) (ILD) are a heterogeneous group of rare disorders of known and unknown aetiology, characterised by derangement of alveolar walls with resultant impairment of gas exchange and diffuse infiltrates on imaging (Fan et al. 2004). The clinical presentation includes chronic tachypnoea, hypoxia, cough and/or crackles.

Sometimes the acronym chILD (childhood interstitial lung disease) is used to describe a group of disorders which have similar presentation though the severity of these diseases and long-term outcomes may be very different. ILD and diffuse paediatric lung disease have also been used synonymously but subsequent lung biopsy often reveals that the pathogenesis of many of these disorders is outside the interstitial compartment in the lungs, often with airway and airspace involvement (Deutsch et al. 2007).

The prevalence rate of idiopathic ILD in UK and Ireland for children aged 0–16 years is estimated to be 3.6 cases/million (Dinwiddie et al. 2002). Conditions included under the umbrella term of

Table 11.3   Severity of illness score (adapted from Fan et al. 2004)

Score	Symptoms	Saturation <90% exercise/sleep	Saturation <90% rest	Pulmonary hypertension
1	No	No	No	No
2	Yes	No	No	No
3	Yes	Yes	No	No
4	Yes	Yes	Yes	No
5	Yes	Yes	Yes	Yes

chronic ILD, as identified by Clement (2004) include pulmonary alveolar proteinosis which is a rare condition with abnormal accumulation of surfactant occurring within the alveoli, affecting gas exchange; hypersensitivity pneumonitis arises as a result of inflammation of the alveoli caused by hypersensitivity to inhaled dusts. Another is Langerhans cell histiocytosis, a rare disease involving growth of abnormal Langerhans cells, deriving from bone marrow, which can affect organs in the body such as the lungs. Finally, sarcoidosis is a disease where the cause is unknown and results in inflammation, affecting various organs in the body.

These conditions are much rarer compared to ILD in adults and at least in children under 2 years of age, the classification system used in adults cannot be applied as the aetiology in some cases, rate of progression and treatment approaches are different and some conditions are unique to early childhood, for example neuroendocrine cell hyperplasia and pulmonary interstitial glycogenosis (Deutsch et al. 2007).

Clinical presentation

Fan et al. (2004) and Clement (2004) state that the onset is often insidious and symptoms may have been present for months to years before the diagnosis of ILD is confirmed. The presentation could be of asymptomatic with radiological features suggestive of ILD. In others, symptoms at presentation include cough which is often dry and tickly, dyspnoea, tachypnoea and chest recession, exercise limitation, tiring during feeding, frequent respiratory infections, haemoptysis and failure to thrive. Parent/carer-reported wheeze is confirmed in some patients on examination but more often inspiratory crackles, tachypnoea and retraction are present.

It is recommended that any child with a normal birth history presenting with the signs and symptoms suggestive of ILD lasting for >3 months should be evaluated for ILD (Table 11.3). Clinical history should include details of relatives or siblings with similar lung conditions, possible precipitating factors, such as feeding history, any acute or severe respiratory infections, environmental exposure to organic and inorganic dust, and use of drugs with pulmonary toxicity.

Diagnosis

Investigations to identify primary disorders that predispose to ILD include:

- immune studies: HIV, immunoglobulins including IgE, skin tests for delayed hypersensitivity, response to immunisations, T- and B-cells
- others as indicated: barium swallow, pH probe
- infectious disease evaluation (cultures, titres, skin tests)
- genetic studies for surfactant dysfunction, serum and urine amino acids.

Pulmonary function tests

The picture may be one of mixed restrictive/obstructive disease. Most patients with mild disease have normal oxygen saturation levels. As the disease progresses or from the outset in severe cases, the patients may desaturate with exercise or during sleep due to ventilation/perfusion mismatch as discussed in Chapter 6. Patients with more advanced disease will be hypoxaemic at rest. Some patients develop pulmonary hypertension and this carries a poor prognosis. Electrocardiogram and echocardiogram will be required to assess development of pulmonary hypertension.

High-resolution computed tomography

This provides information about the extent and distribution of disease and is also helpful in determining the site of lung biopsy. High-resolution computed tomography (HRCT) may demonstrate geographic hyperlucency, where one lung is less dense than the other normal lung, cysts and nodules, and consolidation (Lynch et al. 1999). In infants, sedation is required and the child is hyperventilated by applying positive pressure through a facemask to produce a brief respiratory pause. This will result in motionless HRCT images obtained at either full inflation or resting end-expiration (Long et al. 1999).

Bronchoscopy and bronchoalveolar lavage

These are discussed in more detail in Chapter 4. Bronchoscopy will help to establish opportunistic infection (immunocompromised host) and other abnormalities such as alveolar haemorrhage of any cause including idiopathic pulmonary haemosiderosis (IPH), alveolar proteinosis and surfactant protein deficiency in children.

Lung biopsy

This is performed as either an open or thoracoscopic procedure to provide a tissue diagnosis.

Treatment

Fan et al. (2004) suggest that treatment should be based around the following factors.

Oxygen

To treat hypoxaemia.

Nutrition

Should be optimised as poor growth (weight) is an adverse prognostic factor.

Corticosteroids

Certain aspects of chILD will respond very well to corticosteroids, including hypersensitivity pneumonitis. Other conditions thought to be steroid responsive include chILD associated with connective tissue disease. Steroids are preferably given as intravenous pulse therapy rather than oral daily or alternate-day therapy because it is associated with fewer side-effects. The recommended dose of methylprednisolone is 30 mg/kg with a maximum of 1 g, given intravenously over 1 h, daily, for 3 consecutive days and repeated monthly.

Steroid-sparing agents

These include hydroxychloroquine, azathioprine, cyclophosphamide, methotrexate, ciclosporin, and intravenous gammaglobulin, and will be required in some children with ongoing active disease despite steroid therapy or if they develop unacceptable side-effects with corticosteroids.

Lung transplantation

More children are receiving lung transplantation for end-stage chILD and the survival rates are at least as good for chILD as they are for cystic fibrosis and pulmonary hypertension (for further details see Chapter 13).

Outcome

The prognosis for children with ILD is variable (Fan et al. 2004). Some of these conditions have a better prognosis, such as pulmonary interstitial glycogenosis; these children generally do well, although they may remain symptomatic and require oxygen for years. At the other end of the spectrum, neonates and infants do poorly, as well as older children with ILD and growth failure, pulmonary hypertension and severe fibrosis.

Children with ILD have a better outlook with the advancement of technology, including drug therapy. Although many do require oxygen therapy for a considerable time, support and management to facilitate quality of life from a multidisciplinary perspective are paramount.

Bronchiectasis

Bronchiectasis is defined as dilation of the airways accompanied by inflammatory destruction of the bronchial and peribronchial tissue. Developed countries have seen a decline in infection-related bronchiectasis with the use of antibiotics and implementation of vaccination programmes. However, it still causes significant morbidity in the paediatric population. Children present with chronic productive cough and recurrent chest infections.

Rene Laennac, inventor of the stethoscope, first described bronchiectasis in the early 19th century in patients with tuberculosis and the sequelae of pneumonia in the preantibiotic era. The term bronchiectasis is derived from Greek word *bronchion*, meaning windpipe, and *ektasis*, meaning stretched.

Bronchiectasis is frequently divided into cystic fibrosis (CF) and non-cystic fibrosis types. This section mainly focuses on non-CF bronchiectasis.

Pathogenesis

The pathogenesis is thought to be bronchial obstruction with retention of secretions and infection, ultimately causing bronchial wall destruction. In bronchiectasis there is impairment of the mucociliary function, leading to increased accumulation of secretions which become more viscous, exposing the patient to bacterial infections. Recurrent bacterial colonisation leads to progressive airway injury. There is infiltration with inflammatory mediators, which are molecules that act at the site of infection, for example neutrophils, T-lymphocytes, interleukins, elastase and collagenase, which leads to destruction of elastic and muscular components of the bronchial wall (Sepper et al. 1995). The part of the bronchi affected may become cylindrical, tubular or saccular. Bronchiectasis can present as either focal or diffuse disease involving both lungs. The diameter of the bronchi becomes bigger than the adjacent pulmonary artery which is a characteristic sign seen on HRCT scan.

Box 11.1   Causes of bronchiectasis

Infections

Bacterial: *Streptococcus pneumoniae*, staphylococcus, *Bordetella pertussis*, pseudomonas
Viral: adenovirus, influenza, respiratory syncytial virus
Mycobacterium: tuberculosis
Fungal: aspergillosis

Immunodeficiency

Immune deficiency syndromes
Post chemotherapy
Post HIV infection
Post lung transplantation

Hereditary disorders

Cystic fibrosis
Primary ciliary dyskinesia
Kartagener's syndrome (bronchiectasis, sinusitis, situs inversus)

Bronchial obstruction

Foreign body
Lymph node
Mucus plug
Tumour

Inhalational injuries/aspiration

Gastro-oesophageal reflux
Noxious gases

Syndromes

Yellow nail syndrome: abnormal nails, lymphoedema, pleural effusion
Young's syndrome: azoospermia, sinobronchial infection

Aetiology

The incidence has reduced worldwide with the implementation of immunisation programmes which has lead to a reduced incidence of diseases like whooping cough and measles. In developed countries CF-related bronchiectasis is still a major problem. The causes can be congenital or acquired. Infection is the most common cause for non-CF disease.

Other causes are immune system abnormalities, obstruction of a bronchus due to inhalation of foreign body and inherited disorders like primary ciliary dyskinesia. Multiple lobe involvement can be seen after viral infections, immune deficiency or primary ciliary dyskinesia. Focal bronchiectasis is seen in foreign body inhalation, tumour or extrinsic compression by a lymph node. Bilateral lower lobe involvement suggests aspiration. Box 11.1 summarises the common causes of bronchiectasis.

Clinical presentation

Children frequently present with chronic productive cough and recurrent chest infections. Other common symptoms are shortness of breath, recurrent wheezing, haemoptysis and pleuritic chest pain. There may be a history suggestive of foreign body inhalation with sudden onset of dyspnoea and cough or a choking episode. Children with primary ciliary dyskinesia and immunodeficiency may present with recurrent and persistent symptoms of rhinitis, sinusitis and otitis media. Younger children may just present with a wet-sounding cough and older children may produce copious amounts of sputum. In acute exacerbations children present with worsening cough, increased sputum production with colour change, shortness of breath and pleuritic chest pain. This may be accompanied with new changes on the chest x-ray. On examination, they may be growth retarded, may have angular nail beds as a result of infections known as finger clubbing, and crepitations can be heard on chest auscultation.

Investigations

Imaging

Chest x-ray (CXR) and HRCT are the most useful methods for diagnosis of bronchiectasis. However, HRCT is considered the gold standard investigation for the diagnosis of bronchiectasis. CXR may show abnormalities like bronchial wall thickening or atelectasis. Eastham et al. (2004) stated that sometimes CXR can be normal and hence CXR is of less diagnostic value in children with bronchiectasis. HRCT has a sensitivity of 97%. A feature of bronchiectasis on HRCT is bronchial wall thickening and internal diameter of bronchus being larger than the adjacent artery (signet ring sign).

Bronchoscopy

This is not always required. It should be carried out when HRCT suggests airway abnormality or in case of focal bronchiectasis to aid the diagnosis.

Microbiology

Close attention to airway infection is vital to prevent any further damage. Treatment is guided by the sputum cultures and past infectious organisms. Samples can be obtained by sputum or a cough swab; bronchoalveolar lavage is rarely needed. This will be explored further below.

Spirometry

Spirometry and pulmonary function testing are discussed in Chapter 5. Children with mild bronchiectasis may have normal lung function. With progressive lung disease, they may develop obstructive lung disease.

Other investigations to consider include:

- full blood count (FBC) with differential count
- sweat test
- immunoglobulin levels
- functional antibodies to vaccinations and response to booster dose if initial response is poor
- ciliary biopsy
- contrast swallow and pH study
- Mantoux test
- HIV text.

Treatment

The aim of treatment is to reduce morbidity by controlling symptoms and preventing the progression of bronchiectasis. Management of these children involves multidisciplinary team work as discussed in Chapter 3, including, paediatricians, physiotherapists, respiratory nurses, community nurses, dietician, psychologists and social worker.

There is now some evidence that bronchiectasis does not involve permanent dilation of the bronchi. Eastham et al. (2004) reviewed 93 children with non-CF bronchiectasis clinically and radiologically. Repeat scans in 18 children showed that in six, there was complete resolution of symptoms after 18 months of treatment. The authors then introduced the concept of stages of bronchiectasis. First stage is prebronchiectasis, which can resolve with treatment; in second stage changes persist or progress, followed by established bronchiectasis.

Antibiotics are the mainstay of treatment. The choice of antibiotic is guided by the microbiology. For mild exacerbations, oral antibiotics are generally given for 2 weeks. Children with more severe lung disease may need hospitalisation and intravenous antibiotics. Antibiotics can be given at home by the respiratory community nurse or parents can be educated to do so (Mighten 2007). Children should also be evaluated for airway hyper-responsiveness or asthma. With inflammatory mucosal changes, an inhaled corticosteroid may be of benefit. Kapur et al. (2009) used the Cochrane database to evaluate the use of inhaled steroids in adults. No significant effects were found but there was an improvement in forced expiratory volume in 1 second (FEV1), forced vital capacity (FVC), quality of life and amount of sputum production. Bronchodilators may be helpful where wheeze is a clinical feature. Anwar et al. (2008) have shown in adults that use of long-term low-dose azithromycin in non-CF bronchiectasis improves the exacerbation frequency, spirometry and sputum microbiology. Mucolytic agents like DNase have no significant role in treatment of non-CF bronchiectasis (Crockett et al. 2001).

In cases of humoral antibody deficiency, intravenous or subcutaneous immunoglobulin should be given. Other measures are chest physiotherapy (Banjar 2006) and surgical procedures. Chest physiotherapy can be done in various ways, depending on the age of the child and preference. Surgery is considered in cases of advanced disease not responding to medical treatment, focal disease or life-threatening haemoptysis. Potential side-effects of surgery include empyema, haemorrhage and poor expansion of the remaining lung.

General measures in managing bronchiectasis include avoidance of smoking, adequate nutrition, immunisations and yearly influenza vaccinations. Children and their families do need psychological and social support as they must make frequent visits to hospital, can often miss school and hence their quality of life is affected.

Outcome

The outcome depends on the underlying aetiology. In most cases treatment should halt the progression of disease but lung damage persists into adult life. It can cause significant morbidity because of obstructive airway disease and recurrent exacerbations. With the evolving evidence, rapid evaluation, diagnosis and treatment are essential in children with recurrent chest infections to prevent any further damage.

Children with bronchiectasis should be seen regularly in outpatient clinics with monitoring of their nutrition, growth and lung functions. There is now an emerging role of nurse-led bronchiectasis clinics in adults, as no difference in the outcome has been seen in nurse-led and doctor-led clinics, although there may be increased cost implications in nurse-led clinics (French et al. 2003).

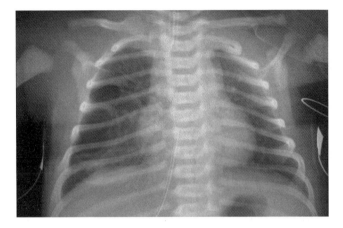

Figure 11.1   Plain chest x-ray of a newborn with CCAM showing three separate cysts in the right lung. Reproduced with permission from Nottingham University Hospitals.

Congenital abnormalities (anomalies)

Congenital anomalies of the lungs are rare but they form an important group of conditions as their presentation may be life threatening and may require urgent surgical intervention. These abnormalities, referred to as malformations, may result from disordered embryological interactions occurring during the course of foetal lung development. They usually present in the newborn period with respiratory distress. Advancements in foetal diagnostic imaging have increased prenatal diagnosis of these anomalies. This section mainly focuses on the common congenital anomalies of the lungs.

- Congenital cystic adenomatoid malformation (CCAM)
- Congenital lobar emphysema (CLE)
- Congenital diaphragmatic hernia (CDH)
- Pulmonary sequestration
- Scimitar syndrome

Congenital cystic adenomatoid malformation

This is the most common cystic congenital anomaly of the lung. The incidence is about 1 in 10,000 to 1 in 35,000 (Duncombe et al. 2002; Laberge et al. 2001; Northway et al. 1967; American Thoracic Society 2003). It usually involves one lobe, with a slight predilection for lower lobes. It affects both lungs equally and is identified equally in both sexes.

Aetiology and pathogenesis

Congenital cystic adenomatoid malformation is the result of abnormal development of terminal bronchioles during the first few weeks of gestation (Figure 11.1). It is characterised by proliferation and cystic dilation of the terminal respiratory bronchioles, which have various types of epithelial lining. Stocker (2002) described three histological types and later two more types were included

(Bancalari et al. 1979; Shennan et al. 1988; Stocker 2002; Stocker et al. 1977). Type 0 CCAM is not compatible with life as it involves all lobes of the lungs. Type 1 CCAM lesions are characterised by single or multiple cysts >2 cm in size, type 2 lesions are <2 cm in size, type 3 lesions are predominantly solid and are <0.5 cm and type 4 are large air-filled cysts. The most common lesion is type 1. CCAM are also classified simply as macrocystic >5 mm and microcystic <5 mm, based on the prenatal imaging (Adzick et al. 1985; Balfour-Lynn et al. 2009). Some CCAMs regress during fetal development but complete resolution is rare. Type 1 CCAM has the best prognosis.

Clinical presentation

The diagnosis is commonly made on the routine antenatal scan at 18–20 weeks of gestation. Large CCAMs may be associated with hydrops foetalis which is a condition in the fetus characterised by polyhydramnios, meaning having too much amniotic fluid in the uterus. The prognostic factors are the size of the lesion and the presence of hydrops foetalis. Ultrasound is the study of choice for follow-up imaging. The most common presentation is with neonatal respiratory distress and later on in life it commonly presents as recurrent pneumonias. Other complications are pneumothorax, haemothorax and haemoptysis. There is a small potential for CCAM to undergo malignant transformation.

Management

Treatment depends on the size of the cystic lesion and the presence of hydrops. If the antenatal scan shows large cystic lesions, delivery should be planned in a specialised tertiary centre. These cases will require urgent radiological evaluation, followed by a surgical excision. If the lesion is small or regressing then delivery should be planned in the referring hospital. In asymptomatic cases postnatal investigations consist of a chest CT scan within a month of birth (Stevenson et al. 1998; Hennessy et al. 2008), followed by elective surgical excision of the lesion between 2–4 months. In view of the potential complications, malignant transformation and the low morbidity and mortality rate of a lung lobectomy, resection of all CCAMs is recommended.

Congenital lobar emphysema

Congenital lobar emphysema is a developmental anomaly of lung characterised by hyperinflation of one or more of the pulmonary lobes. Other terms for CLE include infantile lobar emphysema and congenital lobar overinflation.

Aetiology and pathogenesis

The defect arises from disruption in the bronchopulmonary development. There is abnormal interaction between the embryonic endodermal and mesodermal components of the lung tissue, which may lead to changes in the number and size of airways and alveoli. However, a definitive causative agent cannot be identified in 50% of cases. The most frequent cause is obstruction of airways during lung development, which can be intrinsic or extrinsic. This leads to the creation of a ball-valve mechanism in which a greater volume of air enters the affected lobe during inspiration than leaves during expiration, producing air trapping. Intrinsic obstruction can be due to defects in the bronchial wall cartilage known as intraluminal obstruction due to a mucus plug or meconium. The extrinsic compression is caused by vascular anomalies or an intrathoracic mass. Males are affected more

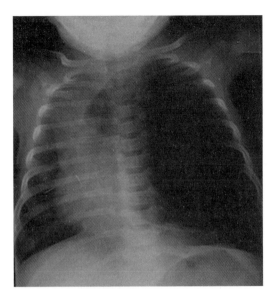

Figure 11.2 Congenital lobar emphysema of left lung. Reproduced with permission from Nottingham University Hospitals.

than females, in the ratio of 2–3/1.The most common site is the left upper lobe (42%) (Figure 11.2), followed by right middle lobe (35%) and right upper lobe (21%). In about 10–15% of CLE cases there is an association with congenital heart disease.

Clinical presentation

The majority of cases present in the first few days or months of life. Most (50%) present in the neonatal period with respiratory distress due to compression by the overdistended lobe. Sometimes CLE may present in childhood with recurrent chest infections. Physical examination may show distension of chest wall with widening of intercostal spaces, chest wall retractions, decreased breath sounds on auscultation over the affected side and hyper-resonance on percussion or increased vibrations, that are normally present with emphysema.

Management

Diagnosis can be made antenatally or postnatally. It is usually evident on plain x-ray, which reveals a markedly hyperlucent lobe which refers to normal or reduced volume during inspiration and air trapping during expiration. There is also mediastinal shift, in which the tissues and organs move the mediastinum to one side of the chest cavity, and compression of the contralateral lung. Thoracic CT scan can be helpful in identifying any cause of external compression. Bronchoscopy is not routinely indicated but can be useful in older children to rule out foreign body or any other compression. For infants with progressive respiratory distress, immediate surgical intervention is indicated (Dogan et al. 1997; Eichenwald and Stark 2007). The surgical treatment of choice is lobectomy. Despite the abnormalities on pulmonary function tests, most surgically treated patients will be asymptomatic and will have normal growth and development (Bancalari et al. 2001; Krummel 1998).

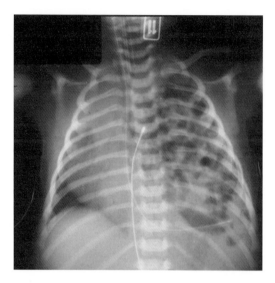

Figure 11.3   Left-sided congenital diaphragmatic hernia in a newborn. Reproduced with permission from Nottingham University Hospitals.

Congenital diaphragmatic hernia

Congenital diaphragmatic hernia (CDH) is an anatomical defect in the diaphragm that permits abdominal contents to herniate into the thoracic cavity. The incidence of CDH has been reported as 1 in 3000–5000 live births (Butler and Claireaux 1962; Jobe and Bancalari 2001). Over the last two decades antenatal diagnosis has increased but despite this and advances in surgery, perinatal mortality remains high.

Pathophysiology

Herniation of abdominal contents occurs most often, from the left posterolateral part of the muscle and is called a Bochdalek hernia. Eighty percent of CDH are left-sided (Figure 11.3) and the rest are right-sided or can be retrosternal, through small areas lying between the costal and sternal attachments of the thoracic diaphragm, known as the foramen of Morgagni (Lally 2002). The diaphragmatic defect results from failed closure of the pleuroperitoneal canals by 8–10 weeks of gestation (embryonic period). Herniation of the abdominal viscera in the thorax results in pulmonary underdevelopment and lung hypoplasia. Isolated CDH is a sporadic condition, with familial cases accounting for less than 2% (Tibboel and Gaag 1996). Chromosomal defects occur in 33% of cases. CDH is often associated with cardiac, gastrointestinal, genitourinary, skeletal or neural anomalies and with trisomies (Kaiser and Rosenfeld 1999; Langham et al. 1996). The major complications are pulmonary hypoplasia and pulmonary hypertension, causing abnormal pulmonary compliance, refractory respiratory failure at birth, hypoxaemia, acidosis and heart failure.

Clinical presentation

Congenital diaphragmatic hernia commonly presents with severe immediate respiratory distress with cyanosis, tachypnoea and tachycardia. On examination, there is prominent hemithorax, with minimal air entry, a displaced apex beat indicating mediastinal shift, and often a scaphoid abdomen. However, 10% of children may present later in life, with a differing clinical picture (Mei-Zahav et al. 2003). The symptoms may be respiratory or gastrointestinal or rarely children may be asymptomatic.

Management

Antenatally CDH is most commonly diagnosed on ultrasound by the presence of abdominal contents within the thoracic cavity. A significant number are detected after 24 weeks of gestation. Right-sided CDH is difficult to detect antenatally as the liver has similar echogenicity to the lung because of the ability to produce more echoes on ultrasound scan due to the firmness of the organ. Subsequent ultrasound examinations are performed to assess the contents of the hernia, evaluate any associated malformations and measure the lung/heart ratio (LHR). Magnetic resonance imaging (MRI) can help to resolve a doubt about the position of liver, to evaluate the volume of lungs or to distinguish a CDH from other lung malformation. Postnatal diagnosis is made by a chest x-ray. Misinterpretation of initial chest x-ray changes occurred in 25%, with pneumothorax or effusion as the most common incorrect diagnosis (Baglaj and Dorobisz 2005).

A multidisciplinary team includes at least neonatologists, obstetricians, paediatric surgeons, geneticists and cardiologists. Delivery should be planned in a tertiary centre. At birth the babies are electively intubated to relieve respiratory distress, and a gastric tube is inserted to decompress the stomach. Ventilation by mask is contraindicated as it may cause distension of the stomach situated in the thoracic cavity. Different modes of ventilation, including conventional ventilation and high-frequency oscillation, are used, aiming for gentle ventilation so as to avoid barotraumas or damage to the tissues because of different pressures, which may precipitate pulmonary hypertension. The role of other interventions, including use of surfactant, nitric oxide and extracorporeal membrane oxygenation, is controversial but they are used in cases with pulmonary hypertension.

These children can have problems with recurrent herniation, delayed growth, chronic lung disease, gastro-oesophageal reflux and neurological impairment so they require long-term multidisciplinary follow-up.

Pulmonary sequestration

Pulmonary sequestrations (PS) are fragments of non-functional lung parenchyma that are not connected to the airway, and are supplied by systemic arterial vessels. The incidence of PS is lower than that of CCAM but the actual numbers are unknown. The availability of prenatal image screening has made the diagnosis of PS more common.

Aetiology and pathogenesis

There are two types of PS, depending on the anatomical features. Intralobar sequestration (ILS, 75–80% of all PS) is surrounded by normal parenchyma and embedded in the normal lobe of lung. Extralobar sequestration (ELS, 10–15% of all PS) consists of a portion of non-functioning lung surrounded by its own pleural sac (Leijala and Louhimo 1987). The remaining 5% can be found in the abdomen, a common site being the upper retroperitoneal area between the lung and the diaphragm. ILS occurs equally in both sexes and is localised in the lower lobes, left more than right. Arterial supply is by the descending thoracic aorta and the venous drainage is via the pulmonary veins. ELS are 3–4 times more common in males. Other anomalies such as congenital diaphragmatic hernia, bronchogenic cysts, cardiac malformations and connections to gastrointestinal tract occur in about 10% of cases. ELS are most commonly found on the left side adjacent to the oesophagus and between the lower lobe and the diaphragm (Stocker 1986). In ELS arterial supply is usually from the descending aorta and venous drainage is to the right heart in 85% of cases and to the left atrium via pulmonary veins in 15%.

Clinical presentation

The most common mode of presentation is recurrent infection. ILS usually presents later in childhood or adulthood. ELS may present with respiratory distress or feeding problems in the first 6 months of life, which may be caused by connection to the oesophagus. Very large feeder blood vessels to the sequestrated lobes can result in heart failure. It may rarely cause haemoptysis.

Management

Contrast-enhanced CT scans will be diagnostic in most cases. The diagnosis of PS is confirmed after a systemic blood supply is demonstrated. Infants with ELS should be investigated for other congenital anomalies. Surgical removal is recommended for all symptomatic cases. Prior to surgery, the extent of the pulmonary lesion should be defined, and the arterial and venous supply should be carefully delineated using contrast-enhanced CT scan and angiography.

Outcome

Outcome usually depends on the degree of pulmonary hypoplasia and the other associated congenital anomalies. With advancements in paediatric thoracic surgery over the last decade, the outcome is good postoperatively. ELS is resected without any functional lung, so there are no functional consequences, and in excess of ILS the functional consequences are insignificant even after the removal of entire lung.

Scimitar syndrome

Scimitar syndrome is a rare congenital lung anomaly consisting in part of right pulmonary venous return to the inferior vena cava. The main feature is the partial abnormal pulmonary venous drainage from a hypoplastic right lung. The right pulmonary artery is often hypoplastic and the right lung may have an arterial supply from the aorta. Symptoms depend on the severity of the pulmonary hypoplasia. Pulmonary function is rarely compromised. With significant shunting, breathlessness or exercise limitation may be a feature. The plain x-ray shows right-sided pulmonary hypoplasia and demonstrates the scimitar sign of a shadow produced from the draining vein. Treatment depends on the associated anatomy; if the shunt is significant it may need surgical correction.

Nursing management of neonatal chronic lung disease and home oxygen

Increased survival of very premature infants has resulted in a greater proportion of infants with neonatal chronic lung disease (NCLD) being discharged home on long-term oxygen therapy (LTOT) (Greenough et al. 2002). Urgent research is needed to identify a safe and effective method of preventing NCLD but until this is achieved, the management of these vulnerable infants must be addressed.

For infants diagnosed with NCLD, surviving the first few months of their lives is only the start of a long and challenging journey. Health professionals need to recognise that each phase of caring for an infant on LTOT brings new burdens in both economic and human terms on parents as primary carers.

The development of specialist nursing services has enabled infants with NCLD to be nursed safely at home by their families with appropriate support and monitoring (Dunbar and Kotecha 2000).

Clinical monitoring at home, including oxygen monitoring, needs to be tailored according to the infant's needs as well as taking into consideration parental anxiety. Oxygen saturation monitoring can be an accurate and effective way to maintain oxygen saturations within target ranges (Smith et al. 2004). In such infants, oxygen saturation levels of less than 92% should be avoided and a target range of at least 94–95% aimed for. This target is consistent with current recommendations as previously discussed.

It must be remembered that effective management of a NCLD infant at home depends on additional factors other than oxygen saturation levels and simply supplying or not supplying a monitor. Excellent multidisciplinary support systems, including medical, technical, psychological and community services, are the backbone to helping these families care for their infant at home to maintain good health and treat ill health (Muir and Dryden 2000). The involvement of the specialist nurse/children's community nurse (CCN) in this process significantly improves the quality of care provision for these families.

A focus on family-centred care requires that parents become educated about their premature infant and their health needs, understanding their own stresses and adaptations, and become active participants in their infant's care. Parental education and teaching of the skills needed to holistically care for their chronically ill child is therefore of greatest importance (Naylor 2003). Empowering parents builds confidence, giving them the ability to provide an achievable degree of normality to family life.

Rather than being solely reliant on the neonatal transitional care nurse, nursing staff with appropriate teaching are in a perfect position to educate parents on a daily basis. The opportunity to continue this teaching and support must then be taken up by the specialist nurse/CCN in the home environment.

Professional education is also essential for safe management of infants with NCLD at home. Primary care clinicians (PCCs) such as GPs and health visitors should be included in the infant's care prior to discharge. It is essential for these clinicians to know what is expected of them. Inviting them to the infant's discharge planning meeting is the first step. Educating and working together with the PCCs gives them the confidence to support these families and, in turn, encourages these families to acquire the needed confidence and competence to take on the responsibility of managing their infant at home without the need for readmission. Increasing professional knowledge will promote a uniform provision of care services. Avoiding contact between the infant with NCLD and other patients whilst visiting the GP surgery or weighing the infant at home and not at baby clinic are simple ways to limit unnecessary exposure to possible infection.

Medical and nursing staff are valuable sources of information and support during the infant's hospitalisation and once home in the community, but the parent's primary source of emotional support is their family/friends. It is important for those who provide the care to acknowledge this and facilitate the transition back to family life prior to discharge through the initiation of an education programme.

Parents are bearing many concerns and duties over a prolonged period to care for their infant with NCLD. The social isolation these families face to avoid exposure to respiratory infections can often have a huge effect on family dynamics. The need for appropriate respite care to reduce feelings of isolation is common amongst these families (Bissell and Long 2003; Brazy et al. 2001; Langley et al.

1999; Manns 2000). The provision of crucial respite care will need to be tailored to fit the needs of each family (Brazy et al. 2001; Manns 2000).

Although oxygen-dependent infants may receive some care from home care nurses, many families do not receive professional home care assistance 24 h a day. Parents need to qualify for these specialist services and suffer the scrutiny of a commissioning board in order to have someone who will care for their infant for brief intervals in their home. Often parents rely on other non-professional caregivers to be available for back-up assistance. The need for such caregivers is more than just practical. Parents faced with a chronically ill infant require support and relief of their caregiving responsibilities to prevent fatigue, feelings of social isolation and strained family relationships (Robinson 1995).

Family and friends contribute to the learning process as significantly as healthcare professionals (McKellar et al. 2006). Resources should therefore provide for the updating of grandparents/relatives and/or friends. It reinforces the need to nurture parental confidence and empower parents in the learning process, helping them to recognise that they have a variety of learning resources available to them and the intrinsic ability to use them effectively (McKellar et al. 2006). Getting family or friends involved in the infant's care prior to discharge means a great deal more work for the neonatal unit, paediatric wards and/or CCNs but also relieves some of the anxiety parents feel on discharge about being the only people able to care for their infant.

Secondary caregivers are capable of caring for the infant in the absence of parents. Family or close friends commonly serve in this capacity. These individuals must be committed to providing continuity of care for the infant. Most importantly, they must be able to perform the necessary technical aspects of the infant's care while providing a nurturing environment. Knowledge and confidence in caretaking skills are required for secondary caregivers to possess a necessary comfort level. Their education should also be commenced prior to the infant's discharge. Components of their teaching plan should mirror that of the parents, including infant resuscitation, special feeding techniques, positioning, management of oxygen and providing developmentally appropriate care and stimulation (Robinson 1995).

Follow-up educational support is also essential for secondary caregivers. They should receive copies of any printed instructional materials, and they need to be made aware of whom they should call when questions arise. The specialist nurse/CCN can ensure that all caregivers' and PCCs' knowledge is consolidated and remains up to date in all aspects of the care and management of the infant on LTOT. Parents, secondary caregivers and PCCs are all susceptible to some of the same stressors. Supporting these families and professions with access to advice 24 h a day, 7 days a week would be ideal to relieve these stresses (Robinson 1995) and should eliminate frequent and unnecessary visits to hospital.

Stresses are also apparent for parents, as taking an infant home on oxygen often means a change to finances; for example, it is not recommended that an infant attends private nursery so that a parent can return to work. This often results in a parent giving up work to care for their child at home. However, disability living allowance, carer's allowance and tax credits are all available for families caring for a child on LTOT. As the key worker, the specialist nurse/CCN can help in completing the relevant paperwork.

Conclusion

By educating and supporting parents/carers and secondary caregivers, they will be helped to feel confident, less isolated and more in control of their lives. Parents/carers will manage their child's condition and treatment jointly with healthcare professionals. Parents/carers will then be able to use their new skills and knowledge to improve their quality of life. Every member of the family should have the privilege of living in a home where they can develop to their utmost capacity. Fleck (2006) maintains that by fostering an environment for optimal development and continuous growth, parent and child will have richer, fuller and happier lives and make greater contributions to their immediate and wider world.

Questions

1. What are the predisposing factors for developing CLD?
2. What is interstitial lung disease?
3. Why do patients with bronchiectasis retain secretions?
4. What is the most common congenital abnormality of the lung in children?
5. How is congenital lobar emphysema with respiratory distress treated?
6. How can parents of infants with CLD receive financial assistance?
7. What is the professional opinion with regard to the use of oxygen saturation monitors within the home environment?

References

Abman SH, Accurso FJ, Koops BL. (1984) Experience with home oxygen in the management of infants with bronchopulmonary dysplasia. *Clinical Pediatrics (Philadelphia)* **23**, 471–6.

Adzick NS, Harrison MR, Glick PL, *et al.* (1985) Fetal cystic adenomatoid malformation, prenatal diagnosis and natural history. *Journal of Pediatric Surgery* **20**, 483–8.

American Thoracic Society. (2003) Statement on the care of the child with chronic lung disease of infancy and childhood. *American Journal of Respiratory and Critical Care Medicine* **168**, 356–96.

Anwar GA, Bourke SC, Afolabi G, Middleton P, Ward C, Rutherford RM. (2008) Use of low dose azithromycin on long term basis in non-cystic fibrosis bronchiectasis. *Respiratory Medicine* **102(10)**, 1494–6.

Baglaj M, Dorobisz U. (2005) Late-presenting congenital diaphragmatic hernia in children, a literature review. *Pediatric Radiology* **35**, 478–88.

Balfour-Lynn IM, Field DJ, Gringras P, *et al.*, on behalf of the Paediatric Section of the Home Oxygen Guideline Development Group of the BTS Standards of Care Committee. (2009) BTS guidelines for home oxygen in children. *Thorax* **64(suppl II)**, ii1–ii26.

Bancalari E, Abdenour GE, Feller R, Gannon J. (1979) Bronchopulmonary dysplasia, clinical presentation. *Journal of Pediatrics* **95**, 819–23.

Banjar H. (2006) Childhood bronchiectasis, a review. *Bahrain Medical Bulletin* **28(2)**, 1–10.

Bissell G, Long T. (2003) From the neonatal unit to home. How do parents adapt to life at home with their baby? *Journal of Neonatal Nursing* **9(1)**, 7–12.

Brazy J, Anderson B, Becker P, Becker M. (2001) How parents of premature infants gather information and obtain support. *Neonatal Network* **20(2)**, 41–8.

British Thoracic Society (BTS). (2009) *Guideline on the Management of Asthma: a national clinical guideline.* London: British Thoracic Society.

Butler N, Claireaux AE. (1962) Congenital diaphragmatic hernia as a cause of perinatal mortality. *Lancet* **1**, 659–63.

Campbell AN, Zarfin Y, Groenveld M, Bryan MH. (1983) Low flow oxygen therapy in infants. *Archives of Disease in Childhood* **58**, 795–8.

Clement A, for the ERS Task Force. (2004) Task force on chronic interstitial lung disease in immunocompetent children. *European Respiratory Journal* **24**, 686–97.

Coalson JJ. (2000) Pathology of chronic lung disease in early infancy. In: Bland RD, Coalson JJ (eds) *Chronic Lung Disease in Early Infancy.* New York: Marcel Dekker, pp. 85–124.

Crockett AJ, Cranston JM, Latimer KM, Alpers JH. (2001) Mucolytics for bronchiectasis. *Cochrane Database of Systematic Reviews* **1**, CD001289.

Department of Health. (2010) Joint Committee on Vaccination and Immunisation statement on immunisation for respiratory syncytial virus. Available at:www.dh.gov.uk/prod_consum_dh/groups/dh_digitalassets/@dh/@ab/documents/digitalasset/dh_120395.pdf.

Deutsch GH, Young L, Deterding R, *et al.* (2007) Diffuse lung disease in young children: application of a novel classification scheme. *American Journal of Respiratory and Critical Care Medicine* **176**, 1120–8.

Dinwiddie R, Sharief N, Crawford O. (2002) Idiopathic interstitial pneumonitis in children, a national survey in the United Kingdom and Ireland. *Pediatric Pulmonology* **34(1)**, 23–9.

Dogan R, Demircin M, Sarigul A, Passogli I, Gocumen A, Bozer AY. (1997) Surgical managment of congenital lobar emphysema. *Turkish Journal of Pediatrics* **39(1)**, 35–44.

Doyle LW, Halliday HL, Ehrenkranz RA, *et al.* (2005) Impact of postnatal systemic corticosteroids on mortality and cerebral palsy in preterm infants, effect modification by risk for chronic lung disease. *Pediatrics* **115**, 655–61.

Dunbar H, Kotecha S. (2000) Domiciliary oxygen for infants with chronic lung disease of prematurity. *Care of the Critically Ill* **16(3)**, 90–3.

Duncombe GJ, Dickinson JE, Kikiros CS. (2002) Prenatal diagnosis and management of congenital cystic adenomatoid malformation of the lung. *American Journal of Obstetrics and Gynecology* **187**, 950–4.

Eastham KM, Fall AJ, Mitchell L,Spencer DA. (2004) Paediatric lung disease, the need to redefine non-cystic fibrosis bronchiectasis in childhood. *Thorax* **59**, 324–7.

Eichenwald EC, Stark AR. (2007) Are postnatal steroids ever justified to treat severe bronchopulmonary dysplasia? *Archives of Disease in Childhood – Fetal and Neonatal edition* **92**, 334–7.

Fan LL, Deterding RR, Langston C. (2004) Pediatric interstitial lung disease revisited. *Pediatric Pulmonology* **38**, 369–78.

Fleck H. (2006) Learning to live with our children. *Public Health Nursing* **23(6)**, 561–2.

French J, Bilton D, Campbell F. (2003) Nurse specialist care for bronchiectasis. *Cochrane Database of Systematic Reviews* **3**, CD004319.

Giacoia GP, Venkataraman PS, West-Wilson KI, Faulkner MJ. (1997) Follow-up of school-age children with bronchopulmonary dysplasia. *Journal of Pediatrics* **130(3)**, 400–8.

Greenough A, Alexander J, Burgess S, *et al.* (2002) Home oxygen status and rehospitalisation and primary care requirements of infants with chronic lung disease. *Archives of Disease in Childhood – Fetal and Neonatal edition* **86(1)**, 40–3.

Halliday HL, Ehrenkranz RA, Doyle LW. (2003a) Early postnatal (<96 hours) corticosteroids for preventing chronic lung disease in preterm infants. *Cochrane Database of Systematic Reviews* **1**, CD001146.

Halliday HL, Ehrenkranz RA, Doyle LW. (2003b) Moderately early (7–14 days) postnatal corticosteroids for preventing chronic lung disease in preterm infants. *Cochrane Database of Systematic Reviews* **1**, CD001144.

Halliday HL, Ehrenkranz RA, Doyle LW. (2003c) Delayed (>3 weeks) postnatal corticosteroids for chronic lung disease in preterm infants. *Cochrane Database of Systematic Reviews* **1**, CD001145.

Hennessy EM, Bracewell MA, Wood N, *et al.*, for the EPICure Study Group. (2008) Respiratory health in pre-school and school age children following extremely preterm birth. *Archives of Disease in Childhood* **93**, 1037–43.

Hudak BB, Allen MC, Hudak ML, Loughlin GM. (1989) Home oxygen therapy for chronic lung disease in extremely low-birth-weight infants. *American Journal of Diseases of Children* **143**, 357–60.

Jobe AH, Bancalari E. (2001) Bronchopulmonary dysplasia. *American Journal of Respiratory and Critical Care Medicine* **163**, 1723–9.

Kaiser JR, Rosenfeld CR. (1999) A population-based study of congenital diaphragmatic hernia, impact of associated anomalies and preoperative blood gases on survival. *Journal of Pediatric Surgery* **34**, 1196–202.

Kapur N, Bell S, Kolbe J, Chang AB. (2009) Inhaled steroids for bronchiectasis. *Cochrane Database of Systematic Reviews* **1**, CD000996.

Krummel TM. (1998) Congenital malformation of the lower respiratory tract. In: Chernick V, Boat T (eds) *Kendig's Disorders of the Respiratory Tract in Children*, 6th edn. Philadelphia: WB Saunders, pp. 310–11.

Laberge JM, Flageole H, Pugash D, *et al.* (2001) Outcome of the prenatally diagnosed congenital cystic adenomatoid malformation, a Canadian experience. *Fetal Diagnosis and Therapy* **16**, 178–86.

Lally KP. (2002) Congenital diaphragmatic hernia. *Current Opinion in Pediatrics* **14(4)**, 486–90.

Langham MR, Kays DW, Ledbetter DJ, Frentzen B, Sanford LL, Richards DS. (1996) Congenital diaphragmatic hernia, epidemiology and outcome. *Clinics in Perinatology* **23**, 671–88.

Langley D, Hollis S, MacGregor D. (1999) Parents' perceptions of neonatal services within the community: a postal survey. *Journal of Neonatal Nursing* **5(4)**, 7–11.

Leijala M, Louhimo I. (1987) Extralobar sequestration of the lung in children. *Progress in Pediatric Surgery* **21**, 98–106.

Lister P, Iles R, Shaw B, Ducharme F. (2000) Inhaled steroids for neonatal chronic lung disease. *Cochrane Database of Systematic Reviews* **3**, CD002311.

Long FR, Castile RG, Brody AS, *et al.* (1999) Lungs in infants and young children, improved thin-section CT with a non-invasive controlled-ventilation technique – initial experience. *Radiology* **212**, 588–93.

Lynch DA, Hay T, Newell JD, Divgi VD, Fan LL. (1999) Pediatric diffuse lung disease, diagnosis and classification using high-resolution CT. *American Journal of Roentgenology* **173**, 713–18.

Madan A, Brozanski BS, Cole CH, Oden NL, Cohen G, Phelps DL. (2005) A pulmonary score for assessing the severity of neonatal chronic lung disease. *Pediatrics* **115**, e450–e457.

Manns S. (2000) Life after SCBU. The long term effects on mothers at home with a child with bronchopulmonary dysplasia and on home oxygen. *Journal of Neonatal Nursing* **6(6)**, 193–6.

McKellar L, Pincombe J, Henderson A. (2006) Insights from Australian parents into educational experiences in the early postnatal period. *Midwifery* **22(4)**, 356–64.

Mei-Zahav M, Solomon M, Trachsel D, Langer JC. (2003) Bochdalek diaphragmatic hernia, not only a neonatal disease. *Archives of Disease in Childhood* **88**, 532–5.

Mighten J. (2007) Home intravenous therapy training for carers of children and young people. *British Journal of Nursing* **6(5)**, 272–6.

Muir J, Dryden S. (2000) Collaborative planning for children with chronic complex care needs. In: Muir J, Sidey A (eds) *Textbook of Community Children's Nursing*. London: Baillière Tindall, pp. 217–22.

Naylor H. (2003) O2 go home – a home oxygen programme for neonatal graduates with bronchopulmonary dysplasia. *Nurse 2 Nurse* **3(3)**, 35–7.

Northway WH Jr, Rosan RC, Porter DY. (1967) Pulmonary disease following respirator therapy of hyaline-membrane disease. Bronchopulmonary dysplasia. *New England Journal of Medicine* **276**, 357–68.

Robinson T. (1995) Educating secondary caregivers. *Neonatal Network* **14(4)**, 69–70.

Sepper R, Kottinen Y, Ding Y, *et al.* (1995) Human neutrophil collagense identified in bronchiectasis BAL fluid, correlates with severity of disease. *Chest* **107**, 1641–7.

Shennan AT, Dunn MS, Ohlsson A, Lennox K, Hoskins EM. (1988) Abnormal pulmonary outcomes in premature infants, prediction from oxygen requirement in the neonatal period. *Pediatrics* **82**, 527–32.

Smith V, Zupancic J, McCormick M, *et al.* (2004) Rehospitalization in the first year of life among infants with bronchopulmonary dysplasia. *Journal of Paediatric Nursing* **144(6)**, 799–803.

Stevenson DK, Wright LL, Lemons JA, *et al.* (1998) Very low birth weight outcomes of the National Institute of Child Health and Human Development Neonatal Research Network. January 1993 through December 1994. *American Journal of Obstetrics and Gynecology* **179**, 1632–9.

Stocker JT. (1986) Sequestrations of the lung. *Seminars in Diagnostic Pathology* **3**, 106–21.

Stocker JT. (2002) Congenital pulmonary airway malformation, a new name for and an expanded classification of congenital cystic adenomatoid malformation of the lung. *Histopathology* **41(suppl 2)**, 424–31.

Stocker JT, Madewell JE, Drake RM. (1977) Congenital cystic adenomatoid malformation of the lung. Classification and morphologic spectrum. *Human Pathology* **8**, 155–71.

Tibboel D, Gaag AV. (1996) Etiologic and genetic factors in congenital diaphragmatic hernia. *Clinics in Perinatology* **23**, 689–99.

Yuksel B, Greenough A. (1992) Randomised trial of inhaled steroids in preterm infants with respiratory symptoms at follow up. *Thorax* **47**, 910–13.

Chapter 12

Inherited lung disease in children

Alan R. Smyth,[1] Ammani Prasad[2] and Janice Mighten[3]

[1]*Professor of Child Health, School of Clinical Sciences, University of Nottingham; Honorary Consultant in Paediatric Respiratory Medicine, Nottingham Children's Hospital*
[2]*CF Co-ordinatory/Senior Research Physiotherapist, Great Ormond Street Hospital for Children*
[3]*Children's Respiratory/Community Nurse Specialist, Nottingham Children's Hospital*

Learning objectives

After studying this chapter, the reader will:

- understand the inheritance of primary ciliary dyskinesia and cystic fibrosis
- be familiar with the pathophysiology of the conditions
- understand the approach used to diagnose these conditions
- appreciate the importance of early diagnosis and pre-emptive treatment
- understand the range of pulmonary pathogens seen in these conditions and the approach to their treatment
- appreciate the importance of multidisciplinary working, including physiotherapy, nursing management and national standards of care.

Chapter 10 provided an insight into asthma treatment and management. The evidence suggests that there is a strong family link, so we will now move on to look at two other genetically inherited respiratory disorders – primary ciliary dyskinesia and cystic fibrosis.

Primary ciliary dyskinesia

In order to maintain healthy lungs which are free of infection, inhaled particles and micro-organisms must be removed from the respiratory tract. The most effective mechanism for achieving this is the mucociliary escalator. The respiratory tract is lined with cells which have tiny 'hairs', or cilia, on their surface. These cilia move in a co-ordinated fashion, like a 'Mexican wave' at a football match, and waft micro-organisms and other particles up the respiratory tract to the larynx, where fluid and particles are eventually swallowed. In primary ciliary dyskinesia (PCD), the cilia either fail to move at all or they move in an unco-ordinated fashion. As a result micro-organisms are not cleared from the airways and infection occurs.

Primary ciliary dyskinesia occurs in between 1/15,000 and 1/30,000 live births. Most cases are autosomal recessive and the condition is more prevalent in communities where consanguinity is common, notably the Asian community in some parts of the UK (O'Callaghan et al. 2010).

Children's Respiratory Nursing, First Edition. Edited by Janice Mighten.
© 2013 Blackwell Publishing Ltd. Published 2013 by Blackwell Publishing Ltd.

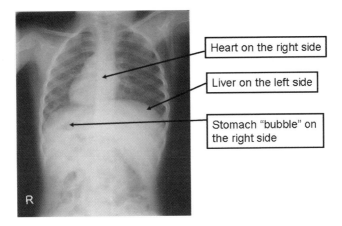

Heart on the right side

Liver on the left side

Stomach "bubble" on the right side

R

Figure 12.1 Chest and abdominal x-ray showing dextrocardia and situs inversus.

Individuals with PCD, as with other types of lung disease where there is chronic infection, are at risk of developing bronchiectasis. This is defined as an irreversible widening of the small airways. This interferes with the mucociliary escalator and allows secretions to accumulate and become secondarily infected.

Approximately half of patients with PCD have dextrocardia (heart on the right side of the chest) and situs inversus (internal organs such as the lungs, liver, spleen and stomach are on the opposite side) (Bush et al. 2007) (Figure 12.1). This occurs because the cilia are responsible for arranging the developing organs in their correct location in the embryo. However, most babies with situs inversus do not have PCD (Bush et al. 2007). Many patients with PCD are diagnosed late, sometimes after lung damage has occurred. The mean age at diagnosis was between 4 and 5 years in one series (Coren et al. 2002). Apart from situs inversus, key clinical clues for PCD are:

- persistent nasal discharge, starting in the newborn period
- respiratory distress (fast laboured breathing) in the newborn period
- a persistent wet cough in older children
- chronically discharging ears (often following grommet insertion).

The diagnosis of PCD is undertaken in a small number of specialised centres in the UK (currently Leicester Royal Infirmary, the Royal Brompton and Southampton University Hospitals NHS Trust). A measurement of the nitric oxide levels at the nose is sometimes used as a screening test (Karadag et al. 1999). (Nitric oxide levels are abnormally low in PCD.) However, the definitive test requires samples of respiratory epithelial cells with cilia, which are taken from the nose using a tiny brush and are examined under the microscope to determine how quickly the cilia beat and whether they do this in a co-ordinated fashion (Stannard et al. 2010). The cilia are also examined using an electron microscope to see if their structure looks abnormal (Stannard et al. 2010).

Much of the treatment of PCD is not based on properly designed clinical trials but rather is borrowed from the treatment used for children with conditions such as cystic fibrosis and asthma. In PCD, the basis of treatment is close monitoring of children, including regular cough swab or sputum samples for microbiology, physical examination and measurement of pulmonary function. Children should have daily chest physiotherapy to help clear respiratory secretions. In young children this will be by percussion and postural drainage ('bash and tip') whereas older patients will use positive airway pressure techniques such as the positive expiratory pressure (PEP) mask or controlled breathing and coughing (active cycle of breathing). These techniques are discussed in more detail in the section below on cystic fibrosis.

Respiratory infection may be detected in cough swab and sputum samples, or suspected when there is a troublesome wet cough. In both instances, children should be treated with antibiotics which may need to be given intravenously in severe cases. The most common organisms found are *Staphylococcus aureus*, *Haemophilus influenzae* and *Pseudomonas aeruginosa*. Therefore annual influenza immunisation should be given. Children are also vulnerable to mucus collection in the middle ear (otitis media with effusion) which can affect hearing and the development of speech. Insertion of grommets should be avoided as this can lead to persistent discharge. The problem usually resolves in the teenage years (Bush et al. 2007). Nasal discharge can be treated by washing out with a 'douche' device (Bush et al. 2007), so in the long term children treated with this approach do well and lung function is better preserved than in patients first diagnosed in adult life (Ellerman and Bisgaard 1997).

Cystic fibrosis

Pathophysiology

Like PCD, lung disease in cystic fibrosis (CF) occurs because of failure of the mucociliary escalator. However, the mechanism is very different. Figure 12.2 shows how the cilia function in the normal lung, compared to PCD and CF. The periciliary layer can be likened to a layer of lubricant in a machine. If the layer is not thick enough the machine cannot run smoothly.

In CF the periciliary or 'lubricant' layer is not as deep as it should be. This layer is composed of salt water. In CF the channel which allows chloride ions to pass out of the cell is not working, whereas the sodium channel, which allows sodium to pass into the cell, is overactive. This means that there is not enough salt (sodium chloride) in the periciliary layer and hence not enough water is drawn in through osmosis. While the periciliary layer allows the cilia to move freely, the mucus is stickier and the cilia become stuck. The mucociliary escalator does not work and particles and micro-organisms build up in the lung. This leads to secondary infection and plugging of small airways with mucus, illustrated in Figure 12.3.

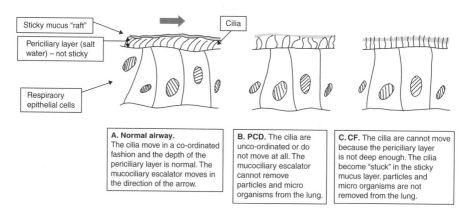

Figure 12.2   Cilia in (A) the normal lung, (B) PCD and (C) CF.

Genetics

Cystic fibrosis is an autosomal recessive condition, which means an individual must have two defective forms of the CF gene to have the condition. In the general population in the UK, 1/25 individuals is a carrier; the CF gene is located on chromosome 7 (Smyth 2008). There are over 1000 different mutations of the CF gene which can cause disease. However, in the UK, one mutation, δ F508, is very common; 50% of UK CF patients have two copies of this gene and 90% have at least one copy. The normal CF gene is responsible for making the chloride channel (cystic fibrosis trans-membrane conductance regulator or CFTR) which maintains the periciliary layer at the correct thickness and hence allows the mucociliary escalator to function. Mutations or defects of the CF gene do not make functioning CFTR. Some mutations of CFTR (such as R117H) are referred to as 'dominant mild mutations'. When one of these genes is present, the CF disease may be less severe.

Diagnosis

Antenatal diagnosis

Close liaison between the clinical genetics and CF teams is essential. If a couple have had a previous baby with CF, and both parents have been genotyped, then chorion villus sampling may be performed in the first trimester to allow genotyping of the fetus. Some parents may opt for termination if CF is diagnosed (Polnay et al. 2002). The first manifestation of CF may be on the 16-week ultrasound scan where echogenic bowel or bowel dilation may be seen. Where both these signs are present there is around a 17% chance of the fetus having CF (Muller et al. 2002). At this point, both parents should have their CF genotype determined and (if the parents wish to proceed) amniocentesis should be performed, allowing genotype testing of the fetus.

Newborn screening

In the UK every newborn infant is now screened for cystic fibrosis and a number of other genetic disorders (UK Newborn Screening Programme Centre 2010). On or around the fifth day of life,

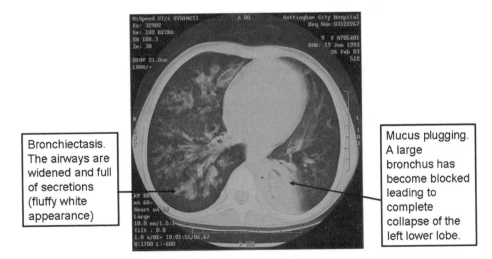

Bronchiectasis. The airways are widened and full of secretions (fluffy white appearance)

Mucus plugging. A large bronchus has become blocked leading to complete collapse of the left lower lobe.

Figure 12.3 A high-resolution CT scan of a 10-year-old girl with CF showing bronchiectasis and the effects of mucus plugging.

a dried blood spot is collected by means of a heel prick, and sent for immune reactive trypsin (IRT) testing (UK Newborn Screening Programme Centre 2010). IRT, an enzyme secreted by the pancreas, is raised in newborns with CF, due to early pancreatic damage. If the IRT is raised, then blood from the same sample is analysed for the four most common CF mutations. If two CF mutations are found, then the child is referred to a paediatrician. If only one mutation is found then further analysis of the same specimen is done, looking for around 30 further mutations. If no further mutations are found then a new blood sample is collected and the IRT test is repeated. If still raised, the child is referred. If no mutations were detected and yet the original IRT was very high, then the IRT is repeated and the child referred if the IRT is still raised. Screening is highly accurate, missing only around one infant in 40,000 screened. Of those missed, many will have meconium ileus (see below) and so will be diagnosed clinically.

The sweat test

The sweat test is the gold standard for diagnosis in CF (Multidisiplinary Working Group 2003). Sweating is induced using the chemical pilocarpine, applied to the smooth surface of the forearm. An electrical current is used to help the pilocarpine enter the skin. The sweat is then collected over a period of 30 min, either using filter paper or in a special device called a Macroduct® (Westcor Biomedical Systems, Utah, US). The collected sweat is then weighed and the sweat chloride level measured.

- >60 mmol/L   Indicates CF
- 40–60 mmol/L   Suspicious – further testing and careful follow-up needed
- <40 mmol/L   Normal

Clinical features and complications

Although we have focused on lung disease so far in this discussion, CF is a multisystem disease. Figure 12.4 shows the effects of CF on other body systems.

Gastrointestinal problems

Meconium ileus

Approximately 15% of babies with CF will come to medical attention, shortly after birth, through failure to pass the first black sticky stool (meconium). This can lead to abdominal distension and vomiting. Treatment is by instilling radiological contrast into the baby's rectum and upward to the level of the obstruction – usually the terminal ileum. The pressure of the radiological contrast may shift the obstruction and x-rays may be taken at the same time to determine if the colon is small ('microcolon'). If this procedure is unsuccessful or if a perforation of the bowel occurs, then surgery with formation of an ileostomy will be needed. In these circumstances, a period of parenteral nutrition may be essential. Both the use of parenteral nutrition and the occurrence of meconium ileus increase the chances of subsequent CF liver disease (see below).

Malabsorption and growth faltering

Most babies diagnosed with CF by newborn screening will already have faltering growth at the time they are referred with a positive screening test. The problems of sticky secretions and obstruction seen in the lungs also occur in the pancreas, leading to a deficiency of pancreatic enzymes and bicarbonate. This means that food (initially milk) is not digested and absorbed, particularly the

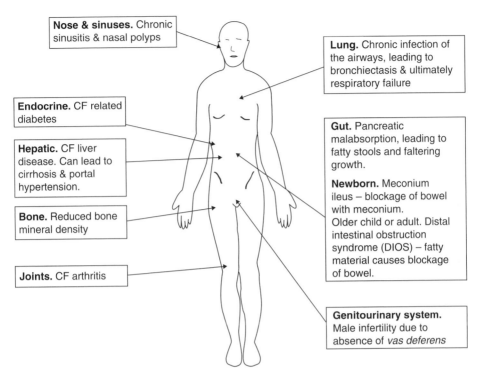

Nose & sinuses. Chronic sinusitis & nasal polyps

Lung. Chronic infection of the airways, leading to bronchiectasis & ultimately respiratory failure

Endocrine. CF related diabetes

Hepatic. CF liver disease. Can lead to cirrhosis & portal hypertension.

Bone. Reduced bone mineral density

Joints. CF arthritis

Gut. Pancreatic malabsorption, leading to fatty stools and faltering growth.

Newborn. Meconium ileus – blockage of bowel with meconium. Older child or adult. Distal intestinal obstruction syndrome (DIOS) – fatty material causes blockage of bowel.

Genitourinary system. Male infertility due to absence of *vas deferens*

Figure 12.4 Complications of CF.

calorie-rich fats. The same applies to the fat-soluble vitamins so supplements of vitamins A and E are given routinely. Vitamins D and K are also given if deficiency is shown or (in the case of vitamin K) there are problems with blood clotting. The enzyme deficiency is overcome by giving enzyme supplements. These can be broken down by acid in the stomach and so enzymes are given as enteric-coated granules. Older children take these in capsules. Younger children and infants will have granules; in the case of babies in the first few weeks of life, these enzyme granules are given with a small amount of fruit puree. The amount of enzyme given is determined by how well the baby grows and the appearance of the stools. Mothers who wish to breastfeed their baby with CF should be encouraged to do so.

In some children malabsorption is difficult to control with enzymes and neutralising gastric acid with drugs such as omeprazole may help. Children with CF also burn more energy (some of this is due to lung disease and infection) and it is recommended they have 120–150% of the recommended dietary intake of calories. In some cases dietary supplements or gastrostomy feeding may be necessary.

Distal intestinal obstruction syndrome

Pancreatic enzyme supplements are not perfect and some of the fatty component of food may not be fully digested, even when the enzyme capsules are taken as prescribed. Children and young people with CF may develop abdominal pain and difficulty passing stool, due to a collection of partially digested food at the narrowest point in the bowel (the ileocaecal valve). This is termed distal intestinal obstruction syndrome. Milder cases respond to laxatives such as lactulose. In more severe cases the radiological contrast medium gastrograffin is given orally.

Respiratory problems

Although CF is a multisystem disorder, most people with CF will die from respiratory failure. Prognosis has improved greatly in the last four decades and life expectancy for babies born in the last decade is around 40 years. This is expected to improve further in future.

In CF there is a vicious circle of infection, inflammation and lung damage which leads to bronchiectasis and ultimately to respiratory failure. Detecting and treating infection early is of paramount importance, if children are to achieve the best possible life expectancy and quality of life. Children with CF admitted to hospital for treatment of respiratory infection may look well compared to the child in the next bed with acute severe asthma. Both are having life-saving treatment – the only difference is that the child with CF sees the benefit of this treatment some years hence.

Treatment

Diagnosis and treatment of infection

As with PCD, a cough swab or sputum sample should be taken at every visit and the child seen at least every 2 months. One of the first organisms found in infants and younger children is *Staph. aureus* and children up to 3 years of age are commonly given prophylactic antistaphylococcal antibiotics (Smyth and Walters 2003). Infection with *H. influenzae* is also common in young children and usually responds to oral antibiotics. More problematic is infection with *P. aeruginosa*. This organism causes chronic infection, is resistant to many antibiotics and may become more resistant as infection in an individual progresses. The key to successful treatment is to eradicate the organism as soon as it is detected. In the UK a combination of the antibiotics ciprofloxacin (orally) and colistin (nebulised) is frequently given, often for 3 weeks initially though courses may need to be as long as 3 months (Langton Hewer and Smyth 2009). In the US nebulised tobramycin (often for 1 month) may be used on its own (Langton Hewer and Smyth 2009). In some children, eradication fails and infection with *P. aeruginosa* becomes chronic. Infection may be controlled (though not eradicated) with long-term treatment with nebulised colistin and intravenous antibiotics given for periods of worsening cough and breathlessness. As with PCD, annual influenza immunisation should be given.

Physiotherapy

As well as antibiotic treatment, chest physiotherapy is crucial to keeping children with CF well, as with PCD. This will be discussed later.

Other respiratory treatment

As the basic problem causing CF lung disease is failure of the mucociliary escalator, it seems sensible to use drugs designed to restore this function. Hypertonic saline (6% or 7%) is given twice daily by nebuliser and this can be shown to restore the function of the mucociliary escalator (Donaldson et al. 2006). Over a period of a year, it reduces by half the number of exacerbations of chest symptoms which patients experience (Elkins et al. 2006a).

Dornase-α is a form of DNase, an enzyme naturally produced by the body to break down DNA. Sputum contains DNA from dead neutrophils (cells that fight bacterial infection) and this makes the sputum sticky. Nebulised dornase-α, given once daily, leads to a small but important improvement in lung function which is maintained for up to 2 years (Jones et al. 2003).

Azithromycin is an antibiotic which, whilst it does kill *P. aeruginosa*, is beneficial in patients with CF who have chronic infection. Over a period of a year it leads to increased weight in CF patients and to fewer exacerbations (again reduced by around 50%) (Saiman et al. 2003). It is effective when taken three times per week.

Steroid treatment (mainly prednisolone) is used sparingly in CF as long-term use leads to unacceptable side-effects (Cheng et al. 1999a). Its main use in current practice is to treat an allergic response to the airborne mould *Aspergillus fumigatus* (allergic bronchopulmonary aspergillosis).

For advanced lung disease, children may need home oxygen, either at night or continuously, most conveniently given with an oxygen concentrator and cylinders. Referral for lung transplantation should be made according to local guidelines (commonly when the forced expiratory volume in 1 s (FEV1) is <30% predicted), and will be discussed further in Chapter 13 (Kerem et al. 1992). Non-invasive ventilation using a nasal or facemask may be helpful at this stage and should be started sooner rather than later, but this is discussed in more detail in Chapter 7.

Nose and sinuses

The respiratory tract includes the nose and paranasal sinuses. The problems of build-up of secretions and secondary infection also occur here, leading to chronic sinusitis in some patients. This may be associated with the formation of fleshy lumps of inflammatory tissue in the nasal passages, called nasal polyps. These respond (after some weeks) to nasal steroid treatment. Occasionally surgery is needed but the polyps tend to recur.

Liver disease

The smaller bile ducts may become blocked with sticky bile in CF, leading to back-pressure and scarring of the liver, a picture known as centrilobular fibrosis. This can cause progressive damage to the liver, leading to cirrhosis – islands of normal liver surrounded by fibrous 'pockets' of scar tissue. This may cause back-pressure in the main blood vessel leading from the gut to the liver (the hepatic portal vein) which leads to 'blisters' in the blood vessels around the oesophagus (oesophageal varices). This can cause life-threatening bleeding, while the damage to the liver cells can prevent the production of adequate amounts of clotting factors, exacerbating the problem. The incidence is just under 2% per 100 patients per year and there is a sharp fall in the risk of liver disease in CF after 10 years of age (Colombo et al. 2002). Screening for CF liver disease is with annual liver function tests and liver ultrasound where the tests abnormal. At the first sign of early liver disease, treatment should be commenced with ursodeoxycholic acid and continued life long (Cheng et al. 1999b). Where liver disease is progressive, referral should be made to a liver unit.

Cystic fibrosis-related diabetes

Just as secretion of enzymes from the pancreas can be impaired, so too production of insulin from the islet cells may reduce over time in people with CF. This can lead to CF-related diabetes which is present in between 12% and 15% of people with CF with an average age of onset of 20 years (Brennan et al. 2004). CF-related diabetes is different from type 1 diabetes in that patients rarely present with drowsiness, acidosis and dehydration (diabetic ketoacidosis). Rather, CF-related diabetes comes on slowly, with poor weight gain or weight loss in older patients. The symptoms may be insidious and so annual screening for CF-related diabetes from the teenage years is essential. This is usually with an annual oral glucose tolerance test. Glucose is given orally with blood glucose measured immediately beforehand and after 2 h. In CF the 2-h level is characteristically raised. In most cases, treatment is with a long-acting insulin analogue such as glargine, which can be administered once daily.

Bones and joints

Cystic fibrosis patients are at risk of reduced bone mineral density because of malabsorption of vitamins D and K, reduced weight-bearing activity, oral steroid use and the effects of chronic infection. From the teenage years, screening should be done every 2 years using dual-energy x-ray absorptiometry. Treatment with vitamin D and calcium is sensible but not of proven benefit. Drugs such as alendronate may improve bone mineral density but have side-effects (such as bone pain) and little is known about their long-term effects (Conwell and Chang 2009).

A specific form of arthritis may be troublesome in patients with CF, often flitting from one joint to the next. This does not cause joint damage and usually responds to simple pain relief. In addition, the frequent use of ciprofloxacin may be associated with joint pain and if this occurs, the antibiotic should be stopped, where possible.

Fertility

Discussions about fertility should commence during adolescence, as part of an annual review (Lyengar and Coleman 2005). Most men with CF are infertile, due to agenesis of the vas deferens (the tube which carries sperm from the testis). However, sexual health advice should still include condom use. Men with CF can father children with specialised fertility treatment. Women with CF, contrary to many older textbooks, have normal fertility, provided they are not severely unwell and their lung function is stable.

The best predictors for pregnancy outcome in women with CF are FEV1 and Body Mass Index (BMI). There is an increased risk of mortality with pregnancy for women with CF who have a decline in lung function, weight and general nutritional status (Lyengar and Coleman 2005). Therefore preconceptual counselling should involve a discussion about the impact of pregnancy on a woman's general health.

Some of the issues that women with CF may face with pregnancy include adapting physiotherapy to a growing 'bump', life issues, i.e. living long enough to see their child grow up, and ultimately general wellbeing (Goddard and Bourke 2009). Goddard and Bourke (2009) also emphasise the need for caution when advising CF women about pregnancy but at the same time respecting their wishes.

Standards of care

It is clear from the above description of multisystem disease that effective care must be multidisciplinary, with a dedicated team comprising a doctor, specialist nurse, physiotherapist, dietician, social worker, psychologist, pharmacist, teacher, play specialist and administrative support. A number of important 'standards of care' documents have been produced with guidance for those providing and commissioning care (Cystic Fibrosis Trust 2001a,b, 2011; Kerem et al. 2005). There is an increasing and appropriate emphasis on quality improvement and recording patient data, confidentially, on national registries such as those in the US and the UK. These registries can measure improvements in survival year on year, allow comparison of outcomes between centres and identify patients who may be suitable to take part in clinical trials.

For both primary ciliary dyskinesia and cystic fibrosis, early diagnosis and timely identification of complications are essential. Careful multidisciplinary management will achieve the best outcome in terms of quality of life and survival. Children are often expected to undergo multiple therapies and any new treatment must be subject to a rigorous comparison with existing therapy so that children have a rational regimen which is as simple as possible. Therefore multidisiplinary working is paramount, including nursing support and care in the community to assist parents with simplifying treatment.

Physiotherapy and promoting independence

As discussed in Chapter 1, anatomical and physiological differences between the respiratory systems of children and adults have important consequences for the physiotherapy management of children with respiratory disease, in terms of assessment, treatment and choice of techniques. Assessment and treatment of young children, teenagers and young adults require skilful age-appropriate communication with the child, the family and within the multidisciplinary team.

It is essential to include the child, parents, relatives and carers as part of the care team. As age increases, the older child and then the teenager/young adult can be progressively more involved in the decision-making process. Children's awareness of the implications of illness and treatment develops as they grow older and they should be encouraged to take on more responsibility for their treatment. Teenagers, particularly, have a more sophisticated understanding and may be beginning to think about the future and the impact of chronic illness on school, social life and body image.

Respiratory assessment and examination

Assessment

Careful assessment is essential to identify problems requiring physiotherapy intervention. It is based on both a subjective and objective assessment and the results dictate the formulation of an appropriate treatment plan. For those requiring long-term intervention, regular assessment is required to evaluate the ongoing effectiveness of the treatment in relation to problems and goals (Middleton and Middleton 2008).

Discussion with medical staff, nursing staff and the parents/carers is essential to gain information about recent changes. In the acute situation, it is particularly important to ascertain how stable the child is: their ability to tolerate handling, the timing and modality (oral, nasogastric or intravenous route) of feeds and whether the child is sufficiently rested to tolerate a physiotherapy treatment if it is appropriate. Results of investigations and other relevant observations should be referred to as appropriate and relevant information gleaned from the observations charts as usual.

In chronically ill children who require home physiotherapy, good communication between the specialist and primary healthcare teams is essential.

Examination

Examination of the older child is similar to that of the adult. Other relevant observations such as the behaviour of a child can often give important clues about their respiratory status. Agitation or irritability may be a sign of hypoxia, while the child in severe respiratory distress may be withdrawn and lie completely still. It is also important to note muscle tone as there may be an increase in work of breathing and difficulty with coughing and expectoration in those with hypotonia. Hypertonia may also be associated with difficulty in clearing secretions. Abdominal distension may cause or exacerbate respiratory distress, as the diaphragm is placed at a mechanical disadvantage.

Airway clearance

Removal of bronchial secretions is considered to be the primary aim of airway clearance techniques. In the acute situation retained secretions may lead to airway obstruction and atelectasis. In chronic disease such as CF, recurrent infection and inflammation result in damage and destruction of the airways and the mucociliary escalator, as discussed previously; also, retained secretions cause an increase in airway resistance and obstruction.

Box 12.1   Airway clearance techniques

Active cycle of breathing techniques (ACBT)
Autogenic drainage (AD)
High-frequency chest wall oscillation (HFCWO)
Intrapulmonary percussive ventilation (IPV)
Oscillating positive expiratory pressure:

• Flutter®
• R-C Cornet®

Acapella
Positive expiratory pressure (PEP)
High positive expiratory pressure
Postural drainage and percussion

Over the past three decades several different airway clearance techniques (ACT) have been developed, all of which are reported to enhance mucus clearance and are advantageous in that they enable older children and adults to be independent in performing their treatment (Box 12.1). The general aim of all airway clearance techniques is to increase lung volume and enhance airflow. Some may also affect the rheological properties of mucus.

The majority of airway clearance studies have been undertaken in cystic fibrosis, where no single technique has been identified as being superior to others (Elkins et al. 2006b; Main et al. 2005; Morrison and Agnew 2009; van der Schans et al. 2000). A few other comparative studies have been undertaken in non-CF bronchiectasis but again have found little difference between the techniques investigated (Patterson et al. 2005, 2007).

Impaired cough as a consequence of weakness from neuromuscular disease (e.g. Duchenne muscular dystrophy and spinal muscular atrophy) can cause serious respiratory complications, including atelectasis, pneumonia, airway obstruction and acidosis (Miske et al. 2004). Chronic respiratory insufficiency and respiratory failure will ultimately result from chronic weakness of respiratory muscles, shallow breathing and ineffective cough. In these situations, independently performed airway clearance techniques may not be feasible but options such as the mechanical insufflation/exsufflation device ('cough assist') and other non-invasive forms of positive pressure ventilation appear to be safe and well tolerated, with a growing body of evidence to support their efficacy (Chatwin and Simonds 2009; Fauroux et al. 2007; Panitch 2006; Vianello et al. 2005).

Autogenic drainage

Autogenic drainage consists of a three-phase breathing regimen which can be performed in sitting or an appropriate postural drainage position (Schöni 1989). Mucus clearance is facilitated by the adjustment of tidal volume breathing during which the highest possible expiratory airflow is reached without causing airway closure. The three phases consist of a period of breathing at low lung volume when secretions are mobilised from the peripheral areas, followed by breathing at mid lung volume to 'collect' the mobilised secretions, and high lung volume breaths to clear and expectorate (IPGCF 2009; Pryor and Prasad 2008; Schöni 1989). Autogenic drainage should only be taught by an experienced therapist, skilled in the technique.

Active cycle of breathing techniques (ACBT)

The ACBT is a flexible breathing regimen consisting of breathing control, thoracic expansion exercises and the forced expiration technique (Pryor and Prasad 2008; Pryor et al. 1979). Breathing control is quiet, gentle breathing at the patient's own comfortable rate, keeping the upper chest and shoulders relaxed, and is used between the more active parts of the cycle to prevent any increase in airflow obstruction or tiredness. Thoracic expansion exercises are deep breathing exercises emphasising inspiration with a quiet and relaxed expiration. These exercises help to loosen bronchial secretions based on the concept of interdependence and increased collateral flow. The forced expiration technique consists of one or two 'huffs' interspersed with periods of breathing control.

High-frequency chest wall oscillation

High-frequency chest wall oscillation (sometimes know as high-frequency chest wall compression or vest therapy) has been used in the USA for many years but is now becoming more widely available. The equipment consists of an electric air compressor which is connected to an inflatable jacket which fits snugly over the thorax. The air pulse generator delivers intermittent positive pressure (pulses of air) into the jacket, which vibrate the chest wall at oscillatory frequencies of 5–20 Hz. Mucus clearance is facilitated by the airflow oscillation and vibration of the airway walls (Pryor and Prasad 2008; Warwick et al. 2004). A total treatment time of 20–30 min is usually recommended and nebulised hypertonic saline is often used during treatment, which is interspersed by episodes of huffing and coughing.

Intrapulmonary percussive ventilation

The intrapulmonary percussive ventilation (IPV) device consists of a high-flow generator, flow interruption valve and a breathing circuit to which a nebuliser may be attached. IPV delivers a continuous rapid burst of gas flow to the patient's airways via a mouthpiece or, where necessary, a mask or catheter mount. Three forms of therapy are provided during IPV: percussive oscillatory vibrations to loosen retained secretions, aerosol delivery to act as a mucolytic and positive expiratory pressure (PEP) to recruit alveolar lung units and assist in expiratory flow acceleration during a cough manoeuvre. The frequency of oscillation can be varied, as can the pressure. Short periods of breathing with IPV are interspersed with huffing and coughing to clear secretions (Newhouse et al. 1998; Pryor and Prasad 2008; Toussaint et al. 2003). Although IPV has been used in the home setting, it is better established for use in the acute setting, during admission.

Positive expiratory pressure

The application of positive expiratory pressure, applied via a facemask or mouthpiece, is believed to improve sputum clearance by its effect on peripheral airways and collateral ventilation. PEP causes an increase in lung volume, enabling air to move behind secretions, forcing them up the bronchial tree to the more central airways (Falk et al. 1984; Pryor and Prasad 2008).

The PEP mask system consists of a facemask and a one-way valve with inspiratory and expiratory ports (Figure 12.5). A resistor is attached to the expiratory port to achieve PEP. Treatment is performed in the sitting position with elbows on a table and the mask held firmly over the nose and mouth. Ten to twelve tidal breaths are taken through the mask with slight emphasis on expiration and followed by one or two huffs and coughing to clear secretions. The frequency and duration of treatment are adapted to the needs of the individual patient (average 10–20 min).

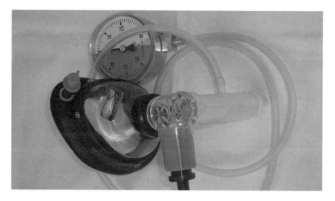

Figure 12.5   Positive expiratory pressure mask.

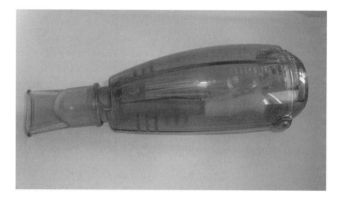

Figure 12.6   Acapella Choice.

Oscillatory positive expiratory pressure

Oscillating PEP devices combine an oscillation of the air within the airways during expiration simultaneously with a variable positive expiratory pressure (Cegla et al. 2002; Konstan et al. 1994; Patterson et al. 2007; Pryor and Prasad 2008). Various devices are available including the Acapella Choice (Figure 12.6) and the incentive spirometer (Figure 12.7). Although the devices differ in their mechanics, all are based on the same physiological principle. The combination of oscillations and intermittent PEP provides both a 'back-pressure', maintaining patency within the airways, and vibrations which enhance mucus clearance.

Postural drainage and percussion

Manual techniques such as percussion and vibrations are usually performed by a parent or assistant but can also be applied by the older child or adult themselves during thoracic expansion exercises (e.g. as part of the ACBT).

Postural drainage or gravity-assisted positioning and manual techniques such as chest percussion are used to assist the clearance of bronchial secretions. Postural drainage uses gravity to assist the drainage of secretions from the more peripheral to central airways (Eaton et al. 2007; Sutton et al.

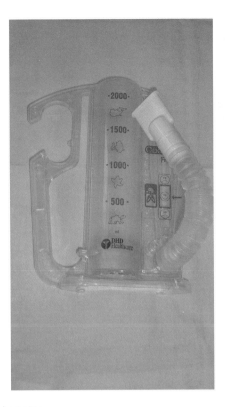

Figure 12.7   Incentive spirometer.

1983) although clearance of secretions is likely to be a result of both drainage and position-related alterations in ventilation (Lannefors and Wollmer 1992).

Postural drainage regimens traditionally included a head-down tipped position, although some studies have shown that secretion clearance is as effective in the flat side-lying position (Cecins et al. 1999) and concerns have also been raised regarding the association between a head-down tip position and gastro-oesophageal reflux (Button et al. 2003, 2004). The head-down tipped position is now far less commonly used in both paediatric and adult populations.

Exercise

Physical activity is an integral part of the physiotherapy regimen for all patients with any respiratory disorder and the benefits of exercise are listed in Box 12.2. In cystic fibrosis, several short-term studies have demonstrated the positive effects of regular physical activity which include increased cardiorespiratory fitness, improved exercise tolerance, reduction in breathlessness, improved performance in activities of daily living and an improved feeling of wellbeing. The long-term benefits of regular exercise include a reduction in the annual rate of decline in lung function, improvements in lung function, fitness and improved quality of life (Bradley and Moran 2008; van Doorn 2009; Wilkes et al. 2009).

It has been suggested that exercise could be used as a replacement for airway clearance in CF but it is generally agreed that when airway clearance is needed on a regular basis, it should be regarded

---

Box 12.2   Benefits of exercise

Improved cardiorespiratory fitness
Increased exercise tolerance
Decreased breathlessness
Improved respiratory muscle strength and endurance
Improved bone health
Improved quality of life
Increased self-esteem/body image/morale
Body composition

---

as complementary to rather than a replacement for it. Physical activity is, however, perceived by some patients with cystic fibrosis (particularly teenagers and adults) as rather different from other routine treatments and some may prefer it as a form of therapy which has multiple benefits and over which they have more control (Abbott et al. 1996).

Although the positive effects of exercise are clear, any benefits of a training programme are short-lived once exercise is discontinued. Sustaining the motivation and commitment required to maintain an adequate level of regular physical activity poses a challenge. Regular encouragement and support from the multidisciplinary team are essential. Varied exercise programmes based on realistic goals and utilising activities which the individual enjoys are more likely to succeed in the long term (Prasad and Cerny 2002).

Types of activity

The general principles of training are very similar to those used in the general population. In younger children it is not usually necessary to prescribe a specific training programme. Instead, children should be encouraged to participate fully in regular physical activity both in and out of school along with their healthy peers. Recommendations for exercise and advice should be individually tailored according to the goals required but any exercise programme should include the following components:

- aerobic (endurance) training
- resistance (strength) training
- anaerobic (sprint) training
- stretching and flexibility.

Physiotherapy management of babies and young children

Airway clearance

Traditionally, for airway clearance in infants and small children with respiratory conditions, including babies with CF, a daily routine comprised a regimen that consisted of postural drainage (with a head-down tip) and percussion. The use of the head-down tipped position is now infrequent but modified postural drainage and percussion remain widely used internationally.

Other techniques such as infant PEP and assisted autogenic drainage along with physical activity have emerged as very feasible alternatives in the infant population (Lannefors et al. 2003;

van Ginderdeuren et al. 2003), although there is no robust scientific evidence to support their use. Ideally treatment should occur before feeds or adequate time should be allowed following a feed to avoid problems associated with vomiting and aspiration.

The toddler stage is a period of transition when the child can begin to play a more active role in their treatment and a wider variety of treatment techniques are available for use. By the age of around 2 or 3 years, most children can begin to participate in breathing exercises in the form of play (using straws and cotton wool balls, party blowers, etc.). Following on from this, they can learn to 'huff' and perform more 'formal' breathing exercises. Forced expiration (huffing) is an important part of many airway clearance techniques modalities. Huffing and other breathing activities, such as blowing cotton wool and musical instruments, often form the basis of airway clearance at this age. By the age of 4 or 5 most children can begin to use some of the independently performed techniques described above, albeit with constant and close supervision.

It is important that when treatment is necessary, it is given. Even when difficulties arise it is important to persevere, as co-operation with treatment in future years may be influenced by how things are handled in the toddler years. In chronic disorders, it is essential that a child learns from an early age that physiotherapy is going to play a significant role in their life. Encouraging the child to play an active role in their care and trying to make activities as much fun as possible are essential to keep the child engaged. For example, positive expiratory pressure can be given in the form of bubble PEP, using a system whereby the child blows through a column of water (to the level of PEP required) with a flexible tube (e.g. suction tubing). Adding a small amount of detergent and/or food colouring increases the novelty of treatment.

Physical activity

The importance of regular physical activity in those with chronic disease such as CF should not be underestimated, not only for cardiorespiratory benefits but also for bone health, muscle strength and posture. Physical activity also has several potential benefits to the respiratory system, including altering patterns of regional ventilation to promote ventilation and the enhancement of airway clearance.

Activity can be encouraged through play as the child gets older. Although babies cannot exercise themselves, physical activities should be encouraged from the very beginning. General play activities such as bouncing (e.g. on a Swiss ball) and rolling on a mat can be used even in infants.

Physiotherapy management of older children and teenagers

Airway clearance

A wide range of airway clearance modalities is available for use in older children and these have been described earlier. In the more acute situation, the choice of technique will depend on the presenting signs and symptoms. The general principles are the same as those that apply to adults and the usual considerations and contraindications apply.

In those children who require regular airway clearance for chronic respiratory conditions such as CF, primary ciliary dyskinesia and non-CF bronchiectasis, the formulation of an airway clearance regimen should be based on individual assessment of clinical status and other factors such as age, social circumstances and patient preference.

Children should be reasonably independent in performing airway clearance by the age of 10–12 years, although this does vary depending on the individual, and initially some supervision and support will continue to be needed. Several factors influence a child's willingness and ability to take on the responsibility of treatment and the decision regarding how much and how soon they should begin to be independent in treatment will vary considerably between individuals. Children need time to gain confidence in taking on a greater degree of responsibility while the parents often need even more time to relinquish it; this will be explored further next as part of the transition process.

The performance of routine daily airway clearance in those with chronic respiratory disorders requires considerable time and can impose a significant burden on patients and families. Adherence to routine airway clearance in chronic illness is known to be poor (Arias Llorente et al. 2008; Bucks et al. 2009; Gudas et al. 1991) and the teenage and adolescent years can pose a particular challenge in this respect.

It is therefore most important that the child is involved in discussions and decisions about their therapy from as early an age as appropriate. Continual education in the reasons for and importance of treatment with honest and open discussion regarding the family's and child's ability to cope with the burden of care are essential. As children grow older and want to lead a full and independent life, it is important that they understand the need for treatment and the potential consequences of not doing treatment. This time of transition is also difficult for parents as their ability to influence the teenager's behaviour may change and they realise that they have to 'hand over' their responsibilities. Patient preference is likely to be another important consideration when choosing an appropriate technique.

Other than postural drainage and percussion, all the airway clearance modalities described above are designed to be performed without any assistance. Both the ACBT and autogenic drainage consist purely of breathing techniques and therefore no equipment is necessary. PEP and oscillatory PEP systems are small, lightweight and easily portable. The only issue is that they do need to be kept clean and dry. High-frequency chest wall oscillators (vest systems), although still relatively portable, are somewhat more cumbersome to transport. 'Sleep-overs' and school trips often present a good opportunity for testing independence with treatment. By the time of transition to adult care, the teenager should be fully independent with their airway clearance regimen.

Young people and exercise

Exercise recommendations or programmes, if required, should be individually tailored for the older child and adolescent. Adolescence is known to be a time when physical activity levels fall, particularly in girls. In CF this has been shown to be accompanied by a decline in respiratory status (Selvadurai et al. 2004; Schneiderman-Walker et al. 2005). It is essential that great attention is paid to exercise during this time. The importance of exercise in terms of health status must be emphasised and older children encouraged and supported by the team to continue to participate in regular activity. Recommendations for activities and the general principles of exercise training have been discussed above and participation in regular physical activity should be strongly encouraged into the adult years.

In those with chronic respiratory disease, the physiotherapy regimen should be reviewed on a regular basis and changes made as appropriate. In addition to airway clearance and exercise, attention should also be paid to other issues such as musculoskeletal problems (posture and bone health) and urinary incontinence (Dodd and Webb 2008).

Summary

As previously stated, the ultimate aim for young people is to encourage independence with physiotherapy, in order to promote good quality of life. The transition process poses many problems including that of compliance with physiotherapy for young people with long-term respiratory conditions.

Nursing management for cystic fibrosis

Cystic fibrosis is in the main a challenging disease for parents, who are constantly dealing with the uncertainty and the unpredictable nature of the disease. Parents are also living with the possibility that their child could die early (Bush 2002).

The early part of the chapter alluded to CF as a complex and multisystem disease. In order to care for children with this long-term condition, consideration needs to be given to the impact of the disease on each individual's life and the treatment options available. This section will consider the nursing support required for children and families living with CF and the care pathways available.

The modernisation agenda now mandates that care should be provided as close to home as possible. For many children with CF, this pathway of care is divided between the teams at a specialist CF centre and a local district general hospital.

This pathway is also supported by standards of care which are used as a benchmark for best practice. Practice also reflects a family-centred approach, for patients and their families, who become experts about their condition.

Standards of care

Rapid change throughout health has produced quality assurance frameworks for all healthcare professionals to use as guidance for clinical care. The specialist team needs to be skilled in CF management and ensure that good communication is key. Therefore sufficient time for multidisciplinary team meetings is also paramount (Cystic Fibrosis Trust 2001a) as these meetings give the opportunity to share patient information in a structured and confidential manner.

It is also important to maintain standards within primary care for patients with long-term conditions. Connett (2005) stresses the importance of including professionals in primary care, particularly the general practitioner (GP), in the management of patients from diagnosis. This would also include the provision of adequate information for the GP with, for example, antibiotic prescribing. This can be facilitated by providing GPs with a copy of local CF management guidelines.

The internet provides a huge source of information for families. However, the ideal for families is to access experts in order to ensure that information is accurate and consistent. Therefore an informative and structured approach is needed by professionals. This can assist families to understand the disease process and the care that is required, particularly at key times, as listed in Box 12.3.

Box 12.3   Stressful events for CF carers

Diagnosis
First time in hospital for IV treatment
Starting nursery/school/college
Secondary diagnosis, i.e. CF-related diabetes
Transition
Fertility/pregnancy
Transplant assessment/surgery
Terminal care

Diagnosis

Ideally it is helpful for the nurse specialist to be present at the consultation when the family are given the diagnosis. It is important for professionals to create an appropriate environment and sufficient time for the family. It is also important for the family that professionals do not deliver too much information at once. For many families, how they are introduced to the diagnosis is often one of the most important points, which will be remembered.

National guidance on the management of children and adults with CF produced in 2001, now superseded by the second edition in 2011, also places emphasis on parental feelings that arise on diagnosis of a child with a life-limiting condition. These feelings are often compared to those experienced with the loss of a healthy baby. Therefore, it is essential to offer ongoing support for parents, which is often provided by the nurse specialist and other members of the care-giving team.

The role of the cystic fibrosis nurse specialist

With survival rates increasing daily, care needs to be provided by a specialist team. The concept of such care is to provide screening opportunities so that early diagnosis and treatment will take place, allowing respiratory infections to be treated before lung damage occurs (Murray et al. 1999). Equally important is good nutritional status and ensuring that parents of children with CF recognise that there must be a low threshold for instigating antibiotic treatment. Therefore nursing management is based on the fundamental need for a nurse who has specialist knowledge of CF (Cystic Fibrosis Trust 2001a).

The CF nurse specialist has an important role acting as a facilitator and advocate for care management and patients' wellbeing (Cystic Fibrosis Trust 2001a). Ward-based nurses who work closely with the multidisciplinary team also need to be aware of all treatment regimens, in order to support families with ongoing care. When patients are admitted to the ward for treatment, parents need to feel confident that nurses have sufficient knowledge to provide the necessary care that is required for their child.

When caring for children and families with CF, nurses face many challenges to provide support and guidance. Throughout their life-long management, the nurse specialist will become the key worker for the families. The nurse specialist is also a good resource for nurses caring for children in both primary and secondary care. They can help colleagues to understand the complexities involved in the management of children and young people with CF.

Difficulties can also arise when nurse specialists need to find a balance between acknowledging the burden of care and assisting carers to manage the complex nursing procedures. This is often required to enable the family to carry out day-to-day activities such as administering nebulised antibiotics. The nurse will have the responsibility of educating and assessing the level of confidence and competence of parents and carers to ensure that the standard expected is maintained within the home environment.

Other examples of standards of care in practice include the nurse specialist working closely with nurses in district general hospitals, by providing education and acting as a resource to nurses who do not have the same level of specialist knowledge but are able to manage the children and families effectively at local level. There are many complexities and demands for nurses when caring for CF patients both on a practical and emotional level. Consequently it is vital to develop good working relationships with local teams and the team at the specialist centre.

Decision-making skills are a major part of the overall management for nurses. In order to promote and maintain standards of care, specialist nurses will also educate and empower young people, school nurses and health visitors. This will aid understanding so that care can be given adequately and safely, particularly when support is needed with non-adherence.

Adolescence and cystic fibrosis

The aim of care for adolescents is to encourage shared decision making. Individuals with CF want to be seen as a person first and a patient second. Therefore nurses need to be aware of the importance of non-verbal communication skills. When communicating with young people, for example, it is vital to ensure that the young person's opinions are being considered.

When difficulties with carrying out treatment become apparent, the nurse should always consider the problem using a non-judgmental approach. The difficulties faced by young people living with CF on a daily basis are not only health related; other factors such as body image, in particular with delayed puberty, can cause young people a great deal of anxiety and affect their general well-being. Situations like this require the nurse specialist and multidisciplinary team to work with young people through any difficulties they may be facing with their health and wellbeing.

Young people also require sufficient preparation for transition to adult services. The CF nurse specialist is pivotal in initiating the process that includes a framework for promoting independence. Each area will naturally devise a model of care for transition to suit local need. The CF team's focus is about supporting young people not only with fostering independence but also with preparation for transfer to adult services. The process of transition and various models will be discussed further in Chapter 14. However, when managing young people with such complex care, consideration needs to be given to the most appropriate method and the best time for this to occur.

Many areas have adopted the concept of transition clinics, where professionals attend from both adult and paediatric services. This enables the young person and parents to meet new individuals and become familiar with a new way of accessing services. Preparation is the key component for a successful transition. The parents may also need a lot of support to help them come to terms with 'letting go'.

The nurse also needs to consider a variety of methods when dealing with young people. Using skills of assessment, in order to recognise signs of respiratory deterioration, nurses can provide current knowledge and information on coping strategies to young people about their condition.

Promotion of self-care

The nurse specialist also supports young people through other difficulties such as conflicts with parents or problems with school attendance due to ill health as a result of poor adherence to treatment. It may be necessary to provide education about living with CF and managing in school or college. This will hopefully facilitate the continuation of their education. With permission from the parents and the young person, communicating with school can help to increase awareness about CF amongst education professionals.

Constant reinforcements about treatment and encouragement to take control of their own treatment regimen are always required for young people with CF. The nurse specialist is often involved with assisting young people to create a holistic treatment plan which they can be responsible for, thus promoting independence. For example, creating a chart to aid compliance with the use of favourite football teams.

Parents will also be assisted by the nurse specialist to find coping strategies to deal with psychological issues. However, nurses need to be aware that sometimes parents' coping mechanisms can obstruct treatment (Maddison 2005). This may be because of a parent's inability to carry out physiotherapy, for example due to a physical injury. With a sympathetic, non-judgemental approach from professionals, this situation can be remedied. A physiotherapist can provide an assessment of not only the child but also the parents' capabilities. In most centres this occurs at every clinic appointment and annual review. Utilising a holistic approach enables ongoing assistance with the emotional impact of a CF diagnosis for a family, which will be explored further in Chapter 16.

Summary

Nurses caring for children and families with CF need to understand the impact of the burden of care on the family unit as a whole. It is also vital to have empathy and sufficient knowledge in order to support the children and young people with CF, throughout their life-long health journey.

Care in the community

The concept of care and management in the community for chronic respiratory conditions has been expanding not only in the UK but throughout the world (Sequeiros and Jarad 2009). From a social policy perspective, acts such as *The New NHS: modern, dependable* (Department of Health 1997) set the political agenda based on the ideology of care in the community for those who are disadvantaged. The Community Care Act (Department of Health 1990) also set the agenda for service provision in the UK (Long 2003).

The government states that patients should be allowed to have care that is best suited to them and their family. For many years services provided by children's community nurses (CCNs) have enabled children to stay at home for as long as possible (Walsh and Crumbie 2007). In the 21st century most children now have access to CCNs (Department of Health 2011). Consequently we have seen that nurses are pivotal to supporting families at home with children requiring complex nursing care.

The intention of the modernisation agenda is to aim for provision of systematic high-quality care. This emphasis of care in the community is based on partnership in care, currently illustrated by care management for many long-term conditions. More recently the Department of Health (2011) has described how CCNs can be part of specialist service delivery.

Aims of care in the community

Many complex care procedures (Box 12.4) are the norm for some children with CF. The aim is for nurses to provide appropriate training for parents on many procedures, prior to discharge home. This training will also be continued by the nurse, who is the key worker within the community. When visiting patients at home, the nurse also has a responsibility to ensure that professional boundaries are maintained.

Primary/secondary care: working in partnership

Effective communication between primary and secondary care is vital for supporting patients with long-term conditions (Walsh and Crumbie 2007). This ongoing management in the community requires the involvement of the GP. It is also necessary to provide the required information for the GP to increase their understanding of the treatment regimen and justify the need for often expensive

---

Box 12.4 Treatment carried out at home

Education: medication
Training: prior to oxygen therapy and enteral feeding
Gastrostomy care
Home intravenous antibiotics
Physiotherapy; nebulisers; inhalers

drugs required to treat infections (Pennell 2005). Therefore meetings involving the care-giving team are paramount to facilitate the process of sharing information.

The GP has an important role in the care of children with CF in the community. Many GPs are involved with families at the time of a suspected diagnosis, before their visit to the CF centre. Initially the main role of the GP is to provide repeat prescriptions. However, it is important that the family builds a rapport with their GP, because the care-giving team is very much reliant on the GP to provide support for families in the long term.

Ultimately the family will need the GP alongside the care-giving team to provide the appropriate support at different times (Pennell 2005). This support can be important in situations such as terminal care at home. Often CF centres are some distance from home for many families. The use of GP services to collect microbiology samples such as sputum specimens is also helpful for families. Consequently the CF team needs to acknowledge that their service has limitations, making it crucial to develop relationships with general practice.

Quality of life issues

The aim of managing children with CF is to strive for good health within the remits of the treatment regimens, and some quality of life for the child and family. Kappler et al. (2009) maintain that the complexities of the disease process and rigorous treatment prevent patients from achieving a normal quality of life.

It is essential for nurses to recognise that education is paramount for those agencies involved in the care of children with CF. This often requires school visits from the nurse specialist, who can dispel any myths and misconceptions about CF. It also provides the opportunity for nurses to give teachers a thorough explanation about the need for snacks in school, along with enzyme supplements known as Creon capsules.

The UK Disability Discrimination Act (2005) provides the legal framework for individuals who are disadvantaged, including those with special health needs. Schools have a legal responsibility to provide an education for children with complex health needs. With the permission of the child and family, help can be provided by the nurse specialist with informing peers about their CF. However, sometimes this is not taken up due to fear of bullying. Although it may be beneficial to the child or young person for their peers to have a better understanding about living with CF, the wishes of the family need to be respected.

When a child's condition has progressed to a point where they are considered to have severe lung disease, they will often require oxygen therapy. In this situation the nurse specialist will communicate with the school to ensure that the necessary equipment and treatments are provided in school. This will enable children with CF to continue with their education (Maddison 2005). There are also times when it may be necessary for the child or young person to have home tuition if their physical health deteriorates and they are not able to attend school full time. This would be discussed with the family, education and the team caring for the child or young person, to create a plan of education around the child's health needs.

Home intravenous therapy

Parents who opt for home care require support, training and written information (Mighten 2007). For many years CF patients have had the choice of taking intravenous (IV) antibiotics at home. In order for this care to be delivered safely, risk assessment must be carried out. This assessment involves giving consideration to the appropriateness of the home environment, including the personal safety of employees when undertaking a home visit (Mighten 2007; Pennell 2005).

Box 12.5   Consideration for homecare (adapted from Maddison 2005)

Advantages of home care

Minimise the risk of cross-infection from other CF patients
Keeps the family together
Finances: less travel expenditure

Disadvantages of home care

Less input from members of the hospital team, i.e. doctors, dietician
Decreased level of treatment
Stress; increased burden of care

Steps to ensure success of home care

Assessment of home environment
Practical assessment under supervision; community support, i.e. nurses, physiotherapists
Necessary requirements: telephone, transport to get back to the hospital

---

Assessment of the home environment very much determines the success of home IV therapy (Box 12.5). Therefore when preparing patients for discharge home, it is important that ward nurses communicate with the care-giving team, to ensure that the nurse specialists and the CF team are aware of the situation.

The nurse assessing the parent has a responsibility to highlight the problems associated with home IV antibiotics and provide adequate information for parents to enable them to manage these problems, which include potential anaphylaxis, line blockage and needle dislodgement from portacaths.

There are times when the child may need a hospital admission. This needs to be made very clear in the initial discussion prior to home IV therapy. It is also necessary to communicate clearly that home IV therapy is not an easy option. This is largely due to the fact that families need to continue with other aspects of everyday life, including:

• lack of sleep
• family commitments, i.e. caring for other siblings
• household chores
• continuation of other treatment in addition to IV therapy.

However, home IV therapy is not suitable for all so it is essential that certain criteria are achieved prior to discharge home (Mighten 2007) as well as consideration of the burden of care and the appropriate delegation of such complex procedures to parents. An overall assessment of each individual family's circumstances, as suggested by Maddison (2005), is vital. If parents do not meet the criteria for assessment listed in Box 12.6, these are all good reasons why such complex treatment should not be carried out within the home environment. This is supported by Sequerios and Jarad (2009), who suggest that patients should be selected appropriately.

The nurse carrying out the practical assessment will need to ensure that competence and confidence are attained. This will be done before home IV therapy is undertaken without professional supervision, to ensure safety of the patient (Mighten 2007). Naturally, each area will have its own policy for assessing competency to administer antibiotics at home. Updating skills for parents and reference to the policy need to be revisited each time treatment is undertaken at home to ensure competency is constant.

Box 12.6   Home IV selection criteria

Literacy skills	Competency assessment
Numeracy skills	Successfully met training criteria
Manual dexterity	Home environment suitable
Compliance with treatment	Good eyesight

Monitoring patients having treatment at home is also vital. Antibiotic treatment is an important part of CF management but physiotherapy and good nutrition are also part of the package and equally important (Maddison 2005). Sequeiros and Jarad (2009) highlight concerns that home IV care for CF patients is less effective than hospital care. Therefore the ability to provide support and monitoring by various members of the care-giving team in the community is important, to ensure that there is consistency between home and hospital care. The ultimate aim of monitoring patients at home is to provide the best possible clinical outcome.

Nurses and physiotherapists in some areas will monitor the overall condition of children with CF having home IV treatment. Lung function, weight and crucially compliance with treatment will be assessed throughout the course of treatment. Without such monitoring, care cannot be considered to be similar to that provided in hospital. Therefore the benefits of home care for some patients are questionable, as suggested by Gilchrist and Lenny (2009).

Summary

Home care is now a significant part of the modernised health service. With more choice available for patients, it is paramount that nurses provide constant reinforcement, support and guidance when providing care in the community (as illustrated in the case study).

Case study

Jo was a 15-year-old girl diagnosed at 18 months with CF. Her care was transferred from a previous level one centre, where the family received shared care with their local district general hospital.

Past medical history

Jo had previously received her first course of IV antibiotic treatment at the age of 5. Prior to coming to her new centre she had IVs every 3 months. At the first consultation it was evident that she had severe chronic lung disease. Her lung function was FEV1 37%, FVC 52% predicted, oxygen saturation levels 94% in air, weight 46.9 kg, height 156 cm, both on the 50th centile.

The first approach was to optimise Jo's care which required addition of more treatment. It was also essential to give consideration to the importance of building relationships with Jo and her family, in order for treatment to be carried out effectively.

Within 6 months of transferring to her new centre, a glucose tolerance test identified that Jo also had CF-related diabetes which meant that she need to start on a small amount of insulin. Jo also had a BMI of 18 kg/m², which highlighted the need for insertion of a gastrostomy button to improve her nutritional status. A portacath for regular venous access to give frequent IV antibiotics would also be inserted at the same time.

Ultimately support was needed for Jo and her parents to cope with the huge psychological impact of Jo's rapid decline and a second diagnosis. In addition to the huge burden of care, even more support was necessary for her mother who is hearing impaired.

To add to an already complex situation, it became apparent that it was necessary to broach the subject of transplant assessment. The initial priority was to address all the physical needs and give Jo and her family time to come to terms with the changes to her situation.

Once they had adjusted to all the new treatment regimens, it was appropriate to have the discussion about lung transplantation. Jo and her family also received continual support from the social worker and psychologist. This enabled the family to come to terms with the changes to their daughter's health.

After surgery had taken place for the gastrostomy and portacath, Jo experienced a difficult post-operative period. She required a period in the high-dependency unit and needed non-invasive ventilator support. Despite a long list of treatments there was no improvement in her condition. Therefore following this episode it was felt that the time was right to broach the subject of transplant assessment.

Following discharge, support was provided at home by nurses and the physiotherapist for Jo and her parents. It was necessary to reinforce all the treatment regimens again, such as care of the gastrostomy, nebuliser therapy and how to use the non-invasive ventilator to assist with respiratory function which is often used as a bridge to transplantation. The physiotherapist provided continual support at home with the ventilator.

Weekly visits from the nurses and physiotherapist continued. This provided the family with the opportunity to ask questions about what the process of lung transplantation would entail.

Jo's time at home was very limited because of a chest infection which had to be treated in hospital for 3 weeks. During this time Jo became totally dependent on oxygen with minimal ability to walk long distances. She therefore needed to use a wheelchair and would need to go home on oxygen therapy 24 h a day. This required liaison with the oxygen company to ensure that the oxygen supply was provided throughout the house. Using liquid oxygen for ambulatory use enabled Jo to have some quality of life outside the home environment.

In addition, consideration had to be given to her continued education and how oxygen therapy was going to be facilitated at school, including all the health and safety elements. Following the necessary training, it was arranged with school for her attendance to be limited to 2 h a day. Help and support were also provided in school by a teaching assistant, to help Jo with the wheelchair and oxygen cylinders.

Therefore continued support from the social worker for Jo and her parents was necessary to reinforce how much Jo's condition had deteriorated and the issue of mortality. The overall aim was to prepare Jo both physically and psychologically for what the process of transplantation would entail. A referral was made to the transplant referring centre.

Following her first consultation with the transplant centre, Jo was placed on the transplant list. Within 6 months she successfully received a lung transplant. However, she did develop complications (post-transplant lymphophoproliferative disease, discussed in Chapter 13).

Conclusion

The value of a multidisciplinary approach to care and management cannot be underestimated. With advances in technology it is vital that nurses and other healthcare professionals understand and appreciate the huge burden of care experienced by families living with CF.

Questions

Answer true or false.

1. In primary ciliary dyskinesia:
   a. inheritance is autosomal recessive in most cases
   b. the diagnosis is often made late
   c. all patients have dextrocardia and situs inversus
   d. the diagnosis may be made by newborn screening
   e. respiratory distress in the newborn is an important diagnostic clue.

2. In the diagnosis of primary ciliary dyskinesia:
   a. the test can be done in most hospital laboratories
   b. the test requires a blood sample
   c. the diagnosis can only be made if none of the cilia are moving
   d. electron microscopy may be helpful
   e. measurement of nitric oxide may be helpful.

3. Which of the following are true of the genetics of cystic fibrosis?
   a. CF is an autosomal dominant condition.
   b. Mutations in both copies of the CF gene are needed for an individual to be affected.
   c. Genetic testing is the only reliable way of making a diagnosis.
   d. Genetic testing is included in the UK newborn screening programme.
   e. Genetic testing can help in antenatal diagnosis.

4. Which of the following are true of the diagnosis of cystic fibrosis?
   a. Antenatal diagnosis is possible.
   b. The sweat test is outdated and no longer used.
   c. Without a positive genetic test, the diagnosis cannot be certain.
   d. Newborn screening is routine in the UK.
   e. Newborn screening uses an immune reactive trypsin test.

5. Which of the following are complications of cystic fibrosis?
   a. Diabetes
   b. Inflammatory bowel disease
   c. Reduced bone mineral density
   d. Liver disease
   e. Cardiomyopathy

6. In the treatment of cystic fibrosis lung disease:
   a. physiotherapy is given only during admissions to hospital
   b. nebulised antibiotics are used to treat chronic *P. aeruginosa* infection
   c. regular sputum and cough swab samples should be taken to guide antibiotic treatment
   d. prophylactic antibiotics against *Staph. aureus* are given to young children
   e. *P. aeruginosa* does not cause lung damage or symptoms.

7. Which of the following refer to nutrition in CF?
   a. Pancreatic enzyme supplements can be given.
   b. Children with CF should have 80% of the recommended calorie intake.
   c. Children with CF are at high risk of obesity.
   d. Gastrostomy feeds should never be used.
   e. Treatment is rarely needed in the first year of life.

8. Which of the following refer to infection in CF?
  a. Influenza vaccine should not be given.
  b. Infection with *P. aeruginosa* should be eradicated as soon as it appears.
  c. The lungs may develop an allergic response to *Aspergillus fumigatus*.
  d. Intravenous antibiotics are rarely needed.
  e. Azithromycin may reduce the number of symptomatic exacerbations.

References

Abbott J, Dodd M Webb AK. (1996) Health perceptions and treatment adherence in adults with cystic fibrosis. *Thorax* **51**, 1233–8.

Arias Llorente RP, Bousoño García C, Díaz Martín JJ. (2008) Treatment compliance in children and adults with cystic fibrosis. *Journal of Cystic Fibrosis* **7**, 359–67.

Bradley JM, Moran F. (2008) Physical training for cystic fibrosis. *Cochrane Database of Systematic Reviews* **1**, CD002768.

Brennan AL, Geddes DM, Gyi KM, Baker EH. (2004) Clinical importance of cystic fibrosis-related diabetes. *Journal of Cystic Fibrosis* **3**, 209–22.

Bucks RS, Hawkins K, Skinner TC, Horn S, Seddon P, Horne R. (2009) Adherence to treatment in adolescents with cystic fibrosis: the role of illness perceptions and treatment beliefs. *Journal of Pediatric Psychology* **34(8)**, 893–902.

Bush A. (2002) Cystic fibrosis: cause, concern and treatment. In: Bluebond-Langer M, Lask B, Angst D (eds) *Psychosocial Aspects of Cystic Fibrosis*. London: Arnold.

Bush A, Chodhari R, Collins N, *et al.* (2007) Primary ciliary dyskinesia: current state of the art. *Archives of Disease in Childhood* **92**, 1136–40.

Button BM, Heine RG, Catto-Smith AG, *et al.* (2003) Chest physiotherapy in infants with cystic fibrosis: to tip or not? A five-year study. *Pediatric Pulmonology* **35(3)**, 208–13.

Button BM, Heine RG, Catto-Smith AG, *et al.* (2004) Chest physiotherapy, gastro-oesophageal reflux, and arousal in infants with cystic fibrosis. *Archives of Disease in Childhood* **89(5)**, 435–9.

Cecins NM, Jenkins SC, Pengelley J, Ryan G. (1999) The active cycle of breathing techniques – to tip or not to tip? *Respiratory Medicine* **93**, 660–5.

Cegla UH, Jost HJ, Harten A, *et al.* (2002) Course of severe COPD with and without physiotherapy with the RC–Cornet®. *Pneumologie* **56(7)**, 418–24.

Chatwin M, Simonds AK. (2009) The addition of mechanical insufflation/exsufflation shortens airway clearance sessions in neuromuscular patients with chest infection. *Respiratory Care* **54(11)**, 1473–9.

Cheng K, Ashby D, Smyth R. (1999a) Oral steroids for cystic fibrosis. *Cochrane Database of Systematic Reviews* **4**, CD000407.

Cheng K, Ashby D, Smyth R. (1999b) Ursodeoxycholic acid for cystic fibrosis-related liver disease. *Cochrane Database of Systematic Reviews* **3**, CD000222.

Colombo C, Battezzati PM, Crosignani A, *et al.* (2002) Liver disease in cystic fibrosis: a prospective study on incidence, risk factors, and outcome. *Hepatology* **36**, 1374–82.

Connett G. (2005) Respiratory care. In: Peebles A, Maddison J, Gavin J, Connett G (eds) *Cystic Fibrosis Care: a practical guide*. London: Elsevier Churchill Livingstone.

Conwell LS, Chang AB. (2009) Bisphosphonates for osteoporosis in people with cystic fibrosis. *Cochrane Database of Systematic Reviews* **4**, CD002010.

Coren ME, Meeks M, Morrison I, Buchdahl RM, Bush A. (2002) Primary ciliary dyskinesia: age at diagnosis and symptom history. *Acta Paediatrica* **91**, 667–9.

Cystic Fibrosis Trust. (2001a) *National Consensus Standards for the Nursing Management of Cystic Fibrosis*. London: UK Cystic Fibrosis Nurse Specialist Group.

Cystic Fibrosis Trust. (2001b) *Standards for the Clinical Care of Children and Adults with Cystic Fibrosis in the UK*. London: Cystic Fibrosis Trust.

Cystic Fibrosis Trust. (2011) *Standards for the Clinical Care of Children and Adults with Cystic Fibrosis in the UK*, 2nd edn. London: Cystic Fibrosis Trust.

Department of Health. (1990) Community Care Act. London: HMSO.

Department of Health. (1997) *The New NHS: modern, dependable*. London: HMSO.

Department of Health. (2011) *NHS at Home: community children's nursing services*. London: Department of Health.

Dodd ME, Webb AK. (2008) Bronchiectasis, primary ciliary dyskinesia and cystic fibrosis. In: Pryor JA, Prasad SA (eds) *Physiotherapy for Respiratory and Cardiac Problems*, 4th edn. Edinburgh: Churchill Livingstone, pp. 550–90.

Donaldson SH, Bennett WD, Zeman KL, Knowles MR, Tarran R, Boucher RC. (2006) Mucus clearance and lung function in cystic fibrosis with hypertonic saline. *New England Journal of Medicine* **354**, 241–50.

Eaton T, Young P, Zeng I, Kolbe J. (2007) A randomized evaluation of the acute efficacy, acceptability and tolerability of flutter and active cycle of breathing with and without postural drainage in non-cystic fibrosis bronchiectasis. *Chronic Respiratory Disease* **4**, 23–40.

Elkins MR, Robinson M, Rose BR, *et al.* (2006a) A controlled trial of long-term inhaled hypertonic saline in patients with cystic fibrosis. *New England Journal of Medicine* **354**, 229–40.

Elkins M, Jones A, van der Schans CP. (2006b) Positive expiratory pressure physiotherapy for airway clearance in people with cystic fibrosis. *Cochrane Database of Systematic Reviews* **2**, CD003147.

Ellerman A, Bisgaard H. (1997) Longitudinal study of lung function in a cohort of primary ciliary dyskinesia. *European Respiratory Journal* **10**, 2376–9.

Falk M, Kelstrup M, Andersen JB, *et al.* (1984) Improving the ketchup bottle method with positive expiratory pressure, PEP, in cystic fibrosis. *European Journal of Respiratory Disease* **65(6)**, 423–32.

Fauroux B, Guillemot N, Aubertin G, *et al.* (2007) Physiologic benefits of mechanical insufflation-exsufflation in children with neuromuscular diseases. *Chest* **133(1)**, 161–8.

Gilchrist FJ, Lenny W. (2009) A review of the home intravenous antibiotic service available to children with cystic fibrosis. *Archives of Disease in Childhood* **94(8)**, 647.

Goddard J, Bourke JS. (2009) Cystic fibrosis and pregnancy. *Obstetrician and Gynaecologist* **11(1)**, 19–24.

Gudas LJ, Koocher GP, Wypij D. (1991) Perceptions of medical compliance in children and adolescents with cystic fibrosis. *Journal of Developmental Behavioural Pediatrics* **12**, 236–42.

International Physiotherapy Group for Cystic Fibrosis (IPGCF). (2009) Physiotherapy in the treatment of cystic fibrosis. Available at www.cfww.org/ipg–cf/article/195/Physiotherapy_in_the_Treatment_of_CF.

Jones AP, Wallis CE, Kearney CE. (2003) Dornase alfa for cystic fibrosis. *Cochrane Database of Systematic Reviews* **3**, CD001127.

Kappler M, Kinderlink U, von Haunersches K. (2009) Cystic fibrosis: between normality and disability. *Monatsschrift fur Kinderheilkunde* **157(2)**, 121–8.

Karadag B, James AJ, Gultekin E, Wilson NM, Bush A. (1999) Nasal and lower airway level of nitric oxide in children with primary ciliary dyskinesia. *European Respiratory Journal* **13**, 1402–5.

Kerem E, Reisman J, Corey M, Canny GJ, Levison H. (1992) Prediction of mortality in patients with cystic fibrosis. *New England Journal of Medicine* **326**, 1187–91.

Kerem E, Conway S, Elborn S, Heijerman H. (2005) Consensus Committee. Standards of care for patients with cystic fibrosis: a European consensus. *Journal of Cystic Fibrosis* **4**, 7–26.

Konstan MW, Stern RC, Doershuk CF. (1994) Efficacy of the Flutter device for airway mucus clearance in patients with cystic fibrosis. *Journal of Pediatrics* **124**, 689–93.

Langton Hewer SC, Smyth AR. (2009) Antibiotic strategies for eradicating Pseudomonas aeruginosa in people with cystic fibrosis. *Cochrane Database of Systematic Reviews* **4**, CD004197.

Lannefors L, Wollmer P. (1992) Mucus clearance with three chest physiotherapy regimes in cystic fibrosis: a comparison between postural drainage, PEP and physical exercise. *European Respiratory Journal* **5(6)**, 748–53.

Lannefors L, Dennersten U, Theander K, Jartensson J, Kornfalt R. (2003) Successful treatment of infants and small children. *Journal of Cystic Fibrosis* **2**, S65–S250.

Long A. (2003) Caring in the community: a nursing perspective. In: Basford L, Slevin O. (2003) *Theory and Practice of Nursing: an integrated approach to caring practice*, 2nd edn. London: Campion Press.

Lyengar S, Coleman M. (2005) Fertility. In: Peebles A, Maddison J, Gavin J, Connett G (eds) *Cystic Fibrosis Care: a practical guide*. London: Elsevier Churchill Livingstone.

Maddison J. (2005) Organisation of CF sevices; from national levels to home care. In: Peebles A, Maddison J, Gavin J, Connett G (eds) *Cystic Fibrosis Care: a practical guide.* London: Elsevier Churchill Livingstone.

Main E, Prasad A, van der Schans CP. (2005) Conventional chest physiotherapy compared to other airway clearance techniques for cystic fibrosis. *Cochrane Database of Systematic Reviews* 1, CD002011.

Middleton S, Middleton PG. (2008) Assessment and investigation of patients' problems. In: Pryor J, Prasad SA (eds) *Physiotherapy for Respiratory and Cardiac Problems*, 4th edn. Edinburgh: Churchill Livingstone, pp. 1–21.

Mighten J. (2007) Home intravenous therapy training for carers of children and young people. *British Journal of Nursing* **6(5)**, 272–6.

Miske LJ, Hickey EM, Kolb SM, *et al.* (2004) Use of the mechanical in-exsufflator in pediatric patients with neuromuscular disease and impaired cough. *Chest* **105**, 741–7.

Morrison L, Agnew J. (2009) Oscillating devices for airway clearance in people with cystic fibrosis. *Cochrane Database of Systematic Reviews* 1, CD006842.

Muller F, Simon-Bouy B, Girodon E, *et al.* (2002) Predicting the risk of cystic fibrosis with abnormal ultrasound signs of fetal bowel: results of a French molecular collaborative study based on 641 prospective cases. *American Journal of Medical Genetics* **110**, 109–15.

Multi-Disciplinary Working Group. (2003) *Guidelines for the Performance of the Sweat Test for the Investigation of Cystic Fibrosis in the UK*. Birmingham: Birmingham Children's Hospital.

Murray J, Cuckle HS, Taylor G, Littlewood J, Hewson J. (1999) Screening for CF. *Health Technology Assessment* **3(8)**.

Newhouse PA, White F, Marks JH, Homnick DN. (1998) The intrapulmonary percussive ventilator and flutter device compared to standard chest physiotherapy in patients with cystic fibrosis. *Clinical Pediatrics (Philadelphia)* **37**, 427–32.

O'Callaghan C, Chetcuti P, Moya E. (2010) High prevalence of primary ciliary dyskinesia in a British Asian population. *Archives of Disease in Childhood* **95**, 51–2.

Panitch HB. (2006) Airway clearance in children with neuromuscular weakness. Pulmonology. *Current Opinion in Pediatrics* **18(3)**, 277–81.

Patterson JE, Bradley JM, Hewitt O, Bradbury I, Elborn JS. (2005) Airway clearance in bronchiectasis: a randomized crossover trial of active cycle of breathing techniques versus Acapella. *Respiration* **72(3)**, 239–42.

Patterson JE, Hewitt O, Kent L, Bradbury I, Elborn JS, Bradley JM. (2007) Acapella versus 'usual airway clearance' during acute exacerbation in bronchiectasis: a randomized crossover trial. *Chronic Respiratory Disease* **4(2)**, 67–74.

Pennell S. (2005) Primary care. In: Peebles A, Maddison J, Gavin J, Connett G. (2005) *Cystic Fibrosis Care: a practical guide*. London: Elsevier Churchill Livingstone, pp. 255–8.

Polnay JC, Davidge A, Lyn UC, Smyth AR. (2002) Parental attitudes: antenatal diagnosis of cystic fibrosis. *Archives of Disease in Childhood* **87**, 284–6.

Prasad SA, Cerny FJ. (2002) Factors that influence adherence to exercise and their effectiveness: application to cystic fibrosis. *Pediatric Pulmonology* **34(1)**, 66–72.

Pryor JA, Prasad SA. (2008) Physiotherapy techniques. In: Pryor JA, Prasad SA (eds) *Physiotherapy for Respiratory and Cardiac Problems*, 4th edn. Edinburgh: Churchill Livingstone, pp. 134–218.

Pryor JA, Webber BA, Hodson ME, Batten JC. (1979) Evaluation of the forced expiration technique as an adjunct to postural drainage in treatment of cystic fibrosis. *British Medical Journal* **2**, 417–18.

Saiman L, Marshall BC, Mayer-Hamblett N, *et al.* (2003) Azithromycin in patients with cystic fibrosis chronically infected with Pseudomonas aeruginosa: a randomized controlled trial. *Journal of the American Medical Association* **290**, 1749–56.

Schneidermann-Walker J, Wilkes DL, Strug L, *et al.* (2005) Sex differences in habitual physical activity and lung function decline in children with cystic fibrosis. *Journal of Pediatrics* **147(3)**, 321–6.

Schöni MH. (1989) Autogenic drainage: a modern approach to physiotherapy in cystic fibrosis. *Journal of the Royal Society of Medicine* **82(suppl 16)**, 32–7.

Selvadurai HC, Blimkie CJ, Cooper PJ, Mellis CM, van Asperen PP. (2004) Gender differences in habitual activity in children with cystic fibrosis. *Archives of Disease in Childhood* **89**, 928–33.

Sequeiros IM, Jarad A. (2009) Home intravenous antibiotic treatment for acute pulmonary exacerbations in cystic fibrosis – is it good for the patient? *Ann Thorac Med* **4(3)**, 111–14.

Smyth AR. (2008) Respiratory disorders: cystic fibrosis. In: McIntosh N, Helms P, Smyth R, Logan S (eds) *Forfar and Arneil's Textbook of Paediatrics*, 7th edn. Edinburgh: Churchill Livingstone, pp. 1227–39.

Smyth A, Walters S. (2003) Prophylactic antibiotics for cystic fibrosis. *Cochrane Database of Systematic Reviews* **3**, CD001912.

Stannard WA, Chilvers MA, Rutman AR, Williams CD, O'Callaghan C. (2010) Diagnostic testing of patients suspected of primary ciliary dyskinesia. *American Journal of Respiratory and Critical Care Medicine* **181**, 307–14.

Sutton PP, Parker RA, Webber BA, *et al.* (1983) Assessment of the forced expiration technique, postural drainage and directed coughing in chest physiotherapy. *European Journal of Respiratory Diseases* **64**, 62–8.

Toussaint M, de Win H, Steens M, Soudon P. (2003) Effect of intrapulmonary percussive ventilation on mucus clearance in Duchenne muscular dystrophy patients: a preliminary report. *Respiratory Care* **48**, 940–7.

UK Newborn Screening Programme Centre. (2010) The national standard protocol for CF screening. Available at: http://newbornbloodspot.screening.nhs.uk/nat_std_cf_protocol.

Van Ginderdeuren F, Malfroot A, Verdonk J, Vanlaethem S, Vandenplas Y. (2003) Influence of assisted autogenic drainage (AAD) and AAD combined with bouncing on gastro-oesophageal reflux (GOR) in infants under the age of 5 months. *Journal of Cystic Fibrosis* **2(suppl 1)**, A251.

Van der Schans CP, Prasad A, Main E. (2000) Chest physiotherapy compared to no chest physiotherapy for cystic fibrosis. *Cochrane Database of Systematic Reviews* **2**, CD001401.

Van Doorn N. (2009) Exercise programs for children with cystic fibrosis: a systematic review of randomized controlled trials. *Disability and Rehabilitation* **26**, 1–9.

Vianello A, Corrado A, Arcaro G, *et al.* (2005) Mechanical insufflation–exsufflation improves outcomes for neuromuscular disease patients with respiratory tract infections. *American Journal of Physical Medicine and Rehabilitation* **84(2)**, 83–8.

Walsh M, Crumbie A. (2007) *Watson's Clinical Nursing and Related Sciences*, 7th edn. London: Elsevier.

Warwick WJ, Wielinski CL, Hansen LG. (2004) Comparison of expectorated sputum after manual chest physical therapy and high-frequency chest compression. *Biomedical Instrumentation and Technology* **38**, 470–5.

Wilkes DL, Schneiderman JE, Nguyen T, *et al.* (2009) Exercise and physical activity in children with cystic fibrosis. *Paediatric Respiratory Reviews* **10**, 105–9.

Chapter 13

Lung transplantation in children

Helen Spencer[1] and Katherine Carter[2]

[1] *Consultant in Transplant and Respiratory Medicine*
[2] *Advanced Nurse Practitioner, Transplant Team, Great Ormond Street Hospital for Children, London*

Learning objectives

By the end of the chapter the reader will understand:

- the challenges faced by the patient and family throughout the transplant journey
- the indications and contraindications for transplant
- the nursing care during each stage of the journey.

Introduction

This chapter will give an overview of paediatric lung transplantation. There will be a discussion about the difficulties in deciding the optimal time to list a patient for transplant. Also the assessment process, waiting on the list and the perioperative and long-term shared care of the transplant patient will be described.

Lung transplantation is now an established therapeutic option for children with end-stage pulmonary disease. The first paediatric lung transplant was carried out in 1986 and since then improvements in surgical techniques, intensive care management and immunosuppressive treatment have led to improvements in results. However, unlike other solid organ transplants, long-term survival following lung transplantation remains elusive for most, with international reported 5-year median survival of just over 50% (Aurora et al. 2009). Thus, transplantation is not a cure and has been described by some families as merely trading one chronic medical condition for another. Whether lung transplantation provides a survival benefit remains controversial but it can certainly improve quality of life of the patient and their families (Wray et al. 1992). The International Society for Heart and Lung Transplantation (ISHLT) has reported that 1200 paediatric lung and 550 heart-lung transplants have been completed worldwide since the registry was first established in 1983 (Wray et al. 1992). Approximately 80–90 paediatric lung transplants are carried out annually worldwide, with 8–10 of those carried out in the UK (Aurora et al. 2009).

Indications for lung transplantation

The ISHLT first published guidelines for the selection of adult and paediatric transplant recipients in 1998, and these were updated in 2006 (Maurer et al. 1998; Orens et al. 2006). Although no separate formal paediatric guidelines have been published as evidence-based recommendations are lacking, a consensus statement from the American Society of Transplantation on paediatric lung transplantation is available (Faro et al. 2007).

It is important that children who may benefit from transplantation are referred for assessment in a timely fashion. There remains a shortage of suitable donors and patients may wait for over 2 years to receive a suitable organ. If referred too late, patients may miss their opportunity for transplant and die on the waiting list or become too sick for transplant. Early referral allows children and families time to gain insight into the realities of what having a transplant involves and allows a considered, informed decision-making process to occur which includes the patient, family and multidisciplinary transplant team. Patients may be re-evaluated on several occasions to try and optimise the timing of listing for transplant. The timing of listing remains a difficult decision with the goal of conferring the most survival benefit from transplantation. Patients are usually listed for transplant when they have a predicted 2-year mortality of 50%.

The indications and selection of transplant recipients vart from centre to centre, as do the contraindications to transplant, although there is a move certainly in the UK to establish national referral and acceptance criteria. Paediatric lung transplantation is currently carried out in two paediatric centers in the UK: Great Ormond Street Hospital, London, and the Freeman Hospital, Newcastle. The most common diagnoses of patients undergoing lung transplantation include cystic fibrosis and idiopathic pulmonary hypertension; a more detailed list of diagnoses leading to transplantation is shown in Table 13.1 (Aurora et al. 2009).

Patient selection

Currently in the UK, only children over the age of 3 years or 100 cm in height may be considered and are funded for transplantation, although transplantation of younger patients may be considered in the UK in the future following expanding experience and encouraging results from a few centres in the USA (Elizur et al. 2009).

General considerations

There are a number of generally agreed criteria for paediatric lung transplant.

- End-stage or progressive pulmonary disease or pulmonary vascular disease.
- Patient is declining despite maximal medical therapy and is at risk of dying without transplant.
- Patient has a poor quality of life.
- Patient and family are informed and consent to transplant.
- Patient and family are able and agree to adhere to rigorous surveillance required following transplant.

Disease-specific selection criteria

There are some guidelines regarding specific criteria for transplantation for particular diseases such as cystic fibrosis (CF) and pulmonary hypertension (PHT) (Galiè et al. 2009; Kerem et al. 1992). However, there are few or no data to guide listing criteria for other diagnoses, and even for CF, there

Table 13.1   Indications for paediatric lung transplant (January 1990 to June 2008) (reprinted with permission from Elsevier)

Diagnosis	Age <1 year Number %	Age 1–5 years Number %	Age 6–11 years Number %	Age 12–17 years Number %
Cystic fibrosis	2 2.4%	5 5.1%	124 53.0%	547 69.2%
Idiopathic pulmonary arterial hypertension	11 13.4%	22 22.2%	25 10.7%	60 7.6%
Retransplant: obliterative bronchiolitis (OB)	–	6 6.1%	8 3.4%	25 3.2%
Congenital heart disease	21 25.6%	8 8.2%	4 1.7%	10 1.3%
Idiopathic pulmonary fibrosis	4 4.9%	8 8.1%	10 4.3%	26 3.3%
Obliterative bronchiolitis (not retransplant)	–	9 9.1%	10 4.3%	29 3.7%
Retransplant: not OB	3 3.7%	2 2.0%	7 3.0%	18 0.6%
Interstitial pneumonitis	6 7.3%	11 11.1%	1 0.4%	5 0.6%
Pulmonary vascular disease	8 9.8%	5 5.1%	7 3.0%	1 0.2%
Eisenmenger's syndrome	1 1.2%	5 5.1%	5 2.1%	6 0.8%
Pulmonary fibrosis, other	1 1.2%	1 1.0%	7 3.0%	11 1.4%
Surfactant protein B deficiency	11 13.4%	4 4.0%	–	–
Chronic obstructive pulmonary disease/ emphysema	5 6.1%	2 2.0%	2 0.9%	6 0.8%
Bronchopulmonary dysplasia	2 2.4%	2 2.0%	6 2.6%	–
Bronchiectasis	–	–	4 1.7%	9 1.1%
Other	7 8.5%	9 9.1%	14 6.0%	39 4.9%

have been a number of changes in the medical treatment resulting in improved survival without transplant, making these guidelines somewhat out of date. Disease-specific criteria which are considered prior to listing for transplant are shown in Table 13.2.

What type of transplant?

As part of the assessment process, the transplant team will decide whether a patient is suitable for a bilateral lung transplant or if they will need a heart-lung transplant. In the early days of

Table 13.2   Disease-specific criteria to consider when listing for transplant

Disease	Factors to consider when listing for transplant
All diseases	Poor quality of life
Cystic fibrosis	FEV1 < 30% Hypoxia PaO$_2$ < 7.3 kPa (55 mmHg) Hypercapnia PaCO$_2$ > 7.3 kPa (55 mmHg) Use of non-invasive ventilation Rapid deterioration in FEV1 Female sex Young age Pulmonary hypertension Recurrent pneumothorax Severe haemoptysis Frequent hospitalisations
Idiopathic pulmonary arterial hypertension	Despite maximal vasodilator therapy WHO functional class III or IV 6-min walk test <330 metres Decreasing exercise tolerance Syncope Haemoptysis Absence of left ventricular dysfunction (if present, will need heart-lung transplant)
Eisenmenger's syndrome	Decreasing exercise tolerance
Pulmonary veno-occlusive disease	No medical treatment available and poor prognosis – list when diagnosed
Surfactant protein deficiency	Surfactant protein B and ABCA3 deficiency – at diagnosis Surfactant protein C deficiency – when deteriorating

WHO, World Health Organization.

thoracic transplant, it was usual for patients to receive a heart-lung transplant, with CF patients often then donating their own heart for transplant (domino procedure). However, in the last decade bilateral lung transplantation has become the procedure of choice. Indeed, very few heart-lung transplants are now carried out and because of the donor organ shortage, most blocks will be separated in order to benefit more patients. If the patient needs a heart-lung block (i.e. patients with pulmonary hypertension and left ventricular failure, Eisenmenger's syndrome or complex congenital heart disease), the chances of receiving suitable organs are very small. Living lobar donation has been proposed as an alternative to bilateral lung or single transplantation and is carried out in some centres in the USA and Japan but is completed rarely and only in adults in the UK.

Timing of listing

The timing of listing for transplantation is the most difficult decision to make. The main aim of transplantation is to prolong life with the secondary aim of improving quality of life. A number of factors must be taken into account when making the decision to list, including prediction of prognosis without transplant, patient height, blood group, average waiting time for donor organs and patient quality of life. Shorter, younger patients, blood group other than AB and patients who need a heart-lung block usually wait longer for a suitable donor. It is very important to consider each individual case carefully, taking into account each individual's rate of disease progression to try and predict their prognosis without transplant. The potential risks and benefits of transplantation for each individual must be considered before committing a child to transplant.

There remains some controversy around the survival benefits of lung transplantation. A number of studies have shown definite evidence of survival benefit following lung transplantation, including one from our own centre (Aurora et al. 1999; Hosenpud et al. 1998). However a study published in 2007 suggested that very few children transplanted for cystic fibrosis in the United States over a 10-year period had any survival benefit (Liou et al. 2007). The international transplant community responded firmly to this and pointed out a number of problems with the study, including the high 5-year survival rate on the waiting list (57%) (Aurora et al. 2008). At that time in the USA, organs were allocated to patients who had waited the longest and did not take into account clinical need. It is likely that patients were listed too early for transplant in order to accrue time on the waiting list and may have been transplanted too early. The USA donor allocation system was changed in 2005 with the introduction of the lung allocation score (LAS) for patients 12 years and older. The LAS takes into account those who have the poorest predicted survival without transplant and the best predicted post-transplant survival. This new system appears to have reduced waiting list times and waiting list mortality but patients with higher LAS scores have increased short-term mortality (Yusen et al. 2010).

Currently the tools for predicting prognosis without transplantation are inadequate, and the decision about when to list remains an imperfect one.

Contraindications to lung transplant

The absolute contraindications to lung transplantation are relatively few but there are a number of relative contraindications which need to be taken into consideration when assessing patient suitability for transplant (Box 13.1). It may be that a patient has a number of relative contraindications which would make transplant too high a risk to undertake.

Box 13.1   Absolute and relative contraindications to paediatric lung transplantation

Absolute contradictions

Malignancy within 2 years
Infection
Acute sepsis
Human immunodeficiency virus
Chronic active hepatitis B
Hepatitis C with histological evidence of liver disease
Burkholderia cenocepacia (genomovar 3)
Active tuberculosis
Multiorgan dysfunction
Severe or progressive neuromuscular disease
Severe thoracic scoliosis/deformity
Refractory non-adherence to treatment
Severe psychiatric illness

Relative contraindications

Invasive ventilation
Malignancy within 5 years
Multiple or pan-resistant organisms
Non-tuberculous mycobacterium
Fungal
Gram-negative bacteria
Methicillin-resistant *Staph. aureus*
Severe osteoporosis
Non-adherence to treatment
Poorly controlled insulin-dependent diabetes
Abnormal Body Mass Index <18 or >25
Other organ dysfunction (particularly kidney)
High-dose steroids (>20 mg/day)
Systemic disease, e.g. collagen vascular disease

The lung transplant assessment process

A careful multiprofessional assessment of the child referred for lung transplantation is an essential part of the lung transplant journey. The main aims of the assessment process are:

- for the transplant team to establish whether the child is suitable for and needs a lung transplant either at this stage or in the future
- for the child and family to find out more about lung transplant so they can make an informed decision about whether lung transplant is something they want now or in the future.

The assessment is completed over a 3–4-day period and involves a number of tests and investigations, a detailed clinical assessment of the child by the lung transplant consultant, a nursing assessment and meeting with the child and family, a psychosocial assessment of the child and family, a multiprofessional meeting to discuss the findings of the assessment and finally a meeting with the child and family to explain the outcome (Table 13.3, Box 13.2). The successful communication of all the key information that the child and family need to make an informed decision about lung transplant is critical.

The nursing assessment and consultation

Early in the lung transplant assessment, either the advanced nurse practitioner or one of the clinical nurse specialists meets with the child and family. At the outset, the specialist nurse's aim is to gain sufficient information about the child and family to help them individualise the consultation and assessment process. The key information the specialist nurse will need to establish early in the consultation includes the following.

- What do the child and family understand about the reason for their visit to the transplant centre?
- What do they already know about lung transplant?
- How do the child and parents perceive the child's illness and quality of life at present?
- What do they understand about the prognosis without transplant?

Depending on the age of the child being assessed, the nurse may meet with them separately. This meeting usually takes place after the nurse has met with the parents, giving the nurse the opportunity to negotiate with the family what information to give to the child at this stage.

Table 13.3 Investigations completed as part of transplant assessment

Department	Tests
Haematology	Full blood count Clotting screen Blood group and antibody screen
Biochemistry	Renal function Liver function Bone profile Fasting glucose, cholesterol and triglycerides Glomerular filtration rate
Serology	Cytomegalovirus Hepatitis B + C Epstein–Barr virus Measles Rubella HIV Toxoplasma Herpes simplex 1 + 2 Varicella
Microbiology	Nose and throat swabs Sputum culture Sputum culture for non-tuberculous mycobacterium
Radiology	Chest x-ray Combi CT scan chest DEXA bone density scan Ultrasound scan abdomen
Lung function	Spirometry Lung volumes by plethysmography 6-minute walk test 3-minute step test VO_2 maximal exercise testing for selected patients
Cardiac	Electrocardiogram Echocardiogram
Special tests	Anti-HLA antibodies (panel reactive antibodies)
Other medical examinations	Ear, nose and throat consultant review Dental review Hearing test

CT, computed tomography; DEXA, dual-energy x-ray absorptiometry; HLA, human leucocyte antigen.

What information is given to the child and family?

Information regarding the life expectancy and long-term outcomes after lung transplantation along-side the risks and benefits of lung transplant is given to the parents and child (if they are old enough) early in the assessment. Survival in children after lung transplant at Great Ormond Street Hospital is over 80% at 3 years, approximately 60% at 5 years and 50% at 7 years. The risk for the individual patient may be more or less than this depending on their diagnosis and presence of other co-morbidities and risk factors.

Box 13.2   Key aspects of the transplant assessment process

Professionals involved in multidisciplinary transplant team

- Lung transplant consultant
- Specialist nurses: advanced nurse practitioner and clinical nurse specialists
- Cardiothoracic surgeon
- Psychologist
- Social worker
- Dietician
- Dentist
- Ear, nose and throat consultant
- Physiotherapist
- Radiologist
- Anaesthetist
- Microbiologist
- Infectious disease consultant

Key components of assessment for lung transplantation

- Child and family meet members of the multiprofessional team
- Clinical assessment including examination and investigations
- Assessment and consultation with a clinical nurse specialist or advanced nurse practitioner
- Assessment and consultation with a clinical psychologist
- Assessment and consultation with a social worker if required
- Multiprofessional meeting to discuss individual case suitability for transplant
- Final meeting with the family to discuss multidisciplinary team decision

---

The common complications and causes of death following transplant are discussed, including infection, acute rejection, poor function of the transplanted lungs, chronic rejection, renal impairment and increased risk of malignancy.

This information is hard for the family to hear and needs to be communicated with sensitivity. The referring team may not have discussed life expectancy, either with or without transplant, prior to the assessment. The information about limited life expectancy may come as a huge shock to the family, affecting their capacity to take in further information at this stage.

The nurse needs to explain to the family that the reason for undertaking lung transplant is not just to extend the child's life but to improve their quality of life. Transplant may not be suitable for the child, or the family and child may decide that they do not wish to proceed with this option. However, if it is something they want and they are suitable, the specialist lung transplant team need to make the difficult decision as to the optimal time to put the child on the transplant waiting list. This decision needs to take into account the child's current quality of life, life expectancy without a lung transplant, the waiting time for a suitable organ as well as the child's life expectancy and quality of life after lung transplant. The specialist nurse needs to try to convey to the family the importance of taking all these things into consideration when making a decision about their child's need for lung transplant and why, so that they are fully informed of the assessment process.

How the child's quality of life is likely to improve also needs to be explained. For example, a child with cystic fibrosis may be breathless at rest, have limited exercise tolerance, use a wheelchair and may require an enormous amount of care, with continuous oxygen therapy, non-invasive ventilation, strict regime of physiotherapy, multiple nebulisers and regular admissions to hospital for intravenous antibiotics, as discussed in Chapter 12. They would be considered to have a fairly poor quality of life. After lung transplant, they will no longer need the above treatment and within the

---

Box 13.3   Key messages that the specialist nurse needs to communicate to the child and family about lung transplant during the assessment

- Lung transplant is not a cure and life expectancy remains limited.
- Quality of life significantly improves after lung transplant in most lung transplant recipients, enabling them to undertake most activities of a normal child of their age.
- The shortage of donor organs means there is no guarantee that if a child is listed for a lung transplant a suitable donor will become available in time and the child may die on the transplant waiting list.
- Families may find having their child on the transplant waiting list very stressful.
- Crucial importance of taking lifelong immunosuppressive treatment.
- The family must be able to perform and commit to the rigorous follow-up care and monitoring required after transplant.

---

first few months following lung transplant, they will be able to go back to school and engage in most normal activities with their peer group. Families may find it difficult to adjust to having a healthy child who is no longer completely dependent on them. Most patients will remain on a large number of oral medications that they will need to take for the rest of their lives. The child and family need to be committed to a lifelong routine of taking immunosuppression for the prevention of organ rejection, and other medications, and this has to be clearly explained to them at assessment.

The lung transplant patient journey is explained in detail by the specialist nurse. This includes information about the process of listing, waiting time on the transplant list, the unpredictability of the timing of transplant and the shortage of donor organs, the night or day of transplant, the inpatient stay, the protocol for long-term follow-up and hopefully the transition to an adult centre.

The transplant team's responsibility is to try and give the child and parents all the information that they need in an understandable and unhurried way to enable the child and family to make an informed decision about lung transplantation (Box 13.3).

Psychosocial assessment

This part of the assessment is undertaken by either a clinical psychologist or a social worker or both, depending on the child and family being assessed.

The aims of the consultation and assessment are to establish the following.

- The family structure, including the extended family and the ages of the immediate family.
- What other support networks do the child and parents have other than the family?
- Are one or both parents working or are they on income support? If so, what benefits are they receiving?
- How do the family cope with having a sick child, practically, financially and psychologically?
- How do the child and parents see the child's quality of life currently?
- How do both the child and family cope with the child's current medical regimen of treatment, outpatient appointments and inpatient admissions to hospital?
- Are the child and parents able to adhere to the demands of the child's current treatment regime?
- Are there any indicators of a lack of adherence to current or previous treatment?
- Do the child and family demonstrate coping strategies that may be useful for them in the future if the child undergoes a lung transplant?
- What is the child's and parents' understanding of lung transplant?
- Is lung transplant something that the child and parents want?

As part of the assessment, the psychologist also asks the child and parents to fill in a questionnaire based on a number of quality of life (QOL) and other psychological inventory measures. This gives us baseline data on how both the child and their parents perceive their QOL as well as other information about how the child and parents are coping at this point and the coping strategies that they employ.

There may be financial implications for the family following transplant which the family should be made aware of. It is likely that benefits such as high-level disability living allowance (DLA) will be lost after transplant and families need to consider the cost implications of travel and loss of earnings resulting from frequent visits to the transplant centre after transplantation.

Assessment outcome

There may be a number of different outcomes following the assessment after review by the multi-disciplinary team (MDT) which include:

- patient suitable for transplant and should be listed immediately
- patient suitable for transplant but not sick enough; to be reassessed in a suitable time frame
- patient has a contraindication and is not suitable for transplant
- patient needs further medical treatment, psychological or other input and should be reassessed for suitability
- patient and family do not wish to proceed with transplantation.

The MDT decision is discussed with the family as the final part of the assessment process. The family may need some time to reflect and consider their own decision about proceeding to listing for transplant. As long as the family are informed, then the final decision about proceeding to transplant is up to them.

Listing for lung transplantation and donor allocation

If after lung transplant assessment the conclusion of the multi-professional team is that the child needs a transplant and the child and/or the parents want the child to be listed for a lung transplant then the child will be registered with UK Transplant. UK Transplant (UKT) is part of the NHS blood and Transplant authority (NHSBT) and all recipients and potential donors from the UK need to be registered with UKT. Transplant donors and recipients need to be matched for blood group, height and occasionally tissue typing if recipients have anti-Human Leucocyte Antigens (HLA) antibodies. Donors are allocated according to the matching criteria. At Great Ormond Street Hospital, if there is more than one suitable recipient then the sickest patient will be transplanted first. If there are no differences in the clinical status of potential recipients then organs are allocated to the patient who has been waiting the longest.

Care of the patient on the transplant waiting list

It is very important to try and optimise the well being of the patient on the transplant waiting list. Medical co-morbidities must be treated appropriately, these may include diabetes, osteoporosis and gastroesophageal reflux. Corticosteroids may impair wound and anastamosis healing after transplant and should therefore be reduced to the lowest dose to keep a patient stable. Nutrition should be optimised with the aim of maintaining a normal body mass index. Particular attention should be paid to maintaining good renal health, with avoidance of renal toxic medication (in anticipation of reduced renal function after transplant).

Procedural anxiety and needle phobia are often identified at the transplant assessment and it is important that these issues are addressed by a local psychologist or play specialist prior to transplantation.

At the time of transplant assessment viral serology is checked, if patients are at risk of infections they should be immunised prior to listing where possible and blood should be taken afterwards to ensure an adequate vaccine response.

Patients should continue their usual medical management and remain under the care of the local team. Once listed, patients will be seen by the transplant centre every 6 months for a booster visit when patients are reassessed clinically, listed height and weight may be adjusted (NHSBT register), blood group and antibody screen is repeated and management is reviewed.

Unfortunately some patients will deteriorate whilst awaiting transplant and it is important that they are seen and treated by the symptom control care team at an appropriate time. It may be helpful if the family wishes, for the child to be removed from the transplant list to facilitate the focus on end of life issues. This should be discussed on an individual basis with the transplant team.

Nursing care of the lung transplant patient

The inpatient stage of the lung transplant patient journey involves:

- urgent admission of the child for lung transplant
- lung transplant surgery
- early post lung transplant stay on the intensive care unit (ICU)
- transfer to the ward for recovery, education and preparation for discharge
- discharge to the patient hotel and then home.

The average length of stay at the specialist centre post lung transplant is 4 weeks (range 3–12 weeks).

Nursing care of the pretransplant patient

The specialist transplant nurses co-ordinate the lung transplant which may occur at any time during a 24-h period. When a suitable organ becomes available, the child and family are transferred to the specialist transplant centre. They may only have 15–30 minutes' notice prior to transport arriving to take them to the transplant centre, which is why the child and family need to be carefully prepared at the time of the assessment. The child should be nil by mouth from the point at which the child and family are informed about the transplant.

The process of preparation for theatre needs to be rapid and well co-ordinated. The child needs to have bloods taken, baseline observations, normal preoperative checks, administration of immunosuppression, a brief clinical assessment, assessment by the anaesthetist and consent obtained from the child and parents by the surgeon. Details of the co-ordination, organ retrieval, organ preservation and the transplant surgery are beyond the scope of this book.

The donor lungs are usually implanted by the surgeon while the child is on cardiopulmonary bypass. When the surgery is complete and the patient is stable, they are transferred to the ICU. A detailed handover from the surgical and anaesthetic team is essential. Information about the donor should not be shared by the transplant co-ordinator unless it is of relevance to the recipient's postoperative recovery, ensuring that confidentiality is maintained at all times as discussed in Chapter 15.

Nursing care of the early post lung transplant patient

Key skills and knowledge that a nurse requires to care for an early post lung transplant patient include:

- ICU nursing skills (while the patient is in ICU)
- clinical assessment skills (discussed generally in Chapter 3)

Box 13.4   Postoperative nursing management of lung transplant patient

- Nursing assessment and monitoring of the patient
- Effective immunosuppression of the patient to prevent rejection
- Minimising the risk of infection due to the immunosuppression
- Optimising the function of the newly implanted donor lungs
- Physiotherapy, positioning and early mobilisation
- Optimising other organ function, in particular the kidneys
- Support of the child and family during the stress of lung transplant and intensive care unit stay
- Education of the child and family to prepare them for discharge

---

Box 13.5   Induction and maintenance immunosuppression

Induction therapy

Basiliximab – a monoclonal antibody that binds to the interleukin-2 receptor antibodies on T-cells. The aim of using a monoclonal antibody is to selectively remove all the T-cells that are most likely to cause rejection. Two doses are given: one on the confirmation of transplant and the second on day 4 post transplant.

Methylprednisolone – a corticosteroid that causes a rapid, transient reduction in peripheral blood lymphocytes. It also inhibits T-cell proliferation, T-cell-dependent immunity and the expression of genes coding for interleukins 1, 2 and 6. Methylprednisolone is given in very high doses as an induction agent.

Maintenance therapy

Tacrolimus or iclosporin –calcineurin inhibitors that inhibit T-cell stimulation. Tacrolimus has superseded ciclosporin as the first-line calcineurin inhibitor. It can be given intravenously or orally. The first dose is given preoperatively and then intravenously for the first few days post transplant. Tacrolimus is then given twice daily lifelong.

Mycophenolate mofetil (MMF) or azathioprine – cell cycle inhibitor that interferes with DNA, RNA and purine, thereby inhibiting proliferation of T- and B-lymphocytes. MMF is initially given intravenously on return from theatre but can be given orally as soon as the patient is absorbing. MMF is given twice daily.

Corticosteroid – once the patient is absorbing, the methylprednisolone is changed to daily oral prednisolone. Patients are weaned to a maintenance dose (0.1–0.2 mg/kg).

- knowledge of lung transplantation and immunosuppression medication
- good communication skills.

The ICU and ward nurses should undertake careful assessment of the respiratory, cardiovascular, renal and gastrointestinal systems, as well as assessing the level of consciousness and pain of the post lung transplant patient (Box 13.4).

Effective immunosuppression of the patient to prevent rejection

The main aim perioperatively is to establish effective immunosuppression to prevent early acute rejection of the donor lungs by the recipient's immune system. The immunosuppression that is given pre- and intraoperatively is termed induction therapy and that given postoperatively and long term is called maintenance therapy (Box 13.5). Patients are required to take immunosuppressant medication lifelong after transplant. It is very important that the drugs are taken regularly every day. The calcineurin inhibitor tacrolimus has a narrow therapeutic index – at low levels it is ineffective and at high levels it is toxic. Therefore drug levels are checked very frequently immediately after transplant and should be checked every 6 weeks long term. There are a number of side-effects seen with the drugs taken regularly after transplant (Table 13.4). There are a number of drugs that can interact with the immunosuppressant medication and may either increase or decrease levels. Interactions should be checked before starting any new medication.

Minimising the risk of infection

The induction therapy and other immunsuppressants given perioperatively significantly increase the risk of infection early post lung transplant. Strategies to minimise the risk of infection to the patient at this stage are vitally important and include the following.

- Isolation – patients need to be nursed in a cubicle; visitors are restricted to parents and only essential staff for the first 2 weeks.
- Handwashing – thorough handwashing by all staff and visitors will reduce the incidence of infection.
- Perioperative intravenous antibiotics – using the individualised patient protocol.
- Antimicrobial prophylaxis – prophylactic antibiotics, antifungal and antiviral agents.
- If the recipient is cytomegalovirus (CMV) positive or if there is a CMV mismatch (donor is CMV positive and recipient is CMV negative), give intravenous ganciclovir.
- Care of surgical wound site – the 'clam shell' incision is covered by a clear surgical wound dressing for the first week post transplant so any signs of infection can be observed easily. After a week the wound can be exposed if it is clean and dry.

Infection is an important cause of morbidity and mortality following lung transplant and patients are carefully monitored for signs of infection. Patients should have a full infection screen if signs of an infection develop.

Optimising the function of the newly implanted donor lungs

The lung transplant recipient will be intubated and ventilated on return from theatre and for the first few hours postoperatively but the aim is to extubate them as quickly as possible within the first 24 h. They remain ventilated until postoperative bleeding is controlled, the patient is stable and the transplant and ICU teams are satisfied that the newly transplanted lungs are functioning effectively, as assessed by arterial blood gases, ventilator requirements and chest x-ray (CXR). Delaying extubation should be avoided unless there is a good clinical indication, as this increases the risk of lower respiratory infection (Box 13.6). Regular physiotherapy, positioning and early mobilisation are essential to prevent atelectasis and secondary lower respiratory tract infection.

When the donor lungs are implanted into the recipient, the donor lungs are denervated. As a result, the breathing rate may be slower than expected or may appear poorly synchronised. This abnormal respiratory pattern can be alarming for healthcare professionals not experienced in lung transplantation, which may result in a delay in extubation or reintubation. By 24–48 h the respiratory movements, pattern and rate will gradually normalise. The mechanism for this is not well understood but the central nervous system appears to take over the function of the severed nerves. The cough reflex of the newly transplanted lungs is absent so the nurse should encourage the patient to practise deep breathing exercises and cough once they are extubated.

Table 13.4 Complications arising from transplant drug therapies.

Drug	Common or important side-effects (please consult a pharmacopoeia for complete list)
Corticosteroids	Hypertension Diabetes Gastritis/worsening of gastro-oesophageal reflux Growth suppression Cataracts Osteoporosis A vascular necrosis of femoral head Behaviour effects Muscle wasting (proximal myopathy) Cushing's syndrome – moon facies, striae, acne

Calcineurin inhibitor
  Tacrolimus
  Ciclosporin
	Hypertension
	Diabetes
	Hypomagnesaemia
	Hyperlipidaemia
	Chronic renal impairment
	Hepatic dysfunction
	Neurological – tremor, headaches, burning sensation in hands and feet, seizures, encephalopathy
	Hypertrichosis and gingival hyperplasia (ciclosporin)
	Bone marrow suppression
	Anaemia
	Leucopenia
	Thrombocytopenia
	Susceptibility to lymphoma and other malignancies

Antiproliferative immunosuppressants Mycophenolate mofetil Azathioprine	Gastrointestinal effects Hair loss Bone marrow suppression Anaemia Leucopenia Thrombocytopenia Susceptibility to lymphoma and other malignancies

Antiviral prophylaxis
  Ganciclovir
  Valganciclovir
  Valaciclovir
	Renal impairment
	Bone marrow suppression
	Anaemia
	Leucopenia
	Thrombocytopenia
	Potential carcinogenic and teratogenic (ganciclovir/valganciclovir)

Pneumocystic carinii (*jiroveci*) pneumonia (PCP) prophylaxis Cotrimoxazole	Gastrointestinal effects Stevens Johnson syndrome Blood disorders – neutropenia, anaemia, thrombocytopenia Hepatic dysfunction/necrosis
Fungal prophylaxis Voriconazole	Gastrointestinal effects Hepatic dysfunction Prolonged QT interval Bone marrow suppression Anaemia Leucopenia Thrombocytopenia

---

Box 13.6   Factors that may delay extubation

- Significant reperfusion injury on the chest x-ray or other chest x-ray abnormalities
- Pulmonary oedema
- Postoperative bleeding
- Abnormalities found during the respiratory assessment
- Poor arterial blood gases
- High ventilator requirements
- Cardiovascular instability or evidence of sepsis
- Patient oversedated and unable to maintain airway
- Anxiety of inexperienced staff

Physiotherapy, positioning and early mobilisation

The primary aim of physiotherapy is to mobilise and remove secretions, to recruit any areas of consolidated or collapsed lungs and to prevent lower respiratory tract infections. Suctioning and repositioning of the patient by the ICU nurse are important as well as regular physiotherapy while the patient is intubated. As soon as the child is stable postoperatively, they should be placed in the upright position to facilitate lung expansion. Both the nurse and physiotherapist should monitor for an increase in blood-stained secretions, as this may indicate bleeding at the anastomosis site.

Once the child is extubated, early mobilisation is essential; this not only promotes motor recovery but is an excellent way to move secretions. The physiotherapist will teach the child deep breathing techniques, bubble positive expiratory pressure (PEP) and self-initiated coughing as soon as they are self-ventilating. The physiotherapist may also use other techniques such as percussion and autogenic drainage at this stage to prevent lower respiratory tract infections, as discussed in Chapter 12. Physiotherapy will need to continue until the lungs are clear as assessed at bronchoscopy (discussed in Chapter 4).

Optimising other organ functions

Cardiovascular system

The post lung transplant patient is normally cardiovascularly stable postoperatively. Occasionally patients return from theatre on milrinone for afterload reduction but this can usually be rapidly weaned and discontinued. Occasionally bleeding from the chest drains persists postoperatively on the ICU at a rate of >2 mL/kg, especially if dissection has been difficult. A patient may need fresh frozen plasma or cryoprecipitate to correct any derangement in the clotting screen. The platelets are normally low after cardiopulmonary bypass so transfusion may be required if they are below 60 and bleeding is persistent. Blood transfusions should only be given if clinically indicated or the Hb <8 g/dL.

Renal system

Fluids are usually restricted to 50% of maintenance for the first 2–3 days after transplant and a negative balance is obtained with the use of diuretics. This is to prevent pulmonary oedema developing in the transplanted lungs. Daily urea and electrolytes are required to monitor renal function. A number of the drugs used in the immediate post-transplant period are nephrotoxic, so it is important to observe for any deterioration in renal function. If the urea and creatinine rise significantly, the fluids may need to be liberalised. Occasionally dialysis is required short term.

Support of the child and family during the intensive care unit period

The time of the transplant operation and the postoperative period both in the ICU and on the ward can be extremely stressful for the child and family. It is important that the child and family are given appropriate support to help them through this period. This support is provided by the nurses at the bedside, specialist transplant nurses and other members of the multiprofessional team. To reduce stress, information about progress needs to be communicated regularly, clearly and with sensitivity.

Education of the child and family to prepare them for discharge

Careful discharge planning by the specialist transplant nurse and the transplant team is essential. As part of the discharge planning, the specialist nurse will spend time with the child and family teaching them about their medications, their follow-up care and how to monitor their child when they get home.

Long-term shared care of the transplant patient

After discharge home, there is a strict protocol for follow-up care and monitoring of the post lung transplant patient by the specialist lung transplant team. The aim of this rigorous monitoring is to identify and treat problems early. Routine follow-up care includes regular outpatients appointments, at least 6-weekly tacrolimus blood levels and five surveillance bronchoscopies and biopsies in the first year. Patients will also need to be seen at any time they are unwell. Establishing clearly defined shared care with the local primary and secondary teams is important to provide excellent care of the patient. After the first 6 months, if the patient is clinically well, some outpatient appointments can be completed at the local centre, provided the local respiratory consultant or paediatrician feels confident to provide the level of care required.

At discharge, patients are given a hand-held spirometer and asked to record their lung function every day. If they feel unwell, develop any symptoms of tiredness, fever, cough, shortness of breath or if they notice a 10% fall in their lung function results, they are asked to contact the transplant office. Often the transplant team will request that the patient is initially reviewed by the local team and will require a clinical assessment, chest x-ray, blood test, nasopharyngeal aspirate and formal lung function, if available. It is difficult to distinguish between infection and rejection in the transplant patient, and if a patient fails to respond quickly to treatment, e.g. antibiotics, they will be reviewed by the transplant centre and a diagnostic bronchoscopy, lavage and biopsy undertaken.

A number of common complications seen after transplant are described below.

Acute rejection

Patients with acute rejection may have relatively few symptoms, which include lethargy, fever, cough or shortness of breath. On examination, a patient may have signs of crackles or a pleural effusion. A CXR may show evidence of perihilar infiltrates or pleural effusion or may be normal in up to 50% patients with acute rejection (Kindu et al. 1999). Acute rejection is diagnosed by a transbronchial biopsy and is usually treated with a 3-day pulse of methylprednisolone, followed by a weaning dose of corticosteroids.

Infection

Infection is the most common cause of death in the first year after transplant. Immunosuppressed patients may appear reasonably well even with severe infections. After transplant, patients are at risk of typical and atypical respiratory infections, bacterial, viral and fungal infections. They are particularly vulnerable to opportunistic infections such as *Pneumocystic carinii*. Transplant patients are usually maintained on prophylaxis to prevent CMV, *Pneumocystic carinii*, *Pseudomonas* and fungal infections but these medications may have a number of side-effects (see Table 13.4). Transplant patients with presumed infection should be appropriately assessed, investigated and treated with early advice from the transplant centre.

Chronic rejection or bronchiolitis obliterans syndrome

The major impediment to long-term survival following lung transplant is chronic rejection. The term bronchiolitis obliterans syndrome (BOS) is used to describe an irreversible decrease in lung function after other possible diagnoses have been excluded. Histologically, there is evidence of fibrous obliteration of the bronchioles (obliterative bronchiolitis or OB). Patients can present with insidious onset of cough, shortness of breath, wheeze and decreased exercise tolerance. Patients can also be asymptomatic but show evidence of decreased lung function with irreversible airway obstruction. A CXR is typically normal or may show evidence of hyperinflation. Computed tomography (CT) scan shows evidence of small airways obstruction, with typical patchy black/white mosaic appearances.

Bronchiolitis obliterans syndrome can appear at any time after transplant and is present in 14% of patients at 1 year and 36% 5 years after transplant (Aurora et al. 2009). Although the pathophysiology of BOS is not fully understood, there are a number of immune and non-immune insults which lead to its development, including acute rejection, infections and gastro-oesophageal reflux. It remains very difficult to treat although azithromycin, augmented immunosuppression, statins and total lymphoid irradiation have been used to stabilise patients (Borro et al. 2007; Fisher et al. 2005; Jain et al. 2010; Johnson et al. 2003). Ultimately patients may need to be considered for retransplantation.

Gastro-oesophageal reflux

Gastro-oesophageal reflux (GOR) is commonly seen after transplant with a reported incidence of 73% (Hadjiliadis et al. 2003). The reasons for this are thought to be multifactorial and include presence of pretransplant GOR, postoperative damage to the vagal nerve and side-effects of medications. As stated previously, there is some evidence to suggest that acid and non-acid reflux with presumed microaspiration is associated with the development of BOS. At our centre, after transplant, patients will be started on appropriate antireflux medications and will then undergo investigations for GOR 3 months after transplant. These investigations include an impedance study (looking for acid and non-acid reflux) and a barium study. If there is evidence of only mild GOR patients may be treated medically. If there is evidence of moderate or severe reflux or of small airways disease, patients will usually undergo a laparoscopic Nissen fundoplication at around 6 months after transplant.

Post-transplant lymphoproliferative disease

Patients who are immunosuppressed are at risk of developing post-transplant lymphoproliferative disease (PTLD). This is usually associated with Epstein–Barr virus infection leading to the uncontrolled proliferation of B-cells. The incidence in the paediatric population is approximately 8% in the first year after transplant and 15% at 5 years after transplant (Aurora et al. 2009). Patients may present in a variety of ways depending on the site and extent of the tumour. PTLD most commonly presents after lung transplant as an asymptomatic pulmonary nodule seen on CXR or CT scan, but patients may also show symptoms of glandular fever, airway obstruction, bowel obstruction or lymphoma. The initial treatment for PTLD is reduction of immunosuppression and new studies suggest that the early use of rituximab, an anti-CD20 antibody, improves survival, with a 3-year overall survival of 73% (Evens et al. 2010). Patients who do not respond or who have a highly aggressive monomorphic PTLD need treatment with chemotherapy.

Diabetes mellitus

The medications used after transplant, including corticosteroids and tacrolimus, may promote the development of diabetes. In our experience this has particularly affected patients with cystic fibrosis who may have already been in a prediabetic phase at the time of transplant. It is important to enquire about symptoms of polydipsia, polyuria and weight loss and consider the diagnosis of diabetes in the post-transplant patient. Patients who develop diabetes are usually cared for by their local diabetic team.

Neuromuscular problems

Proximal myopathy is commonly seen in patients on corticosteroids. About a quarter of patients will develop neurological complications resulting from the calcineurin inhibitors. Common manifestations include tremor and headache, which may progress to reversible posterior leucoencephalopathy syndrome with confusion, hypertension, seizures, cortical blindness and encephalopathy. Reversible posterior leucoencephalopathy typically develops early in the post-transplant period and responds to withdrawal/reduction of calcineurin inhibitors.

Osteoporosis

Patients with advanced pulmonary disease often have reduced bone mineral density which is compounded by the use of corticosteroids after transplant. Patients may present with bone pain or fractures. Treatment includes calcium and vitamin D supplements and bsiphosphonates.

Chronic renal impairment

Calcineurin inhibitors can cause acute and chronic nephrotoxicity. Although the exact mechanisms for this are not fully understood, it is thought that they cause vasoconstriction of the small blood vessels of the kidney. Hypertension is seen in 42% and 69% of paediatric patients at 1 and 5 years post transplant respectively. Renal impairment is seen in 10% and 21% patients at 1 and 5 years post transplant. At 5 years 2.2% patients will require renal dialysis and 0.7% will need a renal transplant (Aurora et al. 2009). To maintain good renal health, patients should remain well hydrated, avoid other potentially nephrotoxic medication, maintain good diabetic control, be normotensive and have their tacrolimus level and kidney function monitored every 6 weeks. Patients are referred to see a renal consultant when they have evidence of chronic renal impairment.

Conclusion

Lung transplantation is a final therapeutic option for selected children with end-stage lung disease. Although survival is limited and complications are numerous, the majority of patients will experience a good quality of life which most families feel is worth the difficult journey. It is hoped that continuing research will lead to improvements and make long-term survival after lung transplant a real possibility.

Questions

1. When might a child with end-stage lung disease be considered as needing a lung transplant?
2. What are the two most common conditions referred for lung transplant?
3. What are the generally agreed criteria for paediatric lung transplant?
4. Why are very few heart-lung transplants undertaken in the current era?
5. What factors must be taken into account when making the decision to list a patient for a lung transplant?
6. What is the survival post lung transplant?
7. What are the key messages that the specialist nurse needs to communicate to the child and family about lung transplant during the assessment?
8. What are the most important aspects of nursing care post lung transplant?
9. What strategies should nurses employ to minimising the risk of infection to the patient early after lung transplant?
10. Why is physiotherapy so important post lung transplant?
11. What immunosuppression medications are post-transplant children on for the rest of their lives and why?
12. What is PTLD?
13. How is rejection diagnosed in a post lung transplant patient?
14. What is the most common case of death in the first year post lung transplant?
15. What is the most common cause of renal impairment in children post lung transplant and how can they protect their kidneys?

References

Aurora P, Christie JD, Edwards LB, *et al*. (2009) The Registry of the International Society for Heart and Lung Transplantation: Twelfth Official Pediatric Lung and Heart/Lung Transplantation Report – 2009. *Journal of Heart and Lung Transplantation* **28(10)**, 1023–30.

Aurora P, Spencer H, Moreno-Galdó A. (2008) Lung transplantation in children with cystic fibrosis: a view from Europe. *American Journal of Respiratory and Critical Care Medicine* **177(9)**, 935–6.

Aurora P, Whitehead B, Wade A, *et al*. (1999) Lung transplantation and life extension in children with cystic fibrosis. *Lancet* **354**, 1591–93.

Borro JM, Bravo C, Solé A, *et al*. (2007) Conversion from cyclosporine to tacrolimus stabilizes the course of lung function in lung transplant recipients with bronchiolitis obliterans syndrome. *Transplant Proceedings* **39(7)**, 2416–19.

Elizur A, Faro A, Huddleston CB, *et al*. (2009) Lung transplantation in infants and toddlers from 1990 to 2004 at St Louis Children's Hospital. *American Journal of Transplantation* **9(4)**, 719–26.

Evens AM, David KA, Helenowski I, *et al*. (2010) Multicentre analysis of 80 solid organ transplantation recipients with post-transplantation lymphoproliferative disease: outcomes and prognostic factors in the modern era. *Journal of Clinical Oncology* **28(6)**, 1038–46.

Faro A, Mallory GB, Visner GA, *et al*. (2007) American Society of Transplantation executive summary on pediatric transplantation. *American Journal of Transplantation* **7(2)**, 285–92.

Fisher AJ, Rutherford RM, Bozzino J, *et al*. (2005) The safety and efficacy of total lymphoid irradiation in progressive bronchiolitis obliterans syndrome after lung transplantation. *American Journal of Transplantation* **5(3)**, 537–43.

Galiè N, Hoeper NM, Humbert M, *et al*. (2009) Guidelines for the diagnosis and treatment of pulmonary hypertension. *European Respiratory Journal* **34(6)**, 1219–63.

Hadjiliadis D, Duane Davis R, Steele MP, *et al*. (2003) Gastroesophageal reflux disease in lung transplant recipients. *Clinical Transplantation* **17**, 363–8.

Hosenpud JD, Bennett LE, Keck BM, *et al.* (1998) Effect of diagnosis on survival benefit of lung transplantation for end-stage lung disease. *Lancet* **351**, 24–7.

Jain R, Hachem RR, Morrell MR, *et al.* (2010) Azithromycin is associated with increased survival in lung transplant recipients with bronchiolitis obliterans syndrome. *Journal of Heart and Lung Transplantation* **29(5)**, 531–7.

Johnson BA, Lacono AT, Zeevi A, *et al.* (2003) Statin use is associated with improved function and survival of lung allografts. *American Journal of Respiratory and Critical Care Medicine* **167(9)**, 1271–8.

Kerem E, Reisman J, Corey M, *et al.* (1992) Prediction of mortality in patients with cystic fibrosis. *New England Journal of Medicine* **326**, 1187–91.

Kindu S, Herman SJ, Larhs A, *et al.* (1999) Correlation of chest radiographic findings with biopsy-proven acute lung rejection. *Journal of Thoracic Imaging* **14**, 178.

Liou TG, Adler FR, Cox DR, *et al.* (2007) Lung transplantation and survival in children with cystic fibrosis. *New England Journal of Medicine* **357**, 2143–52.

Maurer JR, Frost AE, Estenne M, *et al.* (1998) International guidelines for the selection of lung transplant candidates. The International Society for Heart and Lung Transplantation, the American Thoracic Society, the American Society of Transplant Physicians, the European Respiratory Society. *Transplantation* **66(7)**, 951–6.

Orens JB, Estenne M, Arcasoy S, *et al.* (2006) International guidelines for the selection of lung transplant candidates: 2006 update – a consensus report from the Pulmonary Scientific Council of the International Society for Heart and Lung Transplantation. *Journal of Heart and Lung Transplantation* **25(7)**, 745–55.

Wray J, Radley-Smith R, Yacoub M. (1992) Effect of cardiac or heart-lung transplantation on the quality of life of the paediatric patient. *Quality of Life Research* **1(1)**, 41–6.

Yusen RD, Shearon TH, Qian Y, *et al.* (2010) Lung transplantation in the Unites States, 1999–2008. *American Journal of Transplantation* **10(4 Pt2)**, 1047–68.

Section IV

Practical elements and governance issues

Chapter 14

Transition to adult services

Donna Hilton

Youth Service Manager, Nottingham Children's Hospital

Learning objectives

After studying this chapter the reader will have an understanding of:

- the process of transition
- models of transition
- young people's experiences of the transition process
- how youth work supports the process of transition.

Introduction

Young people with long-term health conditions face many challenges throughout their adolescent life and with more young people surviving well into adulthood; the issue of transition from a 'safe' familiar paediatric environment into an unknown adult unit remains ever high on the agenda. Consequently, youth work can play an important role in assisting with this process.

Transition as a journey

The Department of Health (Department of Health 2006a) describes transition as 'a purposeful, planned process that addresses the medical, psychosocial and educational/vocational needs of adolescents and young adults with chronic physical and medical conditions as they move from child-centered to adult-oriented health care systems', also reinforced by Blum et al. (1993).

It is no new concept that arranging transfer for young people from paediatric to adult services is a crucial part of care for adolescent patients. With many conditions once deemed as childhood illnesses, such as cystic fibrosis, now continuing well into adulthood (Viner and Keane 1998) and the fact that over 85% of children with chronic illnesses are surviving into adulthood (Betz 1999), it is even more evident that we need to give the area of transition special attention.

When talking about transition, however, it is important to recognise that this is not just a one-off event that sees young people move from one service to another but is in fact a process (Department

---

Children's Respiratory Nursing, First Edition. Edited by Janice Mighten.
© 2013 Blackwell Publishing Ltd. Published 2013 by Blackwell Publishing Ltd.

of Health 2006a). Throughout the process from childhood to adulthood, children are dependent, while adults are independent. Children are developing in competence, whereas adults have achieved this (Batsleer 2008).

The transition process is a journey from one place to another incorporating both personal and social aspects. The personal aspects are associated with biological maturity while the social aspects refer to growth from dependence to independence (Harrison and Wise 2005).

The recommendation for good practice in transition from the Royal College of Paediatrics and Child Health (2003) is that 'Young people should not be transferred fully to adult services until they have the necessary skills to function in an adult service and have finished growth and puberty'.

When going on a journey, especially one that you haven't been on before, you need a guide. Not one that tells you what to do and which path to take but one that gives you the necessary information and advice to choose the right way for yourself (Young 1999).

The guide

Different models of transition are adapted to meet the needs of each specific group in the UK. McDonagh (2007) maintains that there is no evidence to suggest that one model works better than another. The adolescent rheumatology transition process in Birmingham, described in detail by McDonagh (2007), includes a variable age range of 16–18 and is divided into three phases: early, middle and late. However, it is important to ensure that each transition is individualised. The three main models of transition described by Esmond (2000) are:

- primary care based (not always disease specific)
- specialist adolescent health
- disease focused.

While the most successful transition programmes involve both paediatric and adult services, the whole process should also be undertaken in partnership with the wider multiprofessional team including psychosocial support, as previously discussed in Chapter 12. Viner and Keane (1998) suggest that to achieve effective transition, it is important to recognise that there is much more to transition than just focusing on healthcare.

For those young people who have not had a personalised transition plan and have experienced more of a 'transfer' to adult services, words they have used to describe this are: 'dumped', 'sudden', 'thrown out' and 'abandoned' (McDonagh 2007). When young people were asked what they thought was important for their transition, key words that came up were 'preparation', 'support', 'choice', 'planning', 'peer support', 'skills' and 'guidance' (Nottingham University Hospitals Youth Service 2005). In short, youth workers can be described as a 'guide' for young people to help them on their journey into adulthood. 'A key aspect of youth work is to build relationships with young people which enable them to explore and make sense of their experiences, and plan and take action' (Sapin 2009).

Youth workers encourage and challenge young people to think about what they want to achieve in life, reflect on their behaviour and consider whether the choices they make are helping them get where they want to be (National Youth Agency 2007).

According to the Social Exclusion Unit (2005), one of the five key principles that underpin service delivery within transition is to offer young people a trusted adult who can both challenge and support them.

Youth workers primarily work with young people aged 12–19 years and those based within hospital settings are ideally placed to support adolescent patients through the transition process.

Hospital youth work

Youth work can take place in many settings, usually where young people are situated. Youth work within a hospital setting is currently very rare but the evidence that is available for such provision suggests that it is very effective in addressing young people's experiences in hospital and throughout the transition process (Hilton et al. 2004; Yates et al. 2009).

Key aspects of youth work include building personal and social development. Ways of doing this can include arts-based work, ICT and media projects, sport and outdoor activities, accreditation opportunities, participation projects, addressing youth issues (e.g. sexual health, drugs and alcohol), residentials and volunteering (National Youth Agency 2002).

Based on the experiences of Nottingham University Hospitals (NUH) Youth Service, which is known to be the longest running hospital provision in the UK (National Youth Agency 2008), there have been many positive examples of youth work opportunities within a hospital setting. With long periods of absences from school, the hospital youth service offers the opportunity to facilitate and support young people with issues such as those outlined in Box 14.1.

Young people become involved in youth work activities because they want to – the youth worker's role is to make sure that these opportunities contribute to the young people's learning and development (National Youth Agency 2002).

Box 14.1   Examples of youth work

One-to-one support work

- Issues include school, family, health, bullying, self-esteem, bereavement, careers, alcohol, sexual health

Outdoor education

- Day trips to places of interest and challenging activities (e.g. theme parks, rock climbing)

Accreditation

- Youth Achievement Awards, Open College Network, AQAs

Volunteering

- Patient Volunteer Scheme, peer mentoring

Group work

- Support groups, siblings groups, Hospital Youth Club, daily drop-in sessions

Residential

- Condition specific, generic, themed (e.g. self-esteem), transition, volunteer training

Youth participation

- Youth Committee, involving young people in conference presentations, planning and evaluation

Transition

- Residential programmes, Transition Working Group, individual transition plan

---

Youth workers within a hospital setting can really add a unique dimension to the multiprofessional team by being somebody whose ultimate focus is on the adolescent. While doctors/nurses see young people as patients, social workers see them as clients and teachers see them as pupils, youth workers see them as young people (Young 1999).

Youth workers' interaction with young people, their communication skills and social contact enable them to build relationships with young people in a way that health professionals cannot (see Case study 2).

Transition programmes

Residential experiences have long been at the heart of youth work practice and there is endless potential for good youth work to take place with a group of young people away from their everyday environment. Such benefits may include increased independence and self-esteem, new experiences, a broadening of peer relationships, opportunities to explore issues and time to think and plan for the future (UK Youth 1999).

Hospitals also see the potential of residential experiences for patients, more widely known as therapeutic recreation camps. Since the 1930s, these have been active in the UK to help young people cope with chronic illness (Walker and Pearman 2009).

A new concept is the format of a transition residential, which combines the experience of therapeutic recreation with the expertise of youth work residentials. The NUH Youth Service first piloted this in 2004 and has run a total of five transition residential programmes to date.

The format of the residential involves promoting independent healthcare behaviour through a range of interactive workshops covering the following topics: developing teamwork; building trust and support; planning; budgeting; raising self-confidence; developing life skills (communication, independence, work skills, managing stress, managing change); healthy living (diet, exercise, hygiene); health awareness (alcohol, sexual health); introduction to adult services.

Each workshop involves a team challenge linked to each theme, followed by a discussion with relevant professionals. For example, for the dietary workshop, a Ready Steady Cook challenge was set where the young people had to plan and prepare a meal relevant to specific dietary needs. This was followed up with a discussion led by a dietician to help them think about responsibilities and choices.

Adult staff were invited to attend, along with young adults who had already been through transition. This enabled young people to have further support and any questions answered.

Outcomes

A total of 54 young people were involved, aged between 16 and 19 years. The event has been evaluated on each occasion and 50 of 54 young people reported feeling much more confident about transferring to the adult unit (three were unsure and one still felt unprepared).

The Department of Health (2006b) reports that 'Successful transition planning and programmes are crucially dependent on collaboration between children's and adult services'. All 54 of the young people involved commented that having adult staff and young adult patients attend the event was extremely useful and enabled them to have questions answered and any worries addressed.

Whilst it is difficult to measure outcomes in terms of adherence, young people's independent behaviour and increase in knowledge demonstrate the value of youth work input with projects like this.

Thomson and Holland report that 'The more competent young people feel and the more recognition they receive in a particular area, the more they are likely to invest in that aspect of adult identity' (Thomson and Holland 2002).

Conclusion

While it is acknowledged that there is no one specific model for transition, it is also recognised that well-planned transition programmes improve clinical, education and social outcomes for young people (Department of Health 2006a). This all needs to be facilitated with a team approach through the process of collaboration.

Case study 1   (specialist nurse for respiratory services)

A young girl of about 12 with asthma/allergies was having a hard time socialising with young people her age and engaging with school due to poor attendance at school. This had an adverse affect on her confidence levels. This all lead to a vicious circle of poor school attendance, low feelings, poor self-esteem and lack of (physical) activity. This continued to affect her general health too.

A home visit was undertaken by the respiratory nurse and a youth worker, the aim of which was to introduce the idea of attending the hospital youth club to try and increase the girl's self-esteem, confidence levels and socialising skills. This would also, it was hoped, increase her attendance at school. This would happen because she would see that other young people with just as/more complex health issues were still able to achieve, fulfil their potential and attend school.

The girl joined the youth club and has achieved much with the support of the youth workers. The quiet, unconfident girl with no visible friends of her own age has made friends, performed on stage, jumped from a cliff into the sea and had experiences that she would not have imagined possible if she had not joined this fantastic service.

Caring for this girl from a purely medical perspective would never have allowed her to achieve so much. Successful caring for young people with any health problems cannot be achieved without a multidisciplinary team that is able to see the child and family from several different aspects at once, including how they fit in with the community. The experience and skills of youth workers allow them to help the young blossom in this important period of their development.

This girl had not had a hospital admission for years and was being seen as an outpatient, but still her condition adversely affected many aspects of her life. We must not underestimate the impact that having a chronic health condition has on a young person's development and transition into adulthood. Youth work support ensures that other healthcare workers do not forget the normal issues that young people face during this time.

Case study 2   (professor in paediatric respiratory medicine)

I wanted to highlight the enormous amount of input from the Hospital Youth Service in helping this young man deal with his chronic asthma. He has had brittle asthma for a very long time and has been in and out of hospital for a number of years. This has included near death attacks, ending up in the PICU requiring full support.

Since being involved in the youth group he has started to blossom, both medically as well as emotionally. From being a withdrawn young man, he has started to attend school regularly and he has just succeeded in getting an offer at the local college of further education. In addition, with the support of the Youth Service, he has made a number of trips both locally as well as afar which has allowed him to become independent.

With the youth workers' enormous support and style, this has helped turn around this young man. He is now confident and on his way to being a successful, enterprising young man.

The contribution of the Youth Service here will always be recognised.

References

Batsleer JR. (2008) *Informal Learning in Youth Work*. London: Sage.

Betz CL. (1999) Adolescents with chronic conditions: linkages to adult service systems. *Paediatric Nursing* **25**, 473–6.

Blum R, Garell D, Hodgman C. (1993) Transition from child-centred to adult health-care systems for adolescents with chronic conditions. A position paper of the Society for Adolescent Medicine. *Journal of Adolescent Health* **14**, 570–6.

Department of Health. (2006a) *Transition: getting it right for young people*. London: Department of Health.

Department of Health. (2006b) *Our Health, Our Care, Our Say*. London: Stationery Office.

Esmond G. (2000) Cystic fibrosis: adolescent care. *Nursing Standard* **14(52)**, 47–57.

Harrison R, Wise C. (2005) *Working with Young People*. London: Sage.

Hilton D, Watson A, Walmsley P, Jepson S. (2004) Youth work in hospital: the impact of a youth worker on the lives of adolescents with chronic conditions. *Paediatric Nursing* **16(1)**, 36–9.

McDonagh JE. (2007) Transition of care from paediatric to adult rheumatology. *Archives of Disease in Childhood* **92(9)**, 802–7.

National Youth Agency. (2002) *The NYA Guide to Youth Work and Youth Services*. Leicester: National Youth Agency.

National Youth Agency. (2007) *The NYA Guide to Youth Work in England*. Leicester: National Youth Agency.

National Youth Agency. (2008) *Nottingham University Hospitals Youth Service: a Youth Work 4Health case study*. Leicester: National Youth Agency.

Nottingham University Hospitals Youth Service. (2005) Moving On: a DVD production of young people's experiences of transition. Nottingham: Nottingham University Hospitals Youth Service.

Royal College of Paediatrics and Child Health. (2003) *Bridging the Gaps: health care for adolescents*. London: Royal College of Paediatrics and Child Health.

Sapin K. (2009) *Essential Skills for Youth Work Practice*. London: Sage.

Social Exclusion Unit. (2005) *Transitions: a Social Exclusion Unit interim report on young adults*. London: Social Exclusion Unit.

Thomson R, Holland J. (2002) *Inventing Adulthoods: young people's strategies for transition*. Swindon: Economic and Social Research Council.

UK Youth. (1999) Getaway. *UK Youth* **96**, 8–9.

Viner R, Keane M. (1998) *Youth Matters: evidence-based best practice for the care of young people in hospital*. London: Action for Sick Children.

Walker D, Pearman D. (2009) Therapeutic recreation camps: an effective intervention for children and young people with chronic illness? *Archives of Disease in Childhood* **94**, 401–6.

Yates S, Payne M, Dyson S. (2009) Children and young people in hospitals: doing youth work in medical settings. *Journal of Youth Studies* **12(1)**, 77–92.

Young K. (1999) *The Art of Youth Work*. Lyme Regis, Dorset: Russell House Publishing.

Chapter 15

Professional issues

Janice Mighten

Children's Respiratory/Community Nurse Specialist, Nottingham Children's Hospital

---

Learning objectives

After studying this chapter the reader will have an understanding of:

- the legal context of practice
- law and ethics of nursing
- patient safety
- the importance of maintaining a duty of care
- quality assurance frameworks.

Introduction

Practitioners in the National Health Service (NHS) have a professional responsibility to maintain their knowledge of the law and its impact on clinical practice. It is also essential to practise within the law and specific codes of conduct, outlined by the Nursing and Midwifery Council (NMC 2008), which is responsible for professional regulation. This ensures that practice is maintained within specific standards, through competency. As health service employees, nurses have contractual agreements to provide care that will protect the patient and is of the highest standard. Therefore consideration needs to be given to policy and procedure.

The law of negligence emphasises the duty of care that health practitioners must provide. This is reinforced by Griffith and Tengnah (2004) who maintain that a duty of care is a requirement from one person to another, thus ensuring care to prevent harm. Therefore the principles that nurses apply to practice in order to make a judgement on whether a decision is right or wrong relate to the fundamental concept known as ethics (Griffith and Tengnah 2008).

The ideology of ethics is based on the principle of beneficence (Griffith and Tengnah 2008) – in other words, 'do no harm'. This principle is also outlined within the code of conduct as a standard requirement. Beneficence also highlights the professional responsibility to work with others in protecting and promoting individuals' overall health. However, each individual practitioner has ultimate responsibility for any acts or omissions (NMC 2008).

Children's Respiratory Nursing, First Edition. Edited by Janice Mighten.
© 2013 Blackwell Publishing Ltd. Published 2013 by Blackwell Publishing Ltd.

Legal context of practice

A competent nurse is one who is confident to practise with knowledge that is current. This includes the ability to practise skills at the required level (NMC 2008). Modern-day medicine has promoted the notion of competence, accountability and knowledge with the introduction of the NHS Knowledge and Skills Framework (KSF). This sets a framework for competence in line with training and ensures fitness to practise, quality and service provision (Department of Health 2004a).

Within the legal context of practice, practitioners are accountable whether acting on another's instructions or not (Griffith and Tengnah 2008). Inappropriate delegation, in the eyes of the law, would be assessed using a concept known as the Bolam test. This is case law, which puts great emphasis on the fact that a reasonable standard of care must be adhered to. Therefore each individual will be judged according to the ordinary skilled man. In the case of a nurse, individuals will be judged by standards of the ordinary skilled nurse, who is considered to have the same level of skill (Griffith and Tengnah 2008).

Within healthcare, the Bolam test is modified to give consideration to the skill involved (Griffith and Tengnah 2008). For example, if a respiratory nurse specialist delegated a specific task to a nurse who was not a specialist within that field, and the non-specialist chose to accept the responsibility of that delegation, then he/she would be assessed in the same manner as the respiratory nurse specialist. Naturally the same principles apply to all areas of nursing. Putting this further into context, litigation has increased within the modern health service (Griffith and Tengnah 2008) so it is paramount that nurses keep abreast of all developments in relation to the legal context of their practice.

Evidence-based practice

The concept of evidence-based practice enables the provision of care for respiratory patients using the best available evidence. The importance of evidence-based practice is alluded to by the NMC to support practice. Policies such as the BTS guidance are examples of how evidence can be used to support competent practice.

Nurse prescribing

The Crown report outlined the legal framework for nurse prescribing. This gave clear guidance in order for nurses to practise within a legal and ethical framework (Department of Health 1999). In essence, it is common law that regulates prescribing in relation to the standard of care required for patients, who can claim negligence and sue for damages (Griffth and Tengnah 2004). The Bolam principle also applies to nurse prescribing, thus preventing any breach with a duty of care.

Trounce et al. (2004) reiterate the importance of standards in prescribing practice. They also highlight the need for professional and legal accountability for prescribing decisions, irrespective of any set protocols. Although nurse prescribing within children's nursing is very much a specialist role, it is important for ward-based nurses to be aware of such extended roles and the implications for the legal context of practice.

Law and ethics

The basic principle of ethics, which is a duty of care and to do no harm, is very much at the forefront of nurse prescribing. Following legislation, nurse prescribing has become one of the new innovations for modern-day healthcare. The intention is to provide patients with better service provision

(Jones 2009). It is not intended to replace but to complement the role of doctors. Therefore nurses prescribing outside their practice area or specialty is highlighted.

Naturally extended roles require an assessment. Any advice that is given needs to be documented, in particular any prescribed medication and most significantly the correct dose (Griffith and Tengnah 2004). This will ensure not only patient safety but continuity of care for the patient at future consultations.

Record keeping

To ensure patient safety and continuity of care, it is paramount that record keeping is meticulous. It is also necessary to have policies and local guidelines for nurses when prescribing medicines to patients (Jones 2009), to ensure that they are operating within the legal framework. The law is quite clear about the requirements for good record keeping. The general consensus is: if it has not been documented in the patient's notes, then there is no evidence to support any future claim that correct care was provided.

Every area providing health services will have the necessary documentation required to meet local need. It is the responsibility of every practitioner to document information following any encounter with patients. It has been noted in child protection cases that trying to create a chronology of events can be problematic at times because of poor documentation. With increased public awareness about healthcare, nurses need to be more vigilant in relation to professional accountability and accurate documentation.

Nurse-led clinics

National drivers from the Department of Health set the scene for nurses to provide care that is nurse led to meet the needs of patients. Nurse-led initiatives such as nurse-led clinics have also enabled nurses to practise independently. This is also endorsed by the government, giving patients quicker access to specialist treatment (Hatchett 2008).

The ethos of nurse-led clinics is provision of the best possible care for patients (Hatchett 2003). Nevertheless, accountability is paramount and constant consideration to practising within the legal framework is essential to ensure the health and safety of the patient.

Following discharge from hospital, ward-based nurses may refer patients to a nurse-led asthma clinic, for ongoing support and management. Such clinics have given patients more choice. Treatment can be initiated in a nurse-led format by children's respiratory nurses. Care often includes skin prick testing, management plans and commencement of new treatments such as nebulised antibiotics.

A nurse-led clinic provides the opportunity for education and time to support children and families, in order for treatment to continue at home. As with all new initiatives, it is important that services are evaluated, particularly with children because it is important to find out if parents feel that such services benefit their child's healthcare.

Health and safety law

Health and safety law is significant for nurses, in particular the safe use of equipment. This is achieved through a risk assessment culture, which is now commonplace within healthcare. Therefore, training, policies and procedures to guide practice are all necessary. It is also necessary to ensure that health and safety assessment of equipment is a continuous process, for example with nebulisers and infusion pumps that are used over a period of time, when patients carry out complex procedures at home.

An assessment process ensures that equipment is suitable for the environment when caring for a sick child in the community (Dimond 2005). Therefore a risk management strategy needs to be in place prior to discharge. Such safety measures enable practitioners to consider the welfare of the child, which is ultimately part of a nurse's accountability and professional responsibility to do no harm.

Accountability

To be accountable, one is considered to be responsible and answerable for one's actions, as suggested by Griffith and Tengnah (2008). In every situation, healthcare professionals must use their professional judgement at all times. However, each individual is accountable for their own actions within clinical practice. This responsibility is also shared with their employer. Therefore learners should always seek advice from senior colleagues/mentors.

Professional accountability consists of many facets, including:

• an awareness of the important of inappropriate delegation
• the need to be familiar with and adhere to professional boundaries
• the need to maintain confidentiality and to share information only on a need-to-know basis.

Consent

The law relating to the sick child comes from acts of Parliament known as statute. These statutes are divided into case law and common law (Dimond 2008).There are various statutes that relate to the care of the sick child, such as section 8 of the Family Law Reform Act (Department of Health 1969) and the Children Act 1989.

The Children Act 1989, revised in 2004 (Department of Health 2004b), sets the fundamental principles and standards required for consent to treatment. For all areas of nursing, there is a requirement to have knowledge of the Children Act and an awareness of consent and how this can be influenced by others (Dimond 2008). Carey (2009) explored issues surrounding the ability of adolescents to give consent and also highlights the significance of nurses' beliefs, in relation to acting as an advocate for the rights of young people.

The Family Law Reform Act 1969, section 8, states that children aged 16–17 years old can give consent. However, consent can be retracted if evidence suggests that they are not capable of giving consent or if they have reduced mental capacity, witnessed in practice with disabled children who have complex healthcare needs.

Within the busy nature of the NHS, practitioners need to find a way to create a balance with ethics and morals which shape our professional judgement (Carey 2009). There are many issues to consider when assessing a young person's capability to give informed consent. The precedent set by the notion of 'Gillick competence' emphasised that age would not be the only variable that decides the right to consent (Carey 2009; Gillick 1985).

It is also important for nurses to ascertain if a child is deemed mature and capable of understanding the situation, if it is not possible to contact the parents, which very rarely occurs. To ascertain such facts, an assessment needs to be made to decide whether the child is capable of making an informed decision, often referred to as being either Gillick or Fraser competent.

The legal framework of consent for children and young people maintains that a child is competent according to Lord Fraser's guidelines. This is usually implemented in exceptional circumstances (Dimond 2008). The Fraser guidelines give a clear structure for consent in relation to contraception for young people, but are also applicable to any treatment. Although the law states that parents have the power to give or withholdconsent, this is not absolute (Dimond 2008). It is, however, the parent's responsibility to obtain medical treatment for their child. If this duty of care is not carried out, then by law this is considered to be a criminal offence, in particular in a life-threatening situation.

Children and young people are often invited to take part in research. Many studies relating to respiratory conditions can involve frequent blood tests. For any child who has problems with needles (often referred to as needle phobia), it is important that they are not coerced into such studies that ultimately may not be in their best interest. Consequently, it is important that practitioners and students are aware that the principles of consent within the Family Law Reform Act do not apply to research, unless it is related to current treatment. The law recognises shared consent with parents and young people, and many other facets to consent, such as children in the care system, which is beyond the scope of this book.

Safeguarding

The Children Act (Department of Health 2004b) is the legal framework that sets principles for the welfare of the child. As a nurse, it is important to be familiar with local child protection procedures and concepts of the Children Act. The exception to the general rule of information sharing would be if safeguarding the welfare of the child is the main concern. Confidentiality is over-ridden in child protection cases because of the need for all agencies to work together. However, even in these circumstances, information sharing should only be on a need-to-know basis.

The ethos of care for safeguarding teams is collaborative working in order to protect children from harm. With a specialty such as respiratory nursing, consideration needs to be given to care management, for example compliance with treatments, such as inhalers, oxygen therapy or physiotherapy and how this can be improved, before the issue of neglect is considered. In a situation such as this, the multidisciplinary team has the difficult task of deciding when non-compliance becomes a safeguarding issue. Therefore it is vital that all agencies work together, including the parents and primary care professionals. Ultimately the intention is to improve the overall health and wellbeing of the child and family.

The following case study demonstrates how domestic violence can affect a parent's ability to give informed consent to treatment. This is often due to fear of the repercussions, and in this case the child was not of an appropriate age to consent herself. However, in this case the treatment was in the best interest of the child.

Case study

Jane lived with her mother and father. Both their children were under 5 and within the household there was a history of domestic violence. Jane had interstitial lung disease and her health needs included oxygen therapy 24 h a day. She also had a previous history of delayed development, in particular her speech and poor weight gain with a varied appetite, and therefore required nasogastric feeding until she was fully weaned. At each clinic appointment there was a constant refusal by the father for Jane to have blood tests. This was essential to monitor for toxic effects of the medication that Jane was taking.

Following various multiagency meetings, the family was provided with support from the primary care team, in particular the health visitor. Despite intervention from professionals in primary care, the social situation did not improve. This instigated a child protection conference, the outcome of which was the implementation of a child protection plan.

This plan involved intervention from family care workers to assist Jane's mother to care for the children on her own. Jane's mother moved out of the family home and relocated with the children. At subsequent home and clinic visits, it was clear that Jane had started to thrive physically and emotionally.

It was now possible to reduce Jane's oxygen requirements further. Improvements were made with Jane's speech, appetite and weight. She had also started school, although still requiring oxygen 24 h a day. Therefore a planning meeting was organised prior to her starting school, to ensure that school personnel were able to manage her oxygen requirements in school but also to advise them of the previous child protection plan.

The family continued to be monitored by healthcare professionals, such as the school nurse and GP. Collaborative working in this case supported the ethos of *Every Child Matters* (Department for Education 2003) which is to consider at all times what is best for the child.

Summary

Nurses at all levels have a professional responsibility to have an understanding of the law in relation to clinical practice, particularly the aspect of vicarious liability. Ultimately employers will be responsible for any damages awarded for negligence (Griffith and Tengnah 2004). However, it is vital that each practitioner understands the limitations to vicarious liability because the patient can also make a civil claim against individual health care professionals. Such claims may not be covered by an employment contract.

Quality assurance

Political ideology and social policy set the benchmark for quality assurance measures which are now part of the culture within modern-day health services. This section will consider quality assurance measures which help to guide and support care for children and families with health needs.

The constant theme throughout this book is advancement in modern medicine but the most important elements are standards of care, importance of evidence-based practice and the use of protocols to guide practice.

We have already established that nurses and other healthcare professionals are regulated by governing bodies. However, it is the responsibility of each individual to be familiar with the quality assurance framework that is now part of modern healthcare.

The past few years have been plagued by high-profile media coverage of health service failings, in relation to standards of care delivery. The Darzi Report (Department of Health 2008a) set the benchmark for quality assurance measures with reference to the significance of standards. More recently, the aim of 'liberating the NHS' (Department of Health 2010a) outlined by Lord Darzi is to build on the positive future of the NHS.

As professionals, we extract information from various sources. Examples of this include research, quality service frameworks produced by bodies such as the Care Quality Commission, the National Institute for Health and Clinical Excellence (NICE), and British Thoracic Society (BTS), in relation to disease management. Policies such as these are a valuable source of information, which we adopt to devise local and national policy, care management guidelines and procedures. The benefit for professionals at local level is policy that provides a structured framework for day-to-day management of children with respiratory disease.

Management guidelines not only guide practice but are also intended to encourage nurses to work towards quality in care provision. Nurse specialists working at an advanced level need to give consideration to such quality initiatives. In doing so, they are able to guide those with less experience within their specialist areas, based on quality standards that the modern health service now demands.

This is reinforced in *The Nursing Roadmap for Quality* (Department of Health 2010d) which praises nurses for taking the quality initiatives on board, including the impact this will have on care delivery. This is also reiterated by the Prime Minister's Commission (Department of Health 2010b), which stresses the need for an end to poor-quality care for patients. With this stance, the focus is very much on providing training and lifelong learning for nurses, driven by a competency framework.

Care Quality Commission

The aim of the Health and Social Care Act (2008) is modernisation of health services and integration of both social and healthcare (Department of Health 2008b). This initiative is regulated by the Care Quality Commission, ensuring patient safety and the delivery of high-quality services. Reports such as the failings at Mid-Staffordshire NHS Trust (Healthcare Commission 2009) highlighted the need for urgent review of healthcare services. Changes to practice following these reports ensured that quality of care and safety elements were implemented into practice. In addition, it is now even more essential to ensure that robust regulation of healthcare professionals is undertaken.

National documents

National policy also sets the standards for practice relevant to specialist areas, such as the National Service Framework (NSF) (Department of Health 2004c) and NICE. The NSF is a national document that sets the level of service provided for care in specific areas such as children. Nationally, the ethos of the NSF is to provide care and standards for children based on quality and best evidence to promote best practice.

The National Institute for Health and Clinical Excellence is responsible for the provision of guidance at a national level. The role of NICE is to give advice on new technology and medication. This provides patients, health professionals and the general public with robust reliable guidelines based on best practice, in relation to drugs/treatment and services across the NHS.

The objective of NICE guidance is to promote health. NICE is also actively involved with the regulation of public health measures, in particular preventing illness and disease such as TB. In clinical practice healthcare professionals utilise NICE guidance to improve and maintain current service provision within the financial constraints that are currently occurring worldwide.

The Department of Health (2010d) outlined concepts to enable nurses to understand the framework for quality, which will affect all areas of nursing. This ensures that nurses can contribute to the challenges ahead through productivity within a quality framework.

Practice guidelines

The BTS also aims to ensure improvements to the quality and standard of care for people with respiratory conditions.

As respiratory nurses, we measure quality through audit. By measuring practice and service delivery, standards are set. This adds to patient experiences, thus improving care pathways. This is highlighted by Hodges et al.'s (2007) audit and review of the service provided to children in school with severe allergy. Their findings illustrate the need for further development of a multidisciplinary service for children with allergy. Hodges et al. emphasise that this is needed to provide support for teachers, education and management for parents and children with allergy, through the development of an appropriate care pathway.

The main focus of other quality initiatives such as *Essence of Care* (Department of Health 2010c) is benchmarks based on patient care such as nutrition, privacy and dignity. This is all in line with the governance framework that commenced in 2007. The underpinning literature that supports this concept is the *NHS Plan* (Department of Health 2000) reinforcing the importance of 'getting the basics right'.

Hatchett (2003) illustrates how a quality service is measurable and demonstrates the significance of professional development. Other influential political drivers at the heart of the concepts of quality and standards include *High Quality Care for All* (Department of Health 2008a) by Lord Darzi. This very much emphasised the need for investing in the future to enable choice for the public and illustrated the dedication of NHS workers to service improvement.

In order for service development to progress, healthcare professionals need to buy in to the notion of a vision for the future. Darzi also alludes to variation in care. For respiratory nurses, this is also witnessed in practice because some areas have limited service provision for supporting children home with specialist teams (Department of Health 2008a).

As professionals working with children and young people with respiratory disease and their families, our aim is to make a difference, using knowledge skills and expertise, within a multidisciplinary framework. These elements put nurses very much at the forefront of co-ordinating care for patients, across primary and secondary care. Therefore nurses are pivotal to the success of any quality care framework using specific tools as suggested by the Department of Health (2010d).

Conclusion

At the heart of service delivery lie standards and quality to implement the best possible care available for all. Consideration also needs to be given to work-related pressures that can hinder this. The Department of Health (2010d) also maintains that quality care needs to be delivered in an effective and efficient manner. Therefore it is the responsibility of the nurse specialist to demonstrate high standards, in order to be a good role model for the specialist nurses of the future.

Questions

1. What is a duty of care?
2. How does the KSF ensure safe practice?
3. Based on the law, how would inappropriate delegation be assessed?
4. How do healthcare professionals ensure that children are capable of giving consent to treatment?
5. When would it be necessary to over-ride confidentiality with patient information?
6. The *NHS Plan* supports the concepts of basic care; how is this applied in practice?
7. Standards of care for children in clinical practice are supported by which policy?

References

Carey B. (2009) Consent and refusal for adolescents: the law. *British Journal of Nursing* **13(22)**, 1366–8.

Department for Education. (2003) *Every Child Matters*. London: Stationery Office.

Department of Health. (1969) *Family Law Reform Act*. London: Department of Health.

Department of Health. (1999) *Crown Report: review of prescribing, supply and administration of medicines*. London: Department of Health.

Department of Health. (2000) *The NHS Plan: a plan for investment, a plan for reform*. London: Department of Health.

Department of Health. (2004a) *The NHS Knowledge and Skills Framework and Development Review Process*. London: Stationery Office.

Department of Health. (2004b) *Children Act*. London: Stationery Office.

Department of Health. (2004c) *National Service Framework for Children, Young People and Maternity Services. Executive Summary*. London: Stationery Office.

Department of Health. (2008a) *High Quality Care for All: NHS stage review final report (Darzi Report)*. London: Stationery Office.

Department of Health. (2008b) *Health and Social Care Act*. London: Stationery Office.

Department of Health. (2010a) *Equity and Excellence: liberating the NHS*. London: Department of Health.

Department of Health. (2010b) *Front Line Care. Report by the Prime Minister's Commission on the future of nursing and midwifery in England*. London: Stationery Office.

Department of Health. (2010c) *Essence of Care*. London: Department of Health.

Department of Health. (2010d) *The Nursing Roadmap for Quality: a signposting map for nursing*. London: Stationery Office.

Dimond B. (2005) Legal aspects of the community care of the sick child. In: Sidey A, Widdas D (eds) *Textbook of Community Children's Nursing*. London: Elsevier.

Dimond B. (2008) *Legal Aspects of Nursing*, 5th edn. London: Pearson Longman.

Gillick v West Norfolk and Wisbech Area Health Authority (1985) 3 All ER 402.

Griffith R, Tengnah C. (2004) A question of negligence: the law and the standard of prescribing. *Nurse Prescribing* **2(2)**, 90–2.

Griffith R, Tengnah C. (2008) *Law and Professional Issues in Nursing*. Exeter: Learning Matters Limited.

Hatchett R. (2003) *Nurse Led Clinics: practical issues*. London: Routledge.

Hatchett R. (2008) Nurse-led clinics: 10 essential steps to setting up a service. *Nursing Times* **104(4)**, 62–4.

Healthcare Commission. (2009) *Investigation into Mid Staffordshire NHS Foundation Trust*. London: Healthcare Commission.

Hodges B, Clack G, Hodges I. (2007) Severe allergy: an audit and service review. *Paediatric Nursing* **19(9)**, 26–31.

Jones K. (2009) Developing a prescribing role for acute care nurses. *Nursing Management* **16(7)**, 24–8.

Nursing and Midwifery Council (NMC). (2008) *Standards of Conduct, Performance and Ethics for Nurses and Midwives*. London: Nursing and Midwifery Council.

Trounce J, Greenstein B, Gould D. (2004) *Trounce's Clinical Pharmacology for Nurses*, 17th edn. London: Churchill Livingstone.

Chapter 16

Communication: a holistic approach

Phil Brewin

Consultant Clinical Psychologist, Nottingham Children's Hospital

---

Learning objectives

After reading this chapter, the reader will be able to:

- understand that even the most experienced health professional can (and should) improve their communication skills, and that this improves not only patient experience but also physical outcome
- appreciate that active listening is as important as thoughtful, clear talking
- expect, respect and adapt to the individuality of children and their families
- understand open and closed questions and how they can best be used
- understand the nature and management of painful or distressing procedures
- appreciate how to support children and their parents following diagnosis of an inherited disease
- apply this knowledge and these skills in the context of respiratory nursing with children
- appreciate the crucial importance for patients, as well as nurses, of recognising personal and professional limits, and getting support through reflecting on practice with nursing and other colleagues.

Communication in healthcare

> Relational aspects of health care are important to patients. They value good communication and time to ask questions. Better professional-patient relationships will improve trust and health outcomes. (Office for Public Management 2000)

Every nurse, whatever their stage of training or experience, is already skilled in communication. Nurses routinely communicate with patients, families and colleagues as part of their work, and with countless others in their life outside work. Because of the everyday nature of communication, this chapter will often appear to state the obvious but there is strong evidence that communication difficulties underlie some of the most difficult and important problems in healthcare (Audit Commission 1993; Healthcare Commission 2007). The *Essence of Care* benchmarks of patient-focused healthcare in the NHS were modified 2 years after the original publication to include communication as a key focus (Department of Health 2003). The teaching of communication skills to nurses has been

---

Children's Respiratory Nursing, First Edition. Edited by Janice Mighten.
© 2013 Blackwell Publishing Ltd. Published 2013 by Blackwell Publishing Ltd.

criticised (Chant et al. 2002) and it has been argued that communication should be one of the high-priority topics for audit in the nursing profession (Currie and Watterson 2008).

The National Service Framework (NSF) for Children (Department of Health 2003b) lists the following communication skills shown as necessary for staff working with children in hospitals.

- How to listen to and communicate with children, young people, parents, carers, and the need to understand the extent and the limits of children's comprehension at various stages of development.
- Recognition of the role of parents in looking after their children in hospital.
- Providing information that is factual, objective and non-directive about a child's condition, likely prognosis, treatment options and likely outcomes.
- Giving bad news in a sensitive, non-hurried fashion, with time offered for further consultation away from the ward environment.
- Enabling a child and family to exercise choice, taking account of age and competence to understand the implications.

Good communication, and in particular empathy, can have a direct effect on patients' health. Rakel et al. (2009) assigned some patients suffering from colds to see doctors who (following training) made a special effort to be empathic. Other patients saw a doctor making no special effort. Patients seeing empathic doctors had less severe colds, recovered more quickly and even showed measurable changes in their immune system. Note that empathy should not be confused with sympathy. Sympathy is when you show someone you feel sorry for them. Empathy is when you have convinced someone that you have genuinely understood (not guessed or assumed) some part of what they are feeling or experiencing. The importance of checking you have understood is demonstrated by Wheeler et al. (1996), who found that when student nurses, and even their clinical instructors, rated their empathy, it bore little relationship to the empathy perceived by their patients. In short, if we tell someone 'I know just how you feel', we almost certainly don't.

In paediatric respiratory healthcare, as in other health specialties, communication problems have been identified as being of crucial importance. For example, in clinics for children with asthma, Butz et al. (2007) found that the majority of parents and children struggled to communicate basic symptom information to health staff without prompting.

General communication problems

The following are some of the many ways in which spoken communication can go wrong.

- Person listening doesn't understand and knows it (but might find it hard say so).
- Person listening thinks they understand what the person speaking really means but doesn't.
- Person being spoken to is not listening. (There could be many reasons for this.)
- Person listening is offended, bored or shocked.
- Person speaking is unsure what to say.
- Person speaking finds it hard to put thoughts into words.
- Person speaking thinks person listening has understood but they haven't.
- Person speaking changes or limits what they say, because they're worried what the person listening will think or how they will react.
- Person speaking doesn't care whether the person listening understands.

In each of the above, the 'person speaking' could be a patient, a nurse or another colleague and similarly the listener. Note also that the examples could apply to written communication by replacing 'speaking' with 'writing' and 'listening' with 'reading'.

Improving communication

Because communication is natural and instinctive, we usually do it automatically, unaware of the complex and sophisticated skills that we are using. It is often only when we sense communication is failing that we are forced to think about it, and it can start to feel unnatural, difficult, stressful, frustrating and even give rise to a sense of helplessness.

The aim of this chapter is to provide practical ideas on how to get past these difficulties, by developing new understanding and skills which encourage better communication, using examples in the context of paediatric respiratory nursing. Like improving any skill (e.g. driving), changing how you communicate is likely to feel awkward and hard work at first but should become more familiar and easier with practice. 'Common sense' might suggest that some people are naturally good communicators while others are not, and that this cannot be changed. In fact, there is good evidence that health professionals can improve their communication skills with training (Connolly et al. 2010; Lewin et al. 2001).

In business, communications training is very often focused on 'getting your ideas across'. However, in patient-focused support, it is at least as important, if not more so, to learn to actively listen and understand patients, their carers and other professionals.

Key ideas to improve communication

The following are key tips for improving communication with patients, carers and others. The first one, listening, is the most important.

- Listen actively, so that you are thinking hard about what the child or parent is trying to communicate.
- Be genuinely but respectfully curious, and develop the attitude that a wide range of responses, or a change of mind, would be acceptable and reasonable.
- With families, make it clear that different family members will often see things differently and that's OK.
- Avoid leading questions ('Have you done all your treatment?' versus 'How much of your treatment have you done?').
- Avoid unintended judgemental attitudes to parents, children or young people.
- Make explicit that it's OK to ask for clarification
- Avoid or explain jargon. Remember that words that are common and easily understood by yourself and other trained colleagues may be jargon to families.
- Check understanding ('How would you explain what I've told you to a friend?').

Communication with parents

In general, the younger a child is, the more a health professional is likely to communicate via the parents. The older a child is, the more a health professional should communicate directly with the young person themselves.

Parents often have real difficulties in communicating with their children. One of the indirect benefits of communicating honestly, empathically and effectively with parents is that you are teaching, by example, how parents might communicate more effectively with their children.

Communication with colleagues

Most of the ways to improve communication (for example, active listening) also apply to working with colleagues. Clarity of brief spoken and written information to other nurses, doctors and other colleagues can be improved by structuring what is said using the mnemonic SBAR – Situation, Background, Assessment, Recommendation (NHS Institute for Innovation and Improvement 2010).

School is a key environment for children. Effective communication between nurses and school staff (including teaching assistants) is recognised as crucial to management of respiratory diseases such as childhood asthma (Office for Public Management 2004).

Written communication

Written communication can be a useful alternative, or addition, to spoken communication but it is important to recognise that around 16% of adults in the UK lack 'basic literacy' (Department for Education and Skills 2003).

Most of us tend to use more complex words and grammar when we write, compared with when we speak. Complicated writing, with jargon and long, hard-to-read sentences, is actually quite easy to write. It may even impress some people but it often fails in its main aim of *communication*. On the other hand, clear and brief English looks simple but often requires a lot of effort to do well.

The Plain English Campaign (2001) has published a number of free guides to writing clearly for the widest possible audience, including one specifically for medical information .This includes a glossary of medical terms with plain English alternatives. Even commonplace medical terms can usefully be replaced with everyday alternatives without sounding condescending (e.g. 'fracture' can be replaced with 'broken bone'). This makes it easier to read for adults, children and those with reading or learning difficulties. It is also easier to translate accurately into other languages (see below).

Differences in language

English is not the first language at home for 6% of the UK population (Office for National Statistics 2006). When families speak a different language to the nurses caring for them, this clearly magnifies many of the problems already described and adds some new ones but many of the ideas already discussed will help, whether attempting to communicate directly using the patient's limited English or using an interpreter (see below). In particular:

- use simple language, with as little jargon as possible
- provide written information – either prepared leaflets or hand-written at the time. Many families will have friends, family or a support worker who can translate for them
- check understanding by asking the patient or carer to say (or demonstrate) what they have understood (e.g. about how to take medication or use a device)
- remember it is with *the family* that you want to communicate and establish a working relationship, so when using an interpreter, look at the family (not the interpreter) throughout.

The National Register of Public Service Interpreters has a useful guide to working with interpreters, which is available online (Corsellis 2003).

Differences in culture

There is evidence that parents from different ethnic backgrounds tend to have different beliefs and understandings of illness, including asthma (Cane et al. 2001). Differences included beliefs about diet and the extent to which they had deferential trust in 'western' medicine. Awareness of these trends may help nurses to be alert to possible differences in understanding but they should *never* be assumed to apply to any individual child or parent, as the range of attitudes and beliefs within any ethnic or religious group is almost certainly greater than the differences between any two groups as a whole. If you think an attitude or belief might be important then ask but ask in such a way that is curious about them *as individuals*:

> *Nurse: Some parents I see think their child's illness gets worse when they eat certain kinds of food. Do you think Amjal's illness changes when he eats different foods?*

Communication skills in the context of nursing

The above communication issues and skills, along with some new ones, are illustrated below in a number of scenarios frequently encountered in paediatric respiratory nursing. Because of the personal nature of these encounters, all the case examples are created from a mixture of clinical experience rather than from individual patients and their families.

Introductions: first meeting a child and family

A woman, a man, a 7-year-old girl and a 4-year-old boy are in a paediatric asthma clinic and have already seen the doctor, before being asked to see the nurse (in order to be shown how to use a new inhaler).

> *Nurse [to the girl]: You must be Sally.*
> *Sally nods shyly.*
> *Nurse [to the woman]: And you must be Mum.*
> *Woman: That's right.*
> *Nurse [to Sally]: And is this your little brother?*
> *Sally: Uh-huh*
> *Nurse [to the man]: And I take it you're their Dad?*
> *Man [embarrassed]: Um …*
> *Woman: Well he's Billy's dad but not Sally's.*

Initial introductions can hugely influence how well the rest of a meeting and future conversations will go. After very briefly introducing yourself, it's important to check who everyone in the room is. It is often helpful to ask a child to tell you who other people are. Children will often be too shy to say much at first but by asking them, you are starting to engage them. The adults will usually fill in the silences. In the above scenario, the nurse mistakenly assumed the man was Sally's dad. It might have been better if the nurse had asked Sally, 'And who's this?'. Sally would then have had the chance to say 'Billy's dad' or if she said nothing, then a glance to either Mum or Billy's dad would hopefully prompt them to explain.

At an initial meeting, you are likely to have your own agenda of getting more information and explaining things to the family. Before getting involved in this, it is helpful to check what the family's agenda is. Ask them if there's anything in particular *they* want to find out today and either answer it briefly or agree to tell them later. Emphasise there's a lot to take in and it's always OK to ask.

Getting information: open and closed questions

> *Nurse: Are you feeling better?*
> *Teenage boy: No.*

Table 16.1 Open and closed questions

Closed questions	Open questions
Require a simple answer like yes /no, a number or a thing	Cannot be answered with a yes or no. Require an answer which *describes* something (e.g. a feeling, an experience or an event)
Follow the questioner's agenda	Explore the agenda of person being questioned
Answers tend to be short and specific	Answers are longer and less predictable
Usually easier to answer, without much thought or effort	Often harder to answer, requiring more thought and effort
Answers contain little information	Answers contain more information
Useful when you need simple, specific information	Useful when you want to find out more about how someone is thinking or feeling

This nurse has begun with a 'closed' question, i.e. one that has a very limited number of answers – in this case 'yes' or 'no'. Answers to closed questions usually give very little information. In this case the answer is ambiguous, as we don't know if the boy feels he's not completely better or not improved at all. A corresponding open question would be 'How are you feeling today?' which could be answered in many ways, giving more information. Even a grunt would give the information that he doesn't want, or feel able, to say!

Health professionals are often justifiably criticised for using too many closed questions but this criticism can lead to an oversimplified view that 'open questions are good' and 'closed questions are bad'. In practice, both are useful in different ways, as shown in Table 16.1.

The following exchange shows a nurse thoughtfully using a mixture of open and closed questions – adapting the type of question not just according to the information she needs but also to how the conversation is going.

Nurse: Did you come on the bus today? [simple closed question to help relax patient]
Teenager: Yeah. [question was easy to answer with one word]
Nurse: What have you been up to over the past week? [an open question to find out more]
Teenager: Nothing. [open question hasn't really worked. Perhaps teenager isn't yet relaxed enough to get into conversation where he has to think what he wants to say. Maybe try something easier to answer]
Nurse: Did your asthma give you much trouble this last week? [a closed and focused question]
Teenager: A bit. [two-word answer – we're getting somewhere!]
Nurse: What was the worst thing about having asthma this past week? [a more open question again but still focused on the health issue]
Teenager: [after a pause] *I had to stop playing football with my mates when I got a wheeze.*
Nurse: What did it feel like? [an open question again]
Teenager: Tight and aching – like there was a strap around it. [useful information about patient's experience of asthma]
Nurse: What did you do?
Teenager: I took a couple of puffs of my blue inhaler.
Nurse: How much did that help?
Teenager: It helped a bit but I still felt too out of breath to carry on playing. [NB: If the nurse had asked 'Did it help?' that would have invited a yes/no answer, and produced less information.]

Giving information

Giving information is one of the important roles of nurses, often supplementing or explaining information given by medical doctors. Words that are familiar to health professionals may be jargon to

patients and their families. Parents of children with long-term conditions can become very knowledgeable, through frequent consultations, accessing the internet and talking to other parents. But the
risk remains that they have misunderstandings (or different understandings) which nurses might not
be aware of, leading to unforeseen problems in their care. Key points to remember include:

- make sure that the child or parent you are speaking to is in the right frame of mind to listen
- use ordinary-language (Plain English) alternatives to technical words where possible
- when patient/family are going to need to understand medical jargon, explain it in simple terms
- repeat information as necessary
- provide information in written form (either from leaflets,or brief hand-written notes)
- check understanding using open rather than closed questions.

> *Nurse* [after taking time to explain to a parent how to use a new device]*: Do you understand that OK?*
> *Parent: Yes.*

The parent's 'yes' response to this closed question may mean they understand how to use the device
in the way the nurse intended but it could also mean many other things including:

- they *think* they understand it but have actually missed or misunderstood a crucial point
- they don't really understand it but are embarrassed to admit it
- they don't really understand it but don't want to be a nuisance by asking
- they don't really understand it but are keen to get home before the rush hour.

One alternative would be to ask the parent to repeat what you've said but that gives the sense of
challenging and potentially humiliating the parent. Also, repeating parrot-fashion may not indicate
proper understanding.

A better way to check understanding by asking an open question. A particularly helpful one is
'How would you explain this to a friend (or partner, parent)?'. This is less threatening because the
person is being asked to explain to someone else, rather than prove their own knowledge. But
because this requires the person to interpret and explain what you've said, you get a much better
idea of their understanding.

Painful or distressing procedures

Preparation

The term *distressing procedures* has advantages over the more usual *painful procedures* for two
reasons.

- A number of potentially distressing procedures involving little or no physical pain are used in paediatric respiratory medicine. Examples include oxygen masks, inhaler spacers with masks in small
  children and computed tomography (CT) scans. These can all provoke anxiety, fear and distress.
  Although most of the following refers to examples involving pain, most of the understanding and
  management described below apply equally well to these and other 'painless' procedures.
- Even in procedures that do involve some pain, it is often not the main cause of anxiety or distress
  (Duff 2003).

The reassurance that 'it won't hurt' rarely works in children, because:

- children don't believe it (and they are often entirely justified in this)
- whether the procedure involves significant, slight or no pain at all, other factors are often responsible
  for most of their anxiety, including loss of control.

However, pain is often a major cause of distress, so nurses should be vigilant for any indication
of pain and anticipate it in children at all times (Royal College of Nursing 2009). A review by

the Healthcare Commission (2007) concluded that too few nurses were trained in the effective management of pain in children.

Procedural pain can, of course, be anticipated, and there are a number of ways of helping children to cope. Physiological interventions, such as local anaesthetic (e.g. EMLA® cream or ethyl chloride vapo-coolant spray), 'gas and air' (Entonox®; Vater and Hessel 2000), sedatives (e.g. midazolam) and ultimately general anaesthetic, can be effective. Although relatively safe, sedatives and general anaesthetics have additional risks for children with respiratory disorders (Malviya et al. 1997).

Specialist psychological techniques, in particular cognitive behavioural therapy (CBT) (Powers 1999) and hypnosis (Liossi 2002), are also demonstrably effective in reducing, and even overcoming, procedural pain. However, specialist psychological techniques require highly trained and skilled psychological practitioners. As well as being in short supply, these techniques are often only needed when a child's earlier encounters with medical procedures have been poorly managed. It is clearly much better to avoid or minimise this level of distress in the first place, so children do not become so fearful that it becomes a major problem.

Even when children have had difficult previous experiences, nurses can be very effective in helping them to manage procedures with only brief and mild distress by using skilled and sensitive communication. Nurses are in a key position to ensure that best practice is followed. This requires skilled communication not only with children and their carers but also with nursing and medical colleagues, who may need educating and persuading to implement these procedures.

Is pain really the problem?

Although in clinical practice local anaesthetic appears to be effective, there is evidence that when distraction is used, EMLA cream is no more effective than placebo (Lal et al. 2001). Similarly, Ramsook et al. (2001) found that coolant spray was no more effective than placebo for venepuncture and cannula insertion in children. Both studies found wide variation in the reaction of children in both treatment and placebo groups. Note that this does *not* indicate that these local anaesthetics were ineffective in practice. Rather, as anaesthetics and placebo were *equally effective*, it demonstrates that the anaesthetics' effectiveness is not due to their chemical (or cooling) effect. It seems likely that the widely observed benefit is actually due to the way the staff administer the cream or spray (real or placebo), communicating confidence and reassurance to the child.

Advance preparation: setting the scene

If it is known days or weeks in advance that a child will have to have a procedure, and may be distressed, nursing staff, together with parent/carers, have the opportunity to help the child prepare beforehand. The immediate question arises as to whether to (a) warn and prepare the child well in advance to help them become calm and more able to cope with the distress of the procedure or (b) say nothing in advance so they don't build themselves up into a state of anxiety, which could be avoided by 'just getting it over with' quickly when the procedure has to be done.

As is often the case, clinical experience as well as 'common sense' suggests that both can be true. Box 16.1 presents some arguments for and against preparation. The arguments against preparation are often given by parents who are wary of warning their children of difficult procedures.

The evidence is that preparation is effective, particularly if it focuses on developing a child's ability to distract themselves from the procedure (Powers 1999).

Immediate preparation: when it's got to be done now

Whether or not there has been time for advance preparation of the child, there are several ways to minimise the distress to the child, as well as making the process quicker and more pleasant for staff.

Box 16.1   Arguments for and against warning and preparing a child for a procedure in advance

For

Allows child to become desensitised to fears
Allows child to develop a sense of control in the situation, by giving them options in advance
Increases child's trust in staff and parents, by avoiding unpleasant surprises
Helps child develop strategies (relaxation and distraction) they can use themselves again and again

Against

Increases time child has to think, worry and become more anxious
They have no option about doing it, so it's best just to get on with it
Child will be angry with staff or parent for giving them bad news
Increases child's sense of hopelessness if preparation doesn't prevent distress

---

The Royal College of Nursing has produced a practical guide for nurses taking bloods which is available online (Royal College of Nursing 2006).

Location

Where possible, especially when it is suspected that a child will find procedures stressful (including simple ones, such as taking blood), potentially distressing procedures should take place in a separate treatment room. This should not happen in 'safe' areas such as a play room, which should be protected as places where the child can be confident they can relax.

Preparation of the treatment room and equipment

Collier et al. (1993) highlight the importance not just of proper preparation of the child but also practical preparation by health staff to ensure that all equipment is gathered and ready before a child is approached, and certainly before they enter the treatment room. This helps to minimise the time for the child's anxiety to build up as well as the total time of the procedure. As few people as possible should be in the room but the presence of parents helps the majority of children.

Distraction

Distraction has been shown to be effective in reducing perceived pain, by focusing the mind away from the pain (Collier et al. 1993; Duff 2003). Distraction can be facilitated, for example, with toys for smaller children and puzzle books for older children. Passive distraction is less effective than engaging the child in an active task. For this reason, puzzle books where children are set the challenging task of finding one or more characters or objects in a visually busy and complex drawing can be very effective.

After the procedure

After a traumatic procedure, some parents and staff will try to help the child by minimising what happened and encouraging them to forget it. For example, after a 6-year-old child has had a blood sample taken:

> *Nurse: There you are, it wasn't so bad was it? It's all better now. Here's a sticker for being so brave. That's it over for another year. You'll forget all about it soon.*

The child is likely to feel that their distress has not been understood or taken seriously, that they have been silly to be upset but they have been brave (but this doesn't make sense if they were making a fuss about something that didn't hurt much). It's very unlikely they will forget about it, and they are likely to be as or more distressed next time they have to have a similar procedure.

Rather than encouraging a child to forget, it is better to remind them that they have been through a difficult procedure and that they were justified in being upset; remind them that it is over now and they have done really well to cope. With this in mind, the above exchange might have gone something like this:

> *Nurse* [kneeling down to height of child]*: You really didn't like having that done, did you?*
> *Child:* [shakes head]
> *Nurse: Show me where the needle went in.*
> *Child:* [holds up arm]
> *Nurse: Did it hurt?*
> *Child: Yes.*
> *Nurse: Poor you. Does it hurt just the same now, or is it better?*
> *Child: A bit better.*
> *Nurse: So you were really scared and upset, and it hurt when they put the needle in but quite quickly it stopped hurting so much. You've done really, really well. Here's a sticker for being so brave. When you next have a needle like that, I think you'll manage even better.*

> [Note that if the child says it still hurts just as much, don't contradict them, even if you are fairly sure it must be better by now. Instead sympathise, praise them for being so brave and reassure that you think it will feel a bit better soon.]

One of the often quoted advantages of sedation is that even if the child is traumatised during the procedure, they will have little or no memory of it. However, this makes it difficult for them to improve their confidence, as even if they coped well under mild sedation, they are unlikely to remember that either, unless they are told about it.

Parents who witness their child becoming distressed under sedation will sometimes tell them in great detail what happened:

> *The doctors gave you enough sedative to knock out a horse but you fought and fought and wouldn't nod off. It took three nurses and the doctor to hold you down. After you kicked that doctor, I don't think any of them will be volunteering to put a needle in you next time!*

Parents may talk like this to their child because they want to share the sense of being in a difficult situation together and coming through it. As in the above case, it is often done with a mixture of pride and humour but staff should explain (beforehand) that this is not helpful. For a child to hear they behaved in extreme ways, when they have no memory of it, emphasises their lack of control of the situation and, as in the above case, gives the strong message that they would never be able to tolerate the procedure without sedation.

When children have had procedures done under mild sedation, whether the child was still or thrashing about, staff should describe simply and honestly what happened and focus on how the child, even if they don't remember, did well to get through the procedure. Parents should be reminded to do the same. The child above could have been told (by a nurse or parent):

> '*You probably won't remember much because of the medicine the doctors gave you. I think it made you feel a bit funny and you weren't very happy about letting them put the needle in but the doctor got it all done in the end. You did really well.*

This account of what happened, while not as funny, gives an explanation for the child's behaviour and gently implies that the child has achieved something, and might manage even better in the future (with or without sedation).

Following diagnosis of inherited/congenital respiratory disease

Parents are full of anecdotes about the way they learned of their child's condition. Some tell of sensitive, caring hospital staff, who were able to take into account the psychological state of the family when they told of the predicted future. Others recount horror stories of brusque midwives, unfeeling doctors, who fling a label into the air and leave. (Lansdown 1996)

Support of the parents or primary carers

Serious congenital respiratory illnesses, in particular cystic fibrosis, are now usually diagnosed in early infancy. Diagnosis can arise either following investigation of medical symptoms or as a result of a screening programme. In the case of cystic fibrosis, since the universal adoption of screening across the UK, the majority of parents will have taken home an apparently well child, and the diagnosis arises unexpectedly from the screening results. However, a significant minority of children are given (or warned of) a likely diagnosis before screening has been done, following symptoms such as meconium ileus in cystic fibrosis (see Chapter 12). In these circumstances, parents will have already been concerned for their child, so the diagnosis may confirm their worse fears or dash their hopes.

In most centres, the diagnosis and an initial explanation of the symptoms and implications will be communicated to the parents by a medical consultant, perhaps with another member of the multidisciplinary team present. However, parents are almost certainly in a state of shock at this point and unlikely to hear, understand or remember more than a fraction of the information given, particularly as much of it (e.g. the genetics) is quite complex (Brewin 1991, 1996; Bush 2001). Nurses, even if not present at the initial communication of the diagnosis, have an important role in repeating, reinforcing and explaining the information already given (Cystic Fibrosis Trust 2001).

Over time, parents will need to be given a lot of practical information and support, not just about the illness and treatment but also about wider issues, such as benefits, etc. Some services will have a social worker working closely with the team who can fulfil much of this role.

Healthcare professionals (and perhaps other parents) used to be the only significant source of specialist health information for parents but access to the internet and the continuing expansion and availability of books have meant that they now have access to vast amounts of information which is completely outside the control of health professionals. This will include sites created by other hospitals, charities and pressure groups, as well as individual parents and sufferers of a disease in online forums and social networking sites. Although healthcare practitioners are rightly concerned that some of this information may be alarmist, contradictory and even completely misinformed, it is completely unrealistic to expect that parents will not access this. Nurses and other practitioners therefore need to be open about these sources, recommending particular sites but also asking parents what they have read, so that the practitioner has the opportunities to confirm, expand on, check or correct what parents have understood.

Similarly, parents cannot realistically control the information that children will seek out or find on the internet themselves, at an increasingly young age. Parents should be encouraged (directly and by example) to be open and supportive with their children about this, in the same way that health practitioners are with parents, as discussed above.

It is vital for children's wellbeing and development that they are encouraged to live as normal and fulfilling life as possible, with an eye to the future. As discussed elsewhere in this book, children with diseases such as cystic fibrosis are now expected to live well into adulthood.

Support of the child or young person

As noted above, because diagnosis of many congenital respiratory illnesses occurs during infancy, children themselves are not part of the initial communication. For this reason, children are usually told about their diagnosis by their parents. Unsurprisingly, most parents find this incredibly difficult and many will need support from nurses and other members of the multidisciplinary team to do this.

Some parents understandably try to keep the diagnosis hidden from their child for as long as possible, because 'they are too young to understand' or 'they shouldn't have to worry about it yet'. However, while healthcare professionals are keen to encourage children to live as normal and fulfilling lives as possible, children need to develop a clear understanding of their illness in order to deal with it psychologically and practically. A small number of parents are so anxious about telling their children that they are in denial that their children already have regular clinic visits and are listening to conversations their parents have with doctors, and even with each other. Rather than protecting the children from worry, this tends to isolate children by giving the message that their health problem is too scary for them or their parents to talk about.

The parents who manage best are clear about it with their children from the beginning, raising topics and answering questions as they arise. Nurses can help parents, both directly by encouraging them to do this and indirectly through leading by example – talking in a straightforward way to children in front of their parents, using terms like cystic fibrosis naturally as they arise.

Perhaps surprisingly, the really difficult issues are often not those which are unique to a child with a chronic or life-limiting illness. Rather, the most difficult issues (most obviously death) are universal but a seriously ill children and their parents are forced to confront these earlier and more directly.

The decision for families (and for the individuals within them) to talk or not about death is very personal, related to (but not bound by) culture and likely to change over time (Fredman 1997). There is no single right way to do it but families are more likely to struggle at times when their child's age, stage of illness or other circumstances mean that their current approach no longer works.

Reflective practice, self-awareness and boundaries

At times of stress, parents or young people may seek to talk things through with someone, and the person they choose may be a nurse. Working closely with children with lifelong illnesses through-out their childhood leads to nurses developing a close and personal relationship with children and their parents. This can help by making nurses more trusted and approachable but can also make nurses vulnerable to emotional stress themselves. It is vital that nurses, like all professionals, actively reflect on and review their personal and professional practice in this area, and what boundaries are appropriate for them, to protect themselves as well as families. This reflection could take place with their supervisor or a trusted colleague. It is important that members of the multidisciplinary team appreciate and make use of each other's strengths, are open enough to speak about difficulties or concerns about themselves or other members of the team and, most importantly, are supportive of each other when caring becomes difficult.

Conclusion

Communication is a natural, essential process in all human activity, including paediatric nursing, but can be improved through careful thought, training, effort and reflection. Developing a sense of respectful empathy for children and their parents, even when they have different attitudes to yourself, is vital to achieving effective communication and understanding. Using simple and clear language is essential but not as easy as it sounds and requires constant review. Open and closed questions lead to different kinds of answers, and have a different impact on the person questioned. A skilled nurse is likely to use both. Pain is frequently not the main cause of anxiety in distressing procedures and simple psychological and practical preparation can often reduce distress significantly. Supporting families with long-term chronic illness is rewarding but stressful and complicated, so all healthcare staff involved need support and the chance to reflect on their practice.

Questions

The following questions are intended to encourage a sense of empathy for your patients and help you to think about how to apply communication skills in different contexts.

1. Considering your own practice with children and families, what percentage of the time do you spend listening versus talking to them?
2. Does this vary significantly with different families, and if so, could you change this using different kinds of questions?
3. Why is pain not necessarily the main fear in distressing procedures?
4. How can parents be helped to communicate with their children about their illness?
5. Exercise: for each of the general communication problems on page XXX [p.3], think of examples from your practice where:
   a. a nurse is speaking to a parent
   b. a child is speaking to a nurse
   c. a nurse is speaking to a doctor.

For instance, for 'Person listening thinks they understand what the person speaking really means but doesn't', examples might be as follows.

   a. A nurse told a parent that doctors had confirmed that their child with CF had a serious exacerbation. The parent told relatives that the doctors said their child was hopelessly ill.
   b. During a discussion, a child on almost continuous oxygen told a nurse they'd had enough. The nurse initially thought the child wanted to stop treatment but then later understood the child meant they'd had enough of talking about it.
   c. A nurse (to double-check they'd understood) asked a doctor to confirm which antibiotic they would be prescribing. The doctor thought the nurse was questioning the doctor's decision.

References

Audit Commission. (1993) *What Seems to Be the Matter? Communication between hospitals and patients.* London: HMSO.

Brewin TB. (1991) Three ways of giving bad news. *Lancet* **337**, 1207–9.

Brewin TB. (1996) *Relating to the Relatives: breaking bad news, communication and support.* Oxford: Radcliffe Medical Press.

Bush A. (2001) Giving the diagnosis. In: Bluebond-Langer M, Lask B, Angst DB. (eds) *Psychosocial Aspects of Cystic Fibrosis.* London: Arnold.

Butz A, Walker J, Land CL, Vibbert C, Winkelstein M. (2007) Improving asthma communication in high-risk children. *Journal of Asthma* **44(9)**, 739–45.

Cane R, Pao C, McKenzie S. (2001) Understanding childhood asthma in focus groups: perspectives from mothers of different ethnic backgrounds. *BMC Family Practice* **2**, 4.

Chant S, Jenkinson T, Randle J, Russell G. (2002) Communication skills: some problems in nursing education and practice. *Journal of Clinical Nursing* **11**, 12–21.

Collier J, MacKinlay D, Watson AR. (1993) Painful procedures: preparation and coping strategies for children. *Maternal and Child Health* **18**, 282–6.

Connolly M, Perryman J, McKenn,Y. *et al.* (2010) SAGE & THYME™: a model for training health and social care professionals in patient-focussed support. *Patient Education and Counseling* **79(1)**, 87–93.

Corsellis A. (2003) *Guidelines When Working with an Interpreter*. National Register of Public Service Interpreters website: www.nrpsi.co.uk.

Currie L, Watterson L. (2008) *Report on a Scoping Exercise to Identify Priority Topics for National Audit on The Essence of Care*. Oxford: Royal College of Nursing.

Cystic Fibrosis Trust. (2001) *Standards for the Clinical Care of Children and Adults with Cystic Fibrosis in the UK*. Bromley: Cystic Fibrosis Trust.

Department for Education and Skills. (2003) *The Skills for Life Survey: a national needs and impact survey of literacy, numeracy and ICT skills*. Norwich: Stationery Office.

Department of Health. (2003a) *Essence of Care: patient-focused benchmarks for clinical governance*. London: Department of Health.

Department of Health. (2003b) *Getting the RIGHT START: National Service Framework for Children – Standard for Hospital Services*. London: Department of Health.

Duff A. (2003) Incorporating psychological approaches into routine paediatric venepuncture. *Archives of Disease in Childhood* **88(10)**, 931–7.

Fredman G. (1997) *Death Talk: conversations with children and families*. London: Karnac Books.

Healthcare Commission. (2007) *State of Healthcare 2007: improvements and challenges in services in England and Wales*. London: Healthcare Commission.

Lal MK, McClelland M, Phillips J, Taub NA, Beattie RM. (2001) Comparison of EMLA cream versus placebo in children receiving distraction therapy for venepuncture. *Acta Paediatrica* **90(2)**, 154–9.

Lansdown R.(1996) *Children in Hospital: a guide for family and carers*. Oxford: Oxford University Press.

Lewin S, Skea Z, Entwistle VA, Zwarenstein M, Dick J. (2001) Interventions for providers to promote a patient-centred approach in clinical consultations. *Cochrane Database of Systematic Reviews* **4**, CD003267.

Liossi C. (2002) *Procedure-related Cancer Pain in Children*. Oxford: Radcliffe Medical Press.

Malviya S, Voepel-Lewis T, Tait AR. (1997) Adverse events and risk factors associated with the sedation of children by nonanesthesiologists. *Anesthesia and Analgesia* **85**, 1207–13.

NHS Institute for Innovation and Improvement. (2010) *Safer Care – improving patient safety*. Available at: www.institute.nhs.uk/SBAR.

Office for National Statistics. (2006) *Labour Force Survey*. Newport: Office for National Statistics.

Office for Public Management. (2000) *Shifting Gears – towards a 21st century NHS. A report on the NHS National Plan public consultation for the Department of Health*. London: Office for Public Management.

Office for Public Management. (2004) *Managing Childhood Asthma in Schools*. London: Office for Public Management.

Plain English Campaign. (2001) *How to Write Medical Information in Plain English*. Available at: www.plainenglish.co.uk/files/medicalguide.pdf.

Powers SW. (1999) Empirically supported treatments in pediatric psychology: procedure-related pain. *Journal of Pediatric Psychology* **24**, 131–45.

Rakel DP, Hoeft TJ, Barrett BP, Chewning BA, Craig BM, Niu M. (2009) Practitioner empathy and the duration of the common cold. *Family Medicine* **41(7)**, 494–501.

Ramsook C, Kozinetz CA, Moro-Sutherland D. (2001) Efficacy of ethyl chloride as a local anesthetic for venipuncture and intravenous cannula insertion in a pediatric emergency department. *Pediatric Emergency Care* **17**, 341–3.

Royal College of Nursing. (2006) *Capillary Blood Sampling and Venepuncture in Children and Young People: a workbook to assist practitioners in developing competence*. Available at: www.rcn.org.uk/__data/assets/pdf_file/0014/10355/cbs_venepuncture_workbook.pdf.

Royal College of Nursing. (2009) *Recognition and Assessment of Acute Pain in Children*. Available at: www.rcn.org.uk/development/practice/pain/downloads.

Vater M, Hessel D. (2000) Nitrous oxide and oxygen mixture (Entonox®) and acute procedural pain. *Paediatric and Perinatal Drug Therapy* **4(2)**, 35–44.

Wheeler K, Manhart-Barrett EA, Lahey EM. (1996) A study of empathy as a nursing care outcome measure. *International Journal of Psychiatric Nursing Research* **3(1)**, 281–9.

Glossary

Active cycle of breathing	Controlled breathing and coughing
Bacillus Calmette-Guérin	Vaccine given intradermally to individuals at high risk of TB
Bronchoalveolar lavage	0.9% saline is passed down the bronchoscope and sucked back after around 10 s have elapsed
Cystic fibrosis transmembrane conductance regulator	The channel which allows chloride into the periciliary layer, maintaining salt levels in this layer and ensuring it is the correct thickness
Distal intestinal obstruction syndrome	Fatty material causes blockage of bowel
Immune reactive trypsin	The initial newborn screening test for cystic fibrosis
Interferon-γ release assay	Blood test in which T-lymphocytes produce interferon-γ when the cells have been exposed to TB infection
Largyngeal mask airway	A tube attached to 'cushions' which sit above the vocal cords, allowing the bronchoscope to be passed into the trachea
Mantoux test	Intradermal injection of tuberculin. Positive response at 48–72 h indicates TB infection or previous BCG
Meconium ileus	Blockage of bowel with meconium
Mucociliary escalator	The process by which mucus and impurities are 'wafted' up the respiratory passages to the larynx where they are swallowed

Children's Respiratory Nursing, First Edition. Edited by Janice Mighten.
© 2013 Blackwell Publishing Ltd. Published 2013 by Blackwell Publishing Ltd.

Periciliary layer	A non-sticky layer which 'lubricates' the surface of the respiratory epithelial cells, allowing the cilia to beat effectively
***Pneumocystis* pneumonia**	A severe lung infection caused by *Pneumocystis jiroveci* which is seen in children whose immune system is deficient or suppressed by drugs. Can be diagnosed by BAL
Polymerase chain reaction	Highly sensitive test which can detect genetic material (DNA or RNA) from a pathogen
Positive expiratory pressure	Technique where a patient breathes out against resistance (PEP mask) and then performs a 'huff' to clear secretions
Primary ciliary dyskinesia	A condition in which the respiratory cilia do not move in a co-ordinated fashion and so the mucociliary escalator does not work
Seldinger technique	Technique of chest drain insertion which involves pushing the drain into the chest over a flexible wire
Ziehl Neelson staining	Special stain used to detect TB organisms, which are described as acid or alcohol fast

Abbreviations

ABC	airway, breathing, circulation
ACB	active cycle of breathing
ACT	Asthma Control Test/airway clearance technique
AHR	airway hyper-responsiveness
AP	anteroposterior
ASM	airway smooth muscle
ATS	American Thoracic Society
BAL	bronchoalveolar lavage
BCG	bacillus Calmette-Guérin
BDP	beclomethasone dipropionate
BMI	Body Mass Index
BNFc	*British National Formulary for Children*
BOS	bronchiolitis obliterans syndrome
BP	blood pressure
BPD	bronchopulmonary dysplasia
BTS	British Thoracic Society
CCN	children's community nurse
CCAM	congenital cystic adenomatoid malformation
CCN	children's community nurse
CDH	congenital diaphragmatic hernia
CF	cystic fibrosis
CFTR	cystic fibrosis transmembrane conductance regulator
CLD	chronic lung disease of prematurity
CLE	congenital lobar emphysema
CMV	cytomegalovirus
CNLD	chronic neonatal lung disease
CPAP	continuous positive airway pressure
CT	computed tomography
CXR	chest x-ray
DLA	disability living allowance
ECG	electrocardiogram
ELS	extralobar sequestration
ENT	ear, nose and throat
FBC	full blood count

FEF	forced expiratory flow
FEV1	forced expiratory volume in 1 s
FRC	functional residual capacity
FVC	forced vital capacity
GINA	Global Initiative for Asthma
GOR	gastro-oesophageal reflux
HR-CT	high-resolution computed tomography
ICS	inhaled corticosteroids
IGRA	interferon-γ release assay
ILD	interstitial lung disease
ILS	intralobar sequestration
IPH	idiopathic pulmonary haemosiderosis
IPV	intrapulmonary percussive ventilation
IRT	immune reactive trypsin
ISAAC	International Study of Asthma and Allergies in Childhood
ISHLT	International Society for Heart and Lung Transplantation
IV	intravenous
KU	kilounit
LABA	long-acting β2-agonist
LMA	laryngeal mask airway
LSA	learning support assistant
LTOT	long-term oxygen therapy
LTRA	leukotriene receptor antagonist
LTV	long-term ventilation
MDI	metered dose inhaler
MDT	multidisciplinary team
NCLD	neonatal chronic lung disease
NHS	National Health Service
NICE	National Institute for Health and Clinical Excellence
NICU	neonatal intensive care unit
NIV	non-invasive ventilation
NSF	National Service Framework
PA	posteroanterior
PACS	picture archiving and communication system
PCD	primary ciliary dyskinesia
PCP	*Pneumocystis carinii* (*jiroveci*) pneumonia
PCR	polymerase chain reaction
PCT	primary care trust
PEF	peak expiratory flow
PEFR	peak expiratory flow rate
PEP	positive expiratory pressure
PEWS	paediatric early warning system
PHT	pulmonary hypertension
PICU	paediatric intensive care unit
PTLD	post-transplant lymphoproliferative disease
QOL	quality of life
RDS	respiratory distress syndrome
ROP	retinopathy of prematurity
RSV	respiratory syncytial virus

RV	residual volume
RVC	relaxed vital capacity
SABA	short-acting β2-agonist
SDB	sleep-disordered breathing
SEN	special educational needs
SMA	spinal muscular atrophy
SMARD	spinal muscular atrophy with respiratory disease
TA	teaching assistant
TB	tuberculosis
TLC	total lung capacity
TOF	tracheo-oesophageal fistula
TV	tidal volume
VCD	vocal cord dysfunction
ZN	Ziehl Neelson

Answers

Chapter 1

1. The alar nasalis muscle allows the nostrils to flare open during respiratory distress.
2. The function of the conchae is to direct airflow.
3. The left main bronchus is positioned at a more acute angle.
4. Micrognathia, cleft palate and glossoptosis.
5. Stridor.
6. This occurs because upper airway obstruction causes an increase in effort to create airflow and further narrowing of the airways.

Chapter 2

1. F.   2. T.   3. F.   4. T.   5. F

Chapter 3

1. T.   2. F.   3. T.   4. T.   5. T

Chapter 4

1. FTTTF
2. TTTFF
3. FTTFT
4. TTTFF
5. TTFFF
6. TTFFT
7. TFTFT

Children's Respiratory Nursing, First Edition. Edited by Janice Mighten.
© 2013 Blackwell Publishing Ltd. Published 2013 by Blackwell Publishing Ltd.

Chapter 5

1. FEV1 of less than 80% of predicted value; also FEV1/FVC ratio less than 80%.
2. FEV1 and FEF 25-75, that represents the small airways, will be reduced.
3. Good start with a blow, no variable flow, should be reproducible.
4. Verbal encouragement, practical demonstration, praise following their effort.
5. Use of bacteria-filtered mouthpiece, cleaning the machine, use of separate flow heads when children are known to have respiratory infection, patients with infection should have their tests at the end of a clinic.

Chapter 6

1. SpO_2 96–100%; PaO_2 12–15 kPa.
2. V/Q mismatch occurs (1) when areas of the lung that are receiving the blood supply, known as perfusion, are not moving the air in and out, known as ventilation, and (2) there are areas of the lung that are better ventilated than perfused, due to airway obstruction.
3. The three categories of respiratory failure are failure of the central nervous system, failure of the pump, e.g. spinal cord disease, and lung disease and infection.
4. Low SpO_2 90% and below; low PaO_2, below 12 kPa.
5. Does the child require ambulatory oxygen or oxygen in school? Is the home environment suitable for home oxygen? Are the parents competent and confident to care for their child at home with oxygen?

Chapter 7

1. Restrictive lung diseases, e.g. neuromuscular weakness, obstructive airways disease, e.g. tracheomalacia, lack of respiratory drive, e.g. spinal cord injury, Advanced parenchymal lung disease, e.g. cystic fibrosis.
2. Hypoxemia, hypercarbia, lack of sleep.
3. Hypercarbia (abnormally high carbon dioxide levels) that occurs by night only is nocturnal; if it persists into daytime (awake), this is diurnal.
4. Training, equipment, home visits/overnight stay, resuscitation plan.
5. Adequate support, care package, competent parents, trained carers, short breaks.
6. Where life may be judged unbearable or of no purpose; if the child is in a permanent vegetative state or there is no chance of recovery and suffering is prolonged, life-sustaining treatment may be withheld or withdrawn.
7. Home ventilators create a flow of gas for breathing support using room air.
8. Non-invasive ventilation is applied via the mouth and/or nose; invasive ventilation occurs through a tracheostomy.

Chapter 8

1. FTTFT
2. TTFFT
3. FTFFT

4. TTFFT
5. FFTTF
6. TTTTT
7. TTFTF
8. TFTTF
9. FFFFT
10. TFFTT

Chapter 9

1. Factors that affect absorption are gut motility and the pH in the stomach.
2. Salbutamol is a β2-receptor agonist, which acts on all the β2-receptors in the body, producing many unwanted effects.
3. After absorption, drugs are distributed throughout the body but different amounts are taken up by each body tissue.
4. Nephrotoxicity is damage to the kidneys from toxic drugs such as gentamicin.
5. Montelukast is a leucotriene receptor antagonist, which reduces the body's response to inflammation.

Chapter 10

1. T.   **2.** F.   **3.** T.   **4.** T.   **5.** F.   **6.** T.   **7.** F.   **8.** T.   **9.** F.   **10.** T

Chapter 11

1. Lung injury, mechanical ventilation and exposure to high levels of oxygen in the early stages of life all contribute towards the development of CLD.
2. The alveolar walls are disturbed in interstitial lung disease, affecting the process of gas exchange.
3. The mucociliary function in patients with bronchiectasis is impaired, which causes an increase and accumulation of secretions.
4. Congenital cystic adenomatoid malformation (CCAM) is the most common abnormality of the lung in children.
5. Surgery.
6. Parents caring for children with complex needs can apply for lisability living allowance (DLA). Healthcare professionals can assist parents with completing application forms and provide the necessary medical report to support the claim.
7. The general opinion is that it is not recommended. Parents should be taught how to recognise changes in their child's condition. This very much depends on the practitioner's professional judgement but in the main the use of saturation monitors can cause increased anxiety levels for parents.

Chapter 12

1. TTFFT
2. FFFTT
3. FTFTT

4. TFFTT
5. TFTTF
6. FTTTF
7. TFFFF
8. FTTFT

Chapter 13

1. Patients are usually listed for transplant when they have a predicted 2-year mortality of 50%.
2. Cystic fibrosis and idiopathic pulmonary arterial hypertension.
3.
  - End-stage or progressive pulmonary disease or pulmonary vascular disease.
  - Patient is declining despite maximal medical therapy and is at risk of dying without transplant.
  - Patient has a poor quality of life.
  - Patient and family are informed and consent to transplant.
  - Patient and family are able and agree to adhere to rigorous surveillance required following transplant.
4. Very few heart-lung transplants are now carried out because of the donor organ shortage; most blocks will be separated in order to benefit more patients.
5. A number of factors must be taken into account when making the decision to list, including prediction of prognosis without transplant, patient height, blood group, average waiting time for donor organs, patient quality of life. Shorter, younger patients, blood group other than AB and patients who need a heart-lung block usually wait longer for a suitable donor. It is very important to consider each individual case carefully, taking into account each individual's rate of disease progression to try and predict their prognosis without transplant. The potential risks and benefits of transplantation for each individual must be considered before committing a child to transplant.
6. Survival in children after lung transplant at Great Ormond Street Hospital is over 80% at 3 years, approximately 60% at 5 years and 50% at 7 years. The risk for the individual patient may be more or less than this depending on their diagnosis and presence of other co-morbidities and risk factors.
7.
  - Lung transplant is not a cure and life expectancy remains limited.
  - Quality of life significantly improves after lung transplant in most lung transplant recipients, enabling them to undertake most activities of a normal child of their age.
  - The shortage of donor organs means there is no guarantee that if a child is listed for a lung transplant, a suitable donor will become available in time and the child may die on the transplant waiting list.
  - Crucial importance of taking lifelong immunosuppressive treatment.
  - The family must adhere to the rigorous follow-up care and monitoring required after transplant.
8. The early postoperative management of the lung transplant patient on both the ICU and ward focuses on the following aspects of care:
  - nursing assessment and monitoring of the patient
  - effective immunosuppression of the patient to prevent rejection
  - minimising the risk of infection due to the immunosuppression
  - optimising the function of the newly implanted donor lungs
  - physiotherapy, positioning and early mobilisation

- optimising other organ function, in particular the kidneys
- support of the child and family during the stress of lung transplant and ICU stay
- education of the child and family to prepare them for discharge.

9.
- Isolation
- Hand washing
- Perioperative IV antibiotics
- Antimicrobial prophylaxis
- Monitoring for signs of infection
- Screening for infection
- Care of surgical wound site

10. Post lung transplant physiotherapy and early mobilisation are essential to mobilise secretions and to prevent lower respiratory tract infections which are one of the most common complications of early post lung transplant. The post lung transplant patient has no cough reflex so the physiotherapist teaches the patient to cough regularly, to use deep breathing and bubble PEP to help ensure that they clear secretions.

11. Tacrolimus or ciclosporin, MMF or azathioprine and prednisolone. To prevent the immune system rejecting the donor lungs.

12. Post-transplant lymphoproliferative disease. Patients who are immunosuppressed are at risk of developing PTLD. This is usually associated with infection with Epstein–Barr virus leading to the uncontrolled proliferation of B cells.

13. Biopsy.

14. Infection.

15. Tacrolimus. To maintain good renal health, patients should remain well hydrated, avoid other potentially nephrotoxic medication, maintain good diabetic control, be normotensive and have their tacrolimus level and kidney function monitored every 6 weeks.

Chapter 15

1. A duty of care is a requirement from one person to another in order to prevent harm and maintain the safety of patients.

2. The KSF is a framework for competence and ensures fitness to practise, and quality with service provision.

3. Inappropriate delegation would be assessed using a concept known as the Bolam test. This is case law based on standard of care that must be adhered to, based on the ethical principles of 'do no harm'.

4. An assessment of a child's capability to give consent would be required using the concepts of Gillick or Fraser competence. This states that the child should have the mental capacity to make an informed decision.

5. In any situation where there is a need to safeguard the welfare of the child, the decision to over-ride confidentiality would be necessary. It is important for agencies to share information, particularly when it is in the best interest of the child.

6. Practice initiatives are focused on patient care and the importance of nutrition, privacy and dignity.

7. The National Service Framework (NSF) is a national document. The objective of the NSF is to provide care and standards for children based on quality to promote best practice.

Index